Skeletal Trauma Notes

John V. Fowles, M.B., B.S. (Lond.), F.R.C.S.(C)

Professeur agrégé de clinique
Directeur du Programme d'orthopédie
Département de Chirurgie
Université de Montréal
Montréal, Québec, Canada

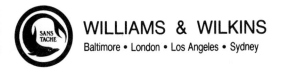

WILLIAMS & WILKINS
Baltimore • London • Los Angeles • Sydney

Editor: Barbara Tansill
Associate Editor: Carol Eckhart
Design: Bert Smith
Illustration Planner: Reginald R. Stanley
Production: Raymond E. Reter

Copyright ©, 1985
Williams & Wilkins
428 E. Preston Street
Baltimore, Md. 21202, U.S.A.

Accurate indications, adverse reactions, and dosage schedules for drugs are provided in this book, but it is possible that they may change. The reader is urged to review the package information data of the manufacturer of the medications mentioned.

Made in the United States of America

Library of Congress Cataloging in Publication Data

Fowles, John V.
  Skeletal trauma notes.

  Bibliography: p.
  Includes index.
  1. Fractures—Handbooks, manuals, etc. 2. Joints—Wounds and injuries—Handbooks, manuals, etc. I. Title. [DNLM: 1. Fractures—handbook. 2. Joints—injuries—handbook. WE 39 F789s]
RD101.F68 1985   617'.15   84–22025
ISBN 0–683–03318–2

Composed and printed at the
Waverly Press, Inc.

85 86 87 88 89
10 9 8 7 6 5 4 3 2 1

To the memory of my Mother;
To my Father;
And to my children, Alison, Nicholas and Claire,
Who look forward to the future.

Preface

Dr. Samuel Johnson said, "It is not sufficiently considered that men more frequently require to be reminded than informed." This book of fractures and joint injuries is not a textbook but rather is designed as an "aide mémoire" for readers already knowledgeable in the subject, orthopaedic and general surgical residents revising for exams, for example, or practicing surgeons who require a small and handy reference work. The book is small and concise and may be consulted during free moments, such as waiting for the next patient in the operating room or before the lights dim in the cinema. A list of textbooks for further reading is found at the end of the book.

The first seven chapters are devoted to general principles of fractures and joint injuries; the remainder deals with skeletal injuries on a regional basis. This is a pragmatic book. Classifications are used only where they are helpful for predicting complications, influencing treatment or evaluating the prognosis. Treatment leans toward non-operative care because the simplest form of satisfactory management is usually the best. Wherever possible the initial treatment should be the definitive treatment. Surgery is advocated only where there is no good closed method available. Remember that overtreatment may be worse than no treatment at all!

Operative techniques are outlined to remind the reader of the important points. For details, s/he should consult the textbooks or the original publications. The illustrations are easy to reproduce on paper or blackboard. Drawing is a good way of learning. The reader may also wish to annotate the text by adding or underlining facts that s/he considers important.

Acknowledgments

This book evolved over several years of teaching in Tunisia and Afghanistan. The stimulus came from the doctors, students and paramedical staff, and from them I learned a great deal. They work in difficult circumstances, both in peace and in war, and yet they maintain their integrity, optimism and sense of humor. These men and women have earned my respect and admiration. I wish to express my gratitude also to CARE-MEDICO for the opportunity of living and working abroad, to the CARE doctors, paramedical staff and administrators for their support, to the volunteers with Orthopaedics Overseas, and to my wife Deirdre who was a constant source of encouragement.

Ted Dewar, Mohamed Kassab and Carroll Laurin are three men with whom I have been associated for many years, and each in his characteristic way has influenced me as colleague, mentor and friend. To them I shall always be indebted.

Finally, I would like to thank Gerda Zaiane in Tunis, Belkise Shah in Kabul, and Carol-Ann Paul and Suzan Senechal in Montreal for typing the manuscript, André Beerenz for his artistic advice, and my colleagues at the Hôtel-Dieu Hospital for their patience and understanding.

Contents

chapter 1

Bone, Fracture Healing and Bone Grafting

Microanatomy and Physiology of Bone

CONSTITUENTS OF MATURE, ADULT BONE

Extracellular

Matrix

Ground substance
- 5% of the matrix;
- glycosaminoglycans, consisting of
  —repeating disaccharides of hexuronic acid linked with
  —hexosamine (an amino sugar) to form an
  —acid mucopolysaccharide. These are usually
  —sulfated. Chondroitin sulfate A is the most common. The sulfated acid mucopolysaccharide is attached to a
  —protein to form a macromolecule called a proteoglycan. These are
  —synthesized by fibroblasts. Matrix also contains
- glycoproteins consisting of several different
  —monosaccharides.

Collagen fibers
- 90–95% of matrix; fibers are
- grouped in bundles and
- embedded in the ground substance;
- this is Type I collagen. Consists of
- three polypeptide alpha chains wound around each other in a

—triple helix. In Type I collagen, one alpha chain differs slightly from the other two.
- collagen contains a high proportion of the amino acids
  —proline and
  —lysine;
  —hydroxyproline and
  —hydroxylysine are only found in collagen.
- molecules of collagen are
  —cross-linked through hydroxylysine.

Mineral salts

- mainly calcium and phosphorus, as hydroxyapatite crystals $Ca_{10}(PO_4)_6(OH)_2$. These are
- 600 Å long and 30 to 50 Å wide;
- crystals lie parallel to collagen fibers in relation to their periodicity;
- smaller quantities of sodium, potassium, carbonates, citrates and other trace elements are also present.

Water

- lies in relation to proteoglycans.

Osteocytes

- derived from
  —osteoblasts which have surrounded themselves with bone. Each osteocyte lies in a
  —lacuna and communicates with adjacent osteocytes and osteoblasts through fine
  —cytoplasmic processes. These lie in
  —canaliculi formed when the bone was laid down around the processes of the osteoblast.
- cell bodies and cytoplasmic processes are bathed in tissue fluid in the lacunae and canaliculi;
- metabolic exchange of nutrients and waste products may occur directly via the
  —cytoplasmic processes, or indirectly via the
  —tissue fluid surrounding the cells, by diffusion through or circulation of the fluid.
- cells are never more than 0.2 mm away from a capillary which could provide the nutrients.
- osteocytes
  —synthesize bone matrix,
  —maintain its integrity, and
  —inhibit the action of osteoclasts.

STRUCTURE OF CORTICAL BONE (Fig. 1.1)

- cortical bone is compact and built of osteones arranged parallel to the long axis of the shaft.

Osteone

- less than 0.5 mm in diameter; the size of osteones is
- limited by the maximum distance over which the osteocytic canalicular system is functional;
- consists of

Haversian canal

- lies parallel to the long axis of the shaft, at the center of the osteone, and
- contains one or two capillaries.

Lamellae

- concentric cylinders of bone centered around the haversian canal;
- crossed by Volkmann's canals containing capillaries which communicate with other haversian canals;
- contain osteocytes also arranged in concentric circles around the haversian canal.

Periosteum

- surrounds the outside of the cortex and consists of two layers:

Internal osteogenic (cambium) layer

- contains multipotential stem cells grouped around the periosteal

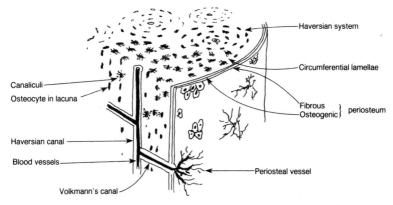

Figure 1.1. Longitudinal and cross section of a long bone cortex. (Modified from Ham AW, Cormack DH: *Histology*, ed 8. Toronto, JB Lippincott, 1979, p 440.)

capillaries. These cells can become osteoblasts, chondroblasts or collagenoblasts;

- determining factors in the differentiation of these multipotential cells include blood supply and oxygenation, pH, the presence of certain mineral salts, movement, stress and maybe other, unknown factors.

External (fibrous) layer

- contains fibroblasts (collagenoblasts) and fibrocytes.

Endosteum

- lines the inside of the cortex; contains
- multipotential cells similar to those of the periosteal cambium layer.

Vascularization of shaft

Medullary vessels

- from nutrient artery and epiphyseal arterial ring;
- vascularize the internal two thirds of the cortex.

Periosteal vessels

- from the rich capillary network in the periosteum which is fed by vessels from muscles attached to the cortex;
- vascularize the outer third of the cortex and
- anastomose with branches from the medullary vessels.

Physiology of cortical bone

- compact bone is perpetually resorbed and renewed.

Resorption

Biochemical changes

- nutritional canalicular system of osteocytes is inefficient and a
- decrease in local
  - —oxygen tension or of availability of
  - —nutrients may produce
  - —degenerative changes in the osteocytes which then die and lyse. The resultant
  - —dead bone which is
- exposed to capillaries or monocytes is then
- resorbed by osteoclasts.

Osteoclast

- A multinucleated giant cell found around the periphery of resorption cavities (Howship's lacunae) in bone;
- formed by fusion of many
  - —monocytes or
  - —macrophages;

- ruffled border of the osteoclast is in
    —intimate contact with the bone surface and probably
    —liberates acid into the tissue fluid bathing both the villous processes of the ruffled border and the bone. This
    —would lower pH locally, but the
    —calcium salts in bone buffer the acids. During this action, the
    —bone salts themselves become acidic and more soluble and
    —pass into solution, leaving
    —collagen fibrils of bone projecting outward to form the
    —"brush border."
- "clear zone" surrounds the ruffled border and may be responsible for
    —attaching osteoclast to bone and
    —delimiting the area of pH changes in the tissue fluid.
- parathormone
    —increases the population of osteoclasts and
    —stimulates them to greater activity;
- calcitonin has the reverse effect;
- osteoclasts are probably attracted to bone areas
    —not covered by osteogenic cells. This
    —membrane of osteogenic cells separates bone from tissue fluid and thus prevents bone matrix from losing its mineral content.
- cannot undergo mitosis.

Reconstruction

Osteoblasts

- basophilic, 15 to 80 μ in diameter, and mononuclear, with fine
- cytoplasmic processes similar to those in an osteocyte. These processes are in contact with
    —other osteoblasts and with
    —osteocytes in the underlying bone. Osteoblasts
- differentiate from
    —osteogenic cells which line and cover all bone surfaces except where osteoclasts are found. They may also differentiate from
    —fibroblasts and
    —pericytes around vessels by osteogenic induction.
- osteoblasts cannot undergo mitosis; they
- manufacture and secrete tropocollagen fibers in the same way that the fibroblasts do. Outside the cell the
- tropocollagen fibers combine to form collagen fibers with a periodicity of 640 Å, which is related to the overlap of the tropocollagen molecules. Their

- orientation is determined by mechanical factors of stress;
- collagen forms the
  —protein matrix of new trabeculae.
- osteoblasts also secrete the
  —ground substance of bone matrix.

Mineralization

- within 24 hours, mineralization of the new protein matrix begins.
- matrix vesicles
  —bud off from osteoblasts and chondroblasts and lie in the osteoid matrix. These vesicles
  —accumulate calcium and contain
  —alkaline phosphatase and
  —pyrophosphatase. The
- alkaline phosphatase may hydrolyze ester phosphate to form
- orthophosphate which could then react with calcium to raise the local Ca x P product and cause precipitation of
- amorphous $Ca_3(PO_4)_2$;
- hydroxyapatite crystals would then form the amorphous calcium phosphate deposits; or these
- crystals may form directly
  —inside the vesicles which then
  —burst and release the crystals. These then
  —continue to grow in the matrix. The
- pyrophosphatase destroys
  —inorganic pyrophosphate, an inhibitor of calcification.

STRUCTURE OF CANCELLOUS BONE

- cortex is thin and weak;
- trabeculae are
  —arranged in a sponge-like lattice with many spaces between the trabeculae. There are
  —no osteones.
- cancellous bone is
  —very vascular and
  —cellular, consisting mainly of osteogenic cells and osteoblasts (makes good osteogenic grafts; e.g., from iliac crest), and is
- susceptible to compression fractures.

Fracture Repair in Cortical Bone

- a fracture is repaired by new tissue which forms between and around the fractured bone. This is the callus. It develops in different ways in different areas and eventually ossifies and remodels.

INITIAL STATE OF FRACTURE SITE

- hematoma
  - —rapidly fills the space between fractured bone ends;
  - —comes from intramedullary, haversian and periosteal vessels and other torn vessels in the surrounding soft tissue;
  - —fat globules from the medulla float in the hematoma.
- periosteum and endosteum are
  - —torn and
  - —lifted off the cortex for a variable distance.
- osteocytes adjacent to the fracture are no longer nourished (due to disruption of blood supply) and die, leaving empty lacunae. The
- injury elicits an acute inflammatory response.

CALLUS FORMATION (Fig. 1.2)

- surgeons call the callus around the outside of the fracture the external callus and that between the bone ends and in the marrow cavity the internal callus, though both are the same.

External callus

Primary callus response

- proliferation (almost a population explosion) of fibroblastic and osteogenic cells starts within 2 days of fracture (sooner in children);
- osteogenic cells come from the cambium layer of the periosteum and appear where periosteum is lifted off the cortex, as well as further

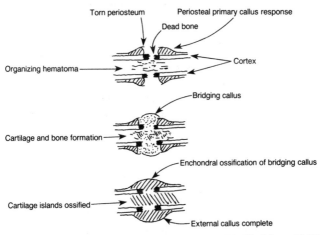

Figure 1.2. Formation of external and internal callus. (Modified from McKibbin B: Repair of fractures. In Wilson JN (ed): *Watson-Jones Fractures and Joint Injuries*, ed 6. Edinburgh, Churchill Livingstone, vol 1, 1982, p 16.)

away from the fracture where periosteum is still attached to bone and has good blood supply;

- most of these cells differentiate into osteoblasts;
- this is the "primary callus response" and is an independent, basic reaction of bone to injury.

Vascular response

- blood supply develops from surrounding soft tissues and participates in the formation of external callus.

Osteoid formation

- from about the sixth day after a fracture, osteoblasts form trabeculae of osteoid tissue (unmineralized bundles of bone collagen) along new capillaries;
- these trabeculae are firmly cemented to fracture fragments, forming a "collar" around the end of each fragment.

Formation of immature bone (provisional or primary callus)

- osteoid is mineralized within hours, by seeding at specific points along the collagen fibers;
- this new, immature ("woven" or "fiber") bone is very cellular, has collagen fibers and trabeculae arranged at random, and is poorly mineralized and weak;
- osteoblasts trapped in this immature bone are transformed into osteocytes.
- if the two "collars" do not soon make contact with each other, this primary callus response stops, and union will depend on the next phase.

External bridging callus

- some osteogenic cells, recruited from surrounding soft tissues by induction, differentiate into chondroblasts and form cartilage, particularly at the level of the fracture line where blood supply may not be so good and oxygen tension is lower than in surrounding bone;
- thus the two collars of immature bone formed around the two ends of the fracture are united by cartilage.
- cartilage and fibrous tissue formation is increased if fracture ends continually move. By
- enchondral ossification of this cartilage in the presence of a microvascular supply from the surrounding soft tissues, bone crosses the fracture from one collar to the other, "glueing" the bone ends together; this is the
- bridging external callus, and the fracture is now
- "sticky." But if a

- cartilage bridge does not form between the two collars of immature bone within a certain period of time, osteogenic activity gradually stops and nonunion may ensue.

Internal callus

Organization of hematoma

- hematoma coagulates;
- within a few hours, fibrin is precipitated, forming the fibrin clot;
- inflammatory cells and collagenoblasts from surrounding mesenchymal tissues invade the clot;
- these cells use the fibrin network as a scaffolding, climbing along its strands;
- new capillary outgrowths from intramedullary and endosteal vessels follow the cells into the clot;
- within 3 days of a fracture, collagenoblasts start depositing collagen fibers in clot;
- this is granulation tissue, and the clot is said to be organized;
- osteogenic cells simultaneously invade the clot, particularly from endosteum lining the marrow cavity and haversian systems.

Direct ossification

- some areas of organized clot ossify directly by transformation of osteogenic cells into osteoblasts;
- these cells form osteoid tissue (bone collagen) which is then mineralized.

Cartilage formation

- islands of cartilage appear in organized clot after approximately 9 days;
- these areas of cartilage become vascularized, then ossify by apparently random enchondral ossification, starting at about 16 days;
- callus is "hard" within 3 or 4 months.

Overall microscopic view of callus

- in young callus the following tissues can be found simultaneously:
  —organized clot (granulation tissue),
  —osteoid,
  —immature bone, and
  —cartilage with areas of
  —enchondral ossification.

Primary bone healing

- is
  —direct healing of immobilized bone ends in close contact

—without the intermediate step of bridging external callus; it occurs after
- compression plating.
- process is slow.
- dead ends of cortical bone are
  —not resorbed but are
  —recanalized by new haversian systems which cross the fracture site from one fragment into the other behind a drilling cone of osteoclasts. Where there is a
  —gap, it is filled with
  —immature bone from haversian endosteum, across which haversian systems are then
  —conducted.
- micromovements prevent this process.

BONE UNION

Continued development of callus
- once the bridging callus is formed, the whole
- callus continues to develop until fractured bone ends are solidly united;
- immature bone formation is usually more advanced at the periphery (external callus) where the vascular response is more rapid than it is in the medulla.

Consolidation and remodeling of callus
- occurs over ensuing months in the
  —presence of vitamin A. Remodeling may be
  —modulated by piezoelectrical phenomena.
- callus of immature bone (weak and bulky) is gradually resorbed by osteoclasts and rebuilt by osteoblasts into mature bone with osteones and haversian systems;
- these osteones, crossing from one fragment to an adjacent one and penetrating both, act like nails or pegs, holding the fracture together;
- trabeculae are oriented along lines of stress;
- dead ends of fractured bone are also replaced by living bone.
- mature bone is strong; therefore, less quantity is required. So mechanically unnecessary parts of the external callus are removed, and a new medullary canal appears because the center of the internal callus is also resorbed;
- new cortex which is formed between the cortices of the fractured bones is as strong as the original and is almost all that remains of the callus;
- new intramedullary, intracortical and periosteal vessels and vascular anastomoses form to replace those destroyed by injury;
- new periosteum covers the new cortex.

Signs of union

Clinical signs (quite reliable)

- no pain on stressing the fracture in angulation and torsion;
- no tenderness on palpation;
- no movement at the fracture site.

Radiological signs

- bone trabeculae crossing the fracture site from one fragment to the other. The fracture line may still be visible;
- later, there is evidence of new cortex formation, reduction in the size of the external callus, and a new medullary canal, and the fracture line is no longer visible.

Chronological summary of callus formation (approximate)

- time of fracture: hematoma forms.
- several hours: fibrin clot forms in hematoma.
- 1 to 2 days: cells proliferate from cambium layer of periosteum; there is also vascular proliferation.
- 3 to 4 days: clot is organized.
- 5 to 7 days: subperiosteal osteoid tissue begins to form and becomes mineralized shortly afterward.
- 8 to 10 days: cartilage formation starts in the organized clot.
- 10 to 12 days: cartilage begins to form in the middle of the external callus in a ring around the fracture line.
- 15 to 16 days: enchondral ossification begins in cartilage.
- 30 to 40 days: external callus (immature bone with ossifying cartilage) is "sticky."
- 16 weeks: hard, internal callus (immature bone) is formed.
- 12 months: remodeling continues.

Fracture Repair in Cancellous Bone

CALLUS FORMATION

External (subperiosteal) callus

- if the fracture is undisplaced or well reduced, there is very little external callus;
- if the fracture is displaced, there is some but not much external callus;
- therefore external callus plays a relatively unimportant role in fracture union (it is more important in children than in adults).

Internal (endosteal) callus

- major method of healing;

- osteogenic cells of endosteum form immature, primary woven bone wherever there is bone contact across the fracture.

BONE UNION
Consolidation and remodeling of callus

- woven bone is replaced by lamellar bone;
- lamellar bone is replaced by trabecular cancellous bone.

Signs of union

Clinical signs

- the most reliable assessment;
- similar to signs with a cortical bone fracture but much more rapid. So
- movement of adjacent joints can be started earlier with a cancellous bone fracture than with a cortical bone fracture.

Radiological signs

- difficult to interpret and rather unreliable;
- compression fracture in cancellous bone can look as though it is healed from the first day!

Factors Which Influence Fracture Healing

GENERAL FACTORS
Age

- from birth to the end of growth, time for a given fracture to heal increases;
- from the end of growth to old age, time for a given fracture to heal remains constant.

Diet

- vitamin C (ascorbic acid) is necessary for formation of protein matrix;
- vitamin D (cholecalciferol) is necessary for mineralization of protein matrix;
- hypoproteinemia retards union;
- vitamin A is necessary for remodeling.

LOCAL FACTORS
Infection

- a major complication of open fracture or surgery;
- a major cause of delayed union and nonunion;
- infected pseudarthrosis is very difficult to treat.

Site, shape and blood supply of fracture

Factors related to rapid union

- cancellous bone heals twice as fast as cortical bone because of its vascularity and large surface area;
- epiphyseal separation heals twice as fast as fracture through the adjacent, cancellous metaphysis;
- oblique or spiral fracture unites faster than transverse fracture because bone surfaces available for callus formation are larger.

Factors related to slow union

- open fracture, Type II or III, implies greater displacement and soft tissue devascularization than occurs with closed fracture, and union may take twice as much time with an open fracture as with a closed fracture;
- open reduction presents a problem similar to that of open fracture;
- displaced fracture heals half as fast as undisplaced fracture;
- comminution slows healing;
- avascularity of one fragment, e.g.,
    - —segmental tibial shaft fracture in which intramedullary blood supply to the middle fragment is cut off at both ends,
    - —subcapital femoral fracture with avascular necrosis of the head, or
    - —fracture of the distal third of the tibial shaft which has no muscular attachments and therefore a poorer blood supply, slows fracture union.

Mobility of fracture site

- continually disrupts the young blood vessels and callus and increases cartilage and fibrous tissue formation, and although moderate mobility may initially stimulate the formation of external callus, delayed union or nonunion may result.

Displacement

- the larger the gap (space) between the ends of the fracture, the more difficult it is for callus to bridge it (contrary to popular opinion, osteoblasts cannot jump!).

Interposition

- pseudarthrosis may develop if soft tissue such as muscle lies between fracture ends.

Pathological bone

- fracture through a tumor may not unite, especially if the tumor is malignant.

Compression

- bone forms in compression and fails in tension. So
- compressed or impacted fracture heals faster.

Physiology of Bone Grafting

TYPES OF BONE AVAILABLE

Cortical

- hard and strong,
- relatively avascular and acellular,
- poorly osteogenic but
- good for fixation when combined with a plate;
- tibia and fibula are usual sources.

Cancellous

- spongy and weak,
- very vascular and cellular,
- good for osteogenesis but
- poor for internal fixation;
- iliac crest, either the anterior or the posterior third, is the usual source.

Autograft (autogenous)

- bone from same individual;
- best graft available.

Isograft (isologous)

- bone from genetically identical individual, e.g., identical twin, with identical histocompatibility antigens.

Allograft (homogenous or homograft)

- from the same species but genetically dissimilar;
- useful in small children, old osteoporotic patients, and patients with large cavities in whom sufficient autogenous bone is not available.

Xenograft (heterologous or heterograft)

- from different species, e.g., bovine bone.

HOW A GRAFT UNITES A FRACTURE

Direct new bone formation by graft cells

- occurs with cancellous graft; very little direct new bone formation occurs with cortical bone graft.
- only the surface osteogenic cells survive; osteocytes die;
- cells must be compatible (autograft or isograft);

- cells must be alive (transfer from donor to host site with minimum delay);
- cells must have immediate access to nutrients in host site, so graft should be placed in well-vascularized area and bathed in tissue fluid.

Bone induction

- all forms of bone graft can induce host osteogenic cells to form bone;
- this may be due to a protein released by the graft.

Replacement of trabeculae

- trabeculae and osteocytes of all transplanted cancellous and cortical bone die;
- new trabeculae form between host bone and the graft, being firmly cemented to both;
- osteoclasts resorb one surface of dead trabeculae of the transplant while osteoblasts deposit new bone on the other surface;
- new capillaries grow into the empty haversian canals of dead bone. Bone resorption and deposition can then occur from inside the canals;
- all trabeculae are thus entirely replaced, faster in cancellous bone (narrow trabeculae) than in cortical bone (wide trabeculae).

IMMUNOLOGICAL RESPONSE

Autografts and isografts

- no immunological response by the host occurs because proteins in the graft are recognized as "self" and are therefore compatible.

Allograft

- fresh allograft evokes strong immunological response;
- after 2 weeks, inflammatory response with T ("killer") lymphocytes kills the graft cells and destroys any tissue that they have made. This is the rejection phenomenon;
- to be accepted, this graft must be modified by
  —freezing or
  —freeze-drying, i.e., by freezing and then drying the bone graft in a vacuum.

GENERAL INDICATIONS FOR GRAFTING

Delayed union and nonunion

- osteogenic, cancellous bone is best for inducing union of a fracture and is
- effective for certain infected nonunions too;
- dual onlay is useful if nonunion is near a joint or bone is very osteoporotic.

Cavities

- cancellous chips are used to fill a cavity after
  —comminuted fracture with loss of part of the bone,
  —excision of a tumor, or
  —saucerization for chronic osteomyelitis.

Arthrodesis

- fusion of a joint, e.g., a wrist or an ankle, in patients with
  —tuberculosis,
  —advanced joint surface destruction, or
  —gross instability;
- use cortical onlay or inlay graft and supplement with cancellous bone.

Bridging defects

- defect exists after loss of part of diaphysis by
  —trauma,
  —infection or
  —tumor. Use
- cortical or cancellous dual onlay or inlay graft (two strips of cortical bone screwed to both ends of the host bone and to each other, with cancellous chips packed between) or
- cancellous chips and strips to fill the gap. A
- free vascularized bone graft with microanastomoses, especially in a relatively avascular area, may be ideal, but this technique is
  —long and difficult and requires a
  —specialized team and special equipment.

Limit motion

- use a block of cortical bone to limit the motion of an unstable joint, e.g., for a
  —recurrent posterior dislocation of the shoulder or for a
  —flail elbow.

Promote rapid union

- some fractures heal poorly, e.g.,
  —subtrochanteric fracture of the femur,
  —ulnar shaft,
  —distal tibia,
  —segmental fracture;
- cancellous bone graft at the time of initial open reduction accelerates union.

Healing in Articular Cartilage

- chondrocytes do not undergo mitosis. A

- wound of articular cartilage alone does not heal. But if underlying bone is injured too, the cartilage defect fills with
- fibrocartilaginous tissue which
- comes from the injured bone. Experiments with
- continuous passive motion show that under certain circumstances the wound may heal with
  —hyaline cartilage which comes from underlying injured bone or with
  —intercellular cartilaginous tissue formed by adjacent chondrocytes.

chapter 2

Fractures in the Adult: Classification and Diagnosis

Classification of Fractures

- a fracture is a complete or incomplete break in the continuity of a bone or of cartilage.

CLOSED OR OPEN

Closed fracture

- there is no break in the skin and no communication between the fracture and the external environment.

Open fracture (compound)

Definition

- skin wound allows communication between the fracture and the external environment.

Contamination

- fracture is contaminated with dirt;
- risk of infection increases with the delay between injury and proper treatment.

Classification

- is based on the nature of the skin wound, as follows:
  Type 1
  - skin wound is punctiform (1 cm or less) and clean;
  - usually caused by sharp fragment of fracture (from within or without);
  - can be dangerous because the inexperienced emergency room physician may
    —ignore it as insignificant and may even
    —suture it immediately in the emergency room!
  Type 2
  - large, relatively clean wound;
  - no extensive soft tissue damage.

Type 3
- dirty wound or a
- wound with extensive loss of skin or soft tissues or with
- impending loss due to a
  —narrow-based skin flap,
  —degloving injury (dermis separated from underlying tissues and therefore devascularized) or
  —associated vascular injury needing repair.

ASSOCIATED VESSEL OR NERVE INJURY (Figs. 31.2 and 32.2)

- major vessel injury takes precedence over fracture for treatment;
- if a nerve or a vascular lesion is not noticed until after treatment is started, you will not know whether it was caused by the injury or by your treatment! So the first examination should be
- neurovascular evaluation of the limb.

COMBINED SKELETAL LESIONS

- fracture associated with other bone or joint injury, e.g., the Monteggia lesion (fracture of the ulna with dislocation of the radial head).

SITE OF FRACTURE (Fig. 2.1)

Epiphysis

- epiphysis is made of cancellous bone with a very thin, weak cortex;
- it carries the cartilaginous surface of the joint;
- fracture of the epiphysis is usually of the compression type;
- fracture is often intra-articular, involving the articular surface;
- anatomic reduction is important to avoid incongruity of joint surfaces and posttraumatic osteoarthritis;
- fractures in the epiphyses heal well because cancellous bone is very cellular and vascular.

Metaphysis

- cancellous bone unites quickly.

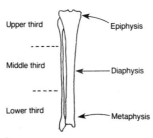

Figure 2.1. Descriptive terms for a long bone.

Diaphysis

- the shaft;
- divided descriptively into proximal, middle and distal thirds;
- made of cortical bone which is hard and relatively acellular and avascular;
- heals slowly.

EXTENT OF FRACTURE

Complete

- bone broken across both cortices;

Incomplete

- one cortex is broken;

Greenstick

- only in children;
- one cortex breaks, the other bends or buckles.

SHAPE OF FRACTURE LINE (Fig. 2.2)

Transverse

- a direct blow;
- usually stable after reduction; i.e., it will not redisplace after reduction.

Oblique

- a direct or indirect blow;
- usually unstable; i.e., it will redisplace after reduction if it is not immobilized.

Spiral

- torsion;
- usually unstable.

Comminuted

- usually caused by greater force, has
- three or more fragments, and is
- unstable;
- special types are

  #### Butterfly fragment

  - caused by direct blow;
  - poses special problems of reduction and fixation.

  #### Segmental fracture

  - two separate fractures in the shaft; the
  - middle segment is deprived of intramedullary blood supply from both ends; the incidence of pseudarthrosis is higher with a segmental fracture than with most other comminuted fractures.

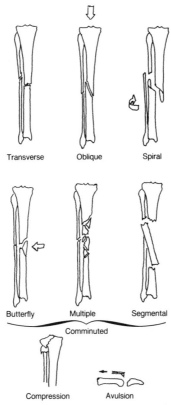

Figure 2.2.   Shape of the fracture line.

- poses special problems of reduction and fixation because the
  —middle fragment cannot be controlled during closed reduction and because
  —open reduction may damage the periosteal blood supply, which will result in the death of the middle segment.

Compression fracture

- occurs in cancellous bone, e.g., the vertebral body or the proximal metaphysis of the tibia.

Avulsion fractures

- corner or flake of bone
- pulled off by ligament or tendon.

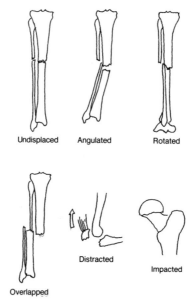

Figure 2.3. Displacement of the fracture fragments.

DISPLACEMENT (Fig. 2.3)

Undisplaced

Angulation

- in anteroposterior (sagittal) plane or
- in lateral (coronal) plane, causing varus or valgus deformity.

Rotation

Overlap

- causes shortening.

Distraction

- caused by muscle pull, e.g., transverse fracture of the olecranon (triceps) or the patella (quadriceps).

Impaction

- one fragment crushed into the other;
- always in cancellous bone, e.g., surgical neck of the humerus, subcapital fracture of hip, or vertebral body.

Combination

- combination of any two or more of the above.

STABILITY

Stable fractures are

- fractures with little or no displacement (but the x-ray made in the hospital may not show the extent of the initial displacement at the time of injury),
- transverse fracture after reduction, and
- fracture of one forearm bone (usually the ulna) or one leg bone (tibia or fibula) with the other bone intact and no adjacent joint injury.

Unstable fractures are

- oblique or spiral fractures,
- comminuted fractures, and
- fracture of one bone with an associated joint or ligament lesion, e.g., a Monteggia fracture.

PARTICULAR KINDS OF FRACTURE

Pathological fractures

General remarks

- a pathological fracture occurs through abnormal bone which is weak and breaks easily, usually after minimal trauma;
- fracture may reveal the underlying disease for the first time;
- closed treatment with plaster cast immobilization is usually adequate, but
- in certain circumstances open reduction and internal fixation, with or without bone grafting, is necessary;
- prophylactic internal fixation, before fracture, may prevent later complications;
- if the bone lesion is a tumor, open reduction and internal fixation of the fracture may be necessary for the patient's comfort;
- at surgery, take a biopsy of the lesion to confirm diagnosis.

Classification of the underlying lesion

Congenital anomalies

- multiple enchondromatosis (Ollier's disease) with fractures through the chondromata;
- osteogenesis imperfecta with fractures through the shaft.

Metabolic bone disease

- rickets and osteomalacia (adult rickets) due to vitamin D deficiency, with fractures through the convex cortex of bent bones;
- scurvy due to vitamin C deficiency, with fractures at the junction of the epiphyseal plate and metaphysis;
- osteoporosis with vertebral compression fractures;

- Cushing's syndrome and steroid therapy which cause osteoporosis and retard fracture healing by suppressing osteogenic activity; and
- hyperparathyroidism and Paget's disease.

Inflammatory disease

- osteomyelitis, either pyogenic or granulomatous; fracture occurs at the junction of dead bone and live bone;
- rheumatoid arthritis.

Neuromuscular disease

- myelodysplasia or
- anterior poliomyelitis with fracture of hypoplastic bone, e.g., the femoral or tibial shaft.

Tumors

- benign
  —solitary bone cyst (before the end of growth);
  —chondroma, especially in the phalanges;
  —giant cell tumor, commonly in the distal radius, in the proximal femur and around the knee joint.
- primary malignant
  —osteosarcoma of the femur or tibia, usually in patients between 15 and 25 years old;
  —myeloma, in patients 40 years of age or older (the vertebral body is a common site of fracture).
- metastatic (older age group)
  —breast (50% to 65% metastasize to bone),
  —prostate (50% to 65%),
  —lungs and bronchi (25% to 30%),
  —kidneys (20% to 25%),
  —cervix and
  —thyroid;
- common sites of metastases are
  —flat bones, the pelvis, ribs and skull,
  —long bones, particularly femoral and humeral shafts, and the
  —skull.

Disorders of unknown etiology

- histiocytosis X and
- polyostotic fibrous dysplasia.

Iatrogenic

- a fractured long bone treated with a plate may refracture through a screw hole;

- taking a cortical graft from a tibia weakens the tibia which may fracture.

Stress (fatigue) fractures

- a fatigue fracture occurs in normal bone which is subjected to unaccustomed repetitive stress;
- clinically, there is pain, local tenderness, and swelling;
- at first, the radiograph may be normal or a hairline crack may be seen; later, the effects of a subperiosteal reaction can be seen;
- examples include
  —metatarsal or femoral neck fractures in soldiers (especially new recruits) on long marches;
  —proximal fibula shaft fractures in parachutists; and
  —tibial shaft fractures in ballet dancers and athletes.
- treatment is protection with crutches and a cast, if necessary.

Clinical Examination

HISTORY

Of the injury

- the five Ws: What, When, Where, Was, Why

  What happened (type of accident)?

  Direct or indirect trauma

  - direct forces cause
    —transverse fractures, sometimes with a butterfly fragment, and
    —comminuted fractures. They are also frequently associated with
    —soft tissue damage (open fracture).
  - indirect forces cause
    —spiral,
    —oblique and
    —avulsion fractures.

  Road accident or fall from a height

  - large forces are generated;
  - multiple injuries are likely, so
  - think of the head, neck, chest, abdomen, spine and pelvis as well as limbs and examine them all.

  Ordinary fall

  - small forces are generated;
  - multiple injuries are unlikely.

Sports injury

- ligaments and muscles.

Skin wound

- clean, incised or
- crushing, tearing injury or
- human or animal bite, particularly on the hand (very dirty).

When did it happen?

- delay between the time of the injury and the time of arrival at the hospital is important if a vascular problem is present or a fracture is open;
- recent fracture is usually reducible by manipulation; but anticipate swelling in the 24 hours following fracture;
- a fracture more than a few days old is usually irreducible by closed manipulation.

Where did it happen?

- especially important if the fracture is open, e.g.,
  —in a field (very dirty, and *Clostridium* spores will be present), on a
  —road (dirty), or in the
  —house (relatively clean). Anticipate
- prolonged convalescence in an industrial or road accident for which compensation is available.

Was it already treated elsewhere?

- what was done?

Why did it happen?

- may help to prevent similar accidents, e.g., work-related, motor vehicle.

General history

Age of patient

- some fractures are more common in young adults, e.g., fracture of the tibia or scaphoid;
- others are more common in older patient, e.g., Colles' or hip fracture.

Present and past medical and surgical history

- other disease may influence treatment, e.g., diabetes mellitus with poor circulation in the injured leg;
- history of carcinoma may suggest pathological fracture. It may be
- important to continue or modify current medication (e.g., digoxin, steroids).

Ocupational and social history

- will influence the treatment and rehabilitation; e.g., acromioclavicular dislocation might be treated differently in a 25-year-old physical education instructor than in a 25-year-old clerk with a desk job.

PHYSICAL EXAMINATION

General condition

Multiple trauma

- the seven Bs of preserving a patient's life are presented in decreasing order of importance:
- Breathing
  —clear airway if blocked;
  —mouth-to-mouth respiration if respiratory arrest;
- Beating heart
  —cardiac massage if cardiac arrest;
- Bleeding
  —shock! So
  —stop the hemorrhage and
  —transfuse fluid (preferably blood) as soon as possible;
- Brain
  —test the level of consciousness;
- Bowel
  —solid or hollow visceral injury;
- Bladder or urethra
  —rupture;
- Bones and joints
  —fractures and dislocations.
- bones may come last, but they are not unimportant!

Local examination of injured part

Musculoskeletal system

Inspection

- look for
  —angulation or rotation,
  —shortening,
  —edema and bruising.

Palpation

- feel gently for
  —tenderness,
  —abnormal movement and crepitus, and

—decreased movement in a joint. Examination is

—painful and may increase soft tissue damage, so do not move the limb unnecessarily.

Function

- reduction or loss of function of the limb usually accompanies injury.

Suspicion

- suspect a fracture, splint the limb, and order appropriate x-rays if the following signs are present:
  —pain,
  —swelling and
  —tenderness.

Associated structures

Vessels

- with major vessel disruption or occlusion and
- compartment syndromes, think of the
- five Ps and see Chapter 32.

Nerves

- motor function is a more objective and reliable test than is a subjective sensory examination. Use this quick
- screening examination for the hand, testing and comparing the strength of the injured side with that of the normal side:
  —radial nerve, extension of the metacarpophalageal (MP) joints;
  —ulnar nerve, spread the fingers (with MP joints extended) or extend the interphalangeal (IP) joints;
  —median nerve, oppose the thumb.

Skin

- open fracture,
- degloving (shear) injury,
- grazes and cuts,
- fracture blisters. Skin damage or gross edema may preclude or delay open reduction because of fear of infection.

Radiographic Examination

- an adjunct to, and not a substitute for, a
- good history and
- physical examination!

TIMING OF RADIOGRAPHIC EXAMINATION

- as soon as the airway has been reestablished,
- shock has been treated, the
- patient's general condition is stable, the
- clinical examination has been completed, and the
- fractured limb has been splinted temporarily,
- the patient can be taken to the x-ray department.

WHEN TO ORDER RADIOGRAPHS

Diagnosis is obvious when there is

- deformity,
- abnormal movement or
- crepitus, so order radiographs for confirmation and as a guide for treatment.

Suspicion of fracture when there is

- pain,
- swelling and
- tenderness, so order radiographs to confirm the presence or absence of fracture or joint injury.

Multiple trauma

- always order anteroposterior (AP) views of the pelvis.

Head injury

- always order x-rays of the cervical spine as well as of the skull.

HOW TO ORDER RADIOGRAPHS

Be precise:
- spell the patient's name correctly;
- indicate the correct side (right or left) of the injury,
- the correct limb (arm or leg), and
- the part of the limb injured, e.g., anteroposterior (AP) and lateral of left tibial shaft.

RULES

Limit irradiation

- x-rays are dangerous to
  —you,
  —the patient, especially a woman of child-bearing age, and
  —anyone in the vicinity. So
    - do not order unnecessary radiographs, make sure of
    - adequate protection for all hospital staff in the vicinity, and whenever possible

- shield the patient's gonads during lower abdominal and pelvic x-rays.

Two x-rays

- always request two x-rays in planes at right angles (AP and lateral) because
- a fracture may be hidden or displacement may not be apparent on one view;
- remember that a fracture or a dislocation is three-dimensional.

Turn the machine, not the limb

- for the two x-ray views, the machine should be turned around the limb:
- if the limb is turned, it will turn through the fracture site, thus causing more
  —displacement,
  —hemorrhage,
  —soft tissue damage, and
  —pain, and
  —the x-rays will not be proper AP and lateral views.

X-ray the entire bone (Fig. 2.4)

- the whole length of the bone must be seen in order not to miss an associated fracture, e.g., a fractured medial malleolus with a fractured neck of the fibula.

X-ray the adjacent joints (Fig. 2.4)

- joints immediately proximal and distal to a fracture must be seen. If they are not,
  —order another x-ray. For example, consider a fracture of the femoral shaft with

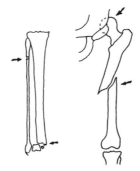

Figure 2.4.   X-ray the whole length of the bone and the adjacent joints.

—dislocation of the same hip. If the dislocation is

—not recognized, the femur will heal in

—malrotation, the

—foot will rotate backward after late open reduction of the hip, and the patient

—will not know whether he is coming or going!

Doubtful cases

- request x-rays of the normal side for comparison,
- obliques, or
- stress films for ligament damage or pseudarthrosis;
- CAT scans are useful especially in vertebral and pelvic injuries;
- scintigraphy may help you to
  —detect stress fractures and
  —evaluate avascular necrosis.

Reading the radiographs

- read all your own radiographs and use Dussault's four-part
- "Playboy" approach by stripping the x-ray to its bare essentials. First look at the
- soft tissues for
  —swelling, displaced fat pads, and air in the tissues. Then think of
- form and line, and examine all the
  —bones for their shape, alignment and interrelationships. Now probe deeper and evaluate the
- denseness and texture of the subject's bones, looking particularly for
  —osteoporosis and
  —lytic or blastic lesions. Finally, you reach the
- core of the problem, the
  —fracture or
  —joint injury itself. Remember that
- displacement of the fracture was greatest at the moment of injury, not necessarily when the radiographs were made; and
- soft tissue damage to
  —skin, vessels and nerves and to
  —muscles, tendons, ligaments and the periosteum is not visible on radiographs. So
  —think of it.

chapter 3
Fractures in Children: Classification and Diagnosis

Similarities with Adult Fractures

CLASSIFICATION

- general terms of classification, e.g., closed and open, intra-articular, oblique and spiral, comminution, angulation and rotation, are applicable to children's fractures;
- differences are considered below.

HISTORY, PHYSICAL AND RADIOLOGICAL EXAMINATION

- equally as important with children as with adults, and should follow the same steps; but
- when the patient is a child, you must explain the problem, the treatment, possible complications and probable outcome to the parents as well.

PATHOLOGICAL AND STRESS FRACTURES

- occur in children too, so keep them in mind.

Special Features of Children's Fractures

- fractures in children are different from fractures in adults because children's bones
  —are resilient,
  —have tough periosteum,
  —grow in length through the epiphyseal plates,
  —heal well and quickly and
  —can remodel.
- these differences in anatomy, physiology and biomechanics result in differences in the
  —pattern of fractures,
  —diagnostic problems,
  —methods of treatment and the
  —prognosis.

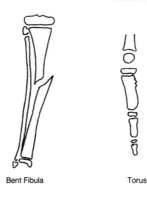

Bent Fibula   Torus

Greenstick

Figure 3.1. Resilience of children's bones.

RESILIENCE (Fig. 3.1)

- elastic resilience results in particular kinds of incomplete fractures:

Bent bones

- a child's bone may bend up to 45° before it breaks; this is
- common in the
  —ulna where it may be associated with dislocation of the radial head, a Monteggia type of lesion, and in the
  —fibula where it may be associated with tibial fracture.

Buckle (torus) fracture

- compression fracture of one cortex (wrinkled on x-ray) without visible injury to the other cortex;
- occurs near the metaphysis in a young child.

Greenstick fracture

- common in the forearm and tibia;
- the bone partly cracks and partly buckles, like young green wood;
- cortex on the convex side is broken (tension), whereas
- cortex on the concave side buckles (compression);
- displacement is greater at the moment of injury than is shown on the x-ray (elastic recoil of the bone and the surrounding soft tissue partly reduces the deformity); but
- beware because
  —muscle pull in the cast can also increase the deformity;

• treatment usually includes completion of the fracture by breaking the other cortex to avoid redisplacement in the cast.

PERIOSTEUM (Figs. 3.2 and 12.8)

• thick and strong;
• usually torn on the convex side of the fracture and intact on the concave side;
• may hinder or prevent reduction unless you know how to use it, e.g.,
• displaced fracture of distal radius with overlap where
  —dorsal periosteum is intact and prevents reduction by traction alone. You must
  —angulate the fracture and engage the fractured margins of the dorsal cortex first;
  —intact dorsal periosteum prevents overcorrection (see Chapter 12). With a
• fracture of the femoral shaft treated in traction, the
  —periosteum and soft tissues guide the fragments into alignment and help
  —prevent distraction;
• supracondylar fracture of the humerus has
  —intact periosteum on one side. This
  —prevents overcorrection and allows you to
  —lock the other side of the fracture to prevent loss of reduction (see Chapter 10).

EPIPHYSEAL GROWTH PLATE INJURIES
Histology of the growth plate (Fig. 3.3)

• the growth plate is responsible for growth in the length of the long bone;
• blood supply comes from the epiphysis;
• the plate is divided into four horizontal zones:
  Zone I
  • resting layer of hyaline cartilage;
  • lies adjacent to the bone of the epiphysis and

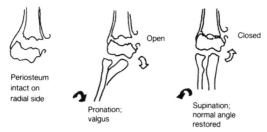

Periosteum
intact on
radial side

Open

Pronation;
valgus

Closed

Supination;
normal angle
restored

Figure 3.2.   Use the periosteal hinge to stabilize the reduction.

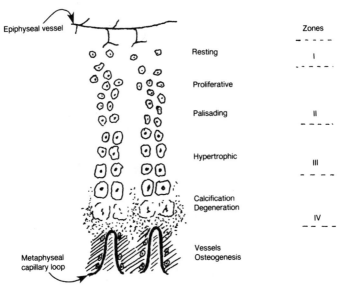

Figure 3.3. Longitudinal section of the growth plate. (Modified from Ham AW, Cormack DH: *Histology*, ed 8. Toronto, JB Lippincott, 1979, p 431.)

- anchors the plate to the epiphysis;
- contains young, immature chondrocytes;
- capillary branches from epiphyseal vessels enter canals in this zone and nourish the first three zones of the plate by diffusion through the cartilage;
- intercellular substance (matrix) contains collagen fibers, mucopolysaccharides and water.

Zone II

- proliferating cartilage cells;
- very active layer;
- young chondrocytes multiply by mitosis and push the epiphysis away from the shaft;
- new cells arranged in longitudinal columns perpendicular to the plate are directed into Zone III;
- contains many cells and less matrix.

Zone III

- hypertrophic cartilage cells;
- cartilage cells near the metaphysis mature and hypertrophy;
- closer to the metaphysis, where the most mature cells lie, they accu-

mulate glycogen, secrete alkaline phosphatase, and liberate matrix vesicles into matrix between adjacent rows of chondrocytes; this zone is

- almost entirely cellular, with little intercellular matrix;
- structurally a weak zone that has few collagen fibers to strengthen it;
- fracture through the plate occurs at the junction between this zone and the zone of calcification (Zone IV);
- in a separation of the epiphyseal plate, therefore, the growth plate stays with the epiphysis and retains its blood supply.

Zone IV

- calcifying cartilage;
- thin zone one to two cells thick;
- intercellular matrix calcifies. (Do not confuse calcification with ossification. This zone is calcified cartilage, not calcified bone.)
- calcification is triggered by chondrocytes which have secreted alkaline phosphatase and liberated vesicles;
- calcified matrix prevents diffusion of metabolites;
- chondrocytes die and disintegrate, leaving empty lacunae;
- calcified matrix between cell columns partly disappears;
- on the metaphyseal side of this zone, empty lacunae are invaded by osteogenic cells and metaphyseal blood vessels bringing nutrients;
- osteogenic cells differentiate into osteoblasts in the presence of capillary loops and lay down
- bone matrix (uncalcified osteoid tissue) on the remains of calcified cartilage columns;
- bone matrix is then calcified to form trabeculae of bone with cartilage cores;
- immature bone and cartilage cores are later resorbed by osteoclasts and rebuilt into mature bone. So the
- growth process is a race between
  —cartilage growth on the epiphyseal side of the plate, which thickens it, and
  —calcification and death of cartilage on the diaphyseal side, which tends to narrow the plate.

Growth plate injuries

General considerations

Diagnosis

- dislocations and ligament injuries are unusual in children because the ligaments and joint capsule are stronger than the epiphyseal plate;
- epiphyses are cartilaginous before ossification and, therefore, transparent to x-rays (radiolucent);

- secondary centers of ossification occur at different times in different bones; you must be aware of these;
- if you are uncertain of the diagnosis, order comparative x-rays of the normal side;
- if you are still uncertain, oblique x-rays (especially for the ankle) and stress views (with the patient under anesthesia) may be helpful;
- an air arthrogram may help in a very young child before secondary ossification centers have appeared, but interpretation is difficult;
- if you
  —still suspect an epiphyseal injury, even though
  —all special examinations are normal,
  —treat the child as though he had an injury. (Your clinical judgment will eventually be superior to radiographs which are only shadows after all!)
- remember that
  —frost bite,
  —electrical and heat burns
  —and irradiation may also damage the plate without visible radiological changes initially.

Treatment

- growth plate injuries more than 1 week old usually cannot be reduced closed;
- open reduction after 2 or 3 weeks is often very difficult. For extra-articular injuries that do not cross the plate, it may be better to
  —wait several weeks and then do corrective osteotomy through the metaphysis. But
  —osteotomy in or too close to the growth plate may damage the plate, so
  —use x-ray control during surgery to see where you are.
- displaced injuries across the growth plate and intra-articular fractures must be reduced even after several weeks delay between injury and treatment;
- all patients with growth plate injuries should be seen at regular intervals for 2 years after injury so that any deformity which develops can be treated early;
- always forewarn parents of the possibility of progressive growth deformity.

Special considerations

- important questions are,
  —is the blood supply to the resting zone of the plate damaged,
  —will new bone growth cover the fractured surface of the plate and

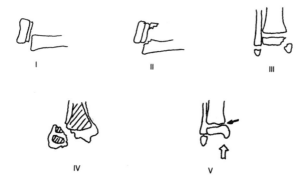

Figure 3.4. Salter-Harris classification of growth plate injuries. (Modified from Salter RB, Harris WR: Injuries involving the epiphyseal plate. *J Bone Joint Surg* 45A:587–622, 1963.)

form a bone bridge from epiphysis to metaphysis (in either case, the future growth of the bone will be altered), and thirdly,
—is the fracture intra-articular?

- the following classification helps predict progressive growth deformity after injury, and, therefore, guides your treatment.

Classification (Salter-Harris) and treatment (Fig. 3.4)

Type I

Pathology

- shear injury with complete separation of the whole plate and epiphysis from the metaphysis without fracture through bone;
- the fracture line undulates horizontally between Zone III and Zone IV (uncalcified and calcified zones) of the plate;
- fracture does not go through articular cartilage;
- periosteum is mostly intact and prevents marked displacement;
- common sites are the distal fibula and the distal radius;
- occurs most often in the very young child.

Treatment

- closed reduction;
- use the periosteal hinge to guide the distal fragment;
- accurate, anatomical reduction is not always necessary, as remodeling may help if angulation is in the plane of movement of the adjacent joint.

Prognosis

- good;

- after reduction, growth usually continues normally. Rarely, if one side of the plate was
- compressed at injury, an osseous bridge may form and deformity will ensue.

Type II

Pathology

- is most common type;
- another shear injury, but the
- fracture line goes
  —horizontally between Zones III and IV (the tension phase), then
  —turns obliquely through one corner of the metaphysis (compression phase);
- x-ray shows the triangular corner of the metaphysis attached to the epiphysis (Thurston-Holland sign);
- fracture does not cross articular cartilage, nor does it cross the growth plate;
- periosteum usually is torn on the tension side only;
- common site is the distal radius.

Treatment

- closed reduction with care and gentleness to avoid further growth plate injury;
- use the periosteal hinge as a guide;
- anatomical reduction is not always necessary if angulation is in the plane of movement of the joint.

Prognosis

- good if properly treated; but
- compression of the plate at the metaphyseal fracture may instigate formation of
  —bone bridge with subsequent
  —deformity.

Type III

Pathology

- rare;
- intra-articular;
- fracture runs horizontally across part of the plate, then crosses the plate, the epiphysis and the articular cartilage vertically or obliquely;
- displacement is common;
- commonest sites are the medial malleolus or the lateral part of the distal tibial epiphysis in the child near the end of growth (Tillaux

fracture), at which time growth deformity is not a problem but congruence of the articular surface is.

Treatment

- accurate open reduction and internal fixation are usually necessary to restore congruent articular surface;
- fragment must not be dissected from its blood supply (capsule, ligament, periosteum);
- reduction should be confirmed by x-ray before wound closure.

Prognosis

- fair, with proper treatment.

Type IV

Pathology

- fairly common;
- intra-articular,
- fracture line is vertical or oblique and crosses the metaphysis, growth plate, epiphysis and articular cartilage;
- diagnosis is difficult if the
  —secondary ossification center has not yet appeared or is still small. In this case, the
  —metaphyseal fragment is the key;
- displacement is frequent and results from the tension of attached muscles;
- common site is the lateral humeral condyle.

Treatment

- open reduction is almost always necessary;
- fixation with two fine, smooth Kirschner wires is best because they do not damage the growth plate;
- do not put threaded wires or screws across the plate. If the
- metaphyseal fragment is large, it may be fixed with a horizontal screw, but this must not cross the plate;
- do not dissect the fragment from its blood supply;
- confirm accurate reduction by x-rays before closure;
- remove wires or screws when fracture has healed.

Prognosis

- uncertain, even when properly treated;
- failure to obtain accurate reduction may result in
  —nonunion,
  —malunion,
  —progressive growth deformity (unlike in the adult in whom the deformity does not increase with time), or

—incongruity of the joint surface with stiffness and eventual osteoarthritis.

Type V

Pathology

- "Jekyll and Hyde" injury because it
  —looks innocent but
  —is not!
- probably rare;
- crush injury of the plate by compression;
- diagnosis is clinical, with
  —history of injury,
  —swelling and
  —maximum tenderness over the growth plate. To determine this point of maximum tenderness, use the pencil test; i.e., press the soft eraser end of a pencil over the growth plate until the point of maximum tenderness is elicited;
- radiographs appear normal;
- premature closure of the plate with progressive shortening or angulation may occur.

Treatment

- cast protection for several weeks.

Prognosis

- poor, in spite of treatment, so warn the parents!

FRACTURE HEALING
Speed of healing

- union is fast, particularly in the young child.

Shaft

fractured femoral shaft will usually unite in
- 3 weeks at birth,
- 8 weeks at 8 years old,
- 12 weeks at 12 years old,
- 20 weeks in the adult.

Metaphysis

- metaphyseal fracture heals twice as fast as shaft fracture in the same age group.

Epiphyseal plate injury

- heals 3 or 4 times as fast as shaft fracture in the same age group.

Nonunion

- rare in children unless the fracture is

—infected or

—open reduction has damaged the blood supply or introduced infection. In general,

- open reduction and internal fixation are seldom indicated in children except for

—displaced intra-articular fractures and

—some growth plate injuries.

REMODELING (Figs. 3.5 and 3.6)

Growth potential

- because of growth potential, a child's bone responds to normal stresses (muscle pull, gravity) by remodeling itself to withstand these stresses (Wolff's law: form follows function).

Correction of deformity

- remodeling may correct the deformity of an incomplete reduction, but
- often remodeling cannot help; you should not accept a poor reduction, hoping that "Mother Nature" and "Father Time" will solve the problem!
- your reduction must at least restore longitudinal and rotational alignment.

Guidelines

- the following guidelines indicate when remodeling can help the patient and when it cannot.

  Remodeling will help:

  - the young patient
    —who has at least 2 years growth left;

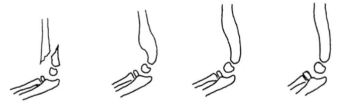

Figure 3.5. Remodeling of unreduced supracondylar fracture by resorption and longitudinal growth.

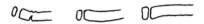

Figure 3.6. Remodeling of angulation by differential apposition and resorption and asymmetrical physeal growth.

—the younger the child, the greater the potential for remodeling;
- metaphyseal fracture because
  —the nearer the fracture is to the growth plate, the greater the potential for remodeling;
- anteroposterior angulation, i.e.,
  —angulation in the plane of movement of the adjacent joint (anteroposterior or sagittal plane), e.g., posterior angulation of fracture of the distal radius;
- shortening because
  —healing bone often overgrows in the child (due to hyperemia) and may correct a shortening of 1 to 2 cm, e.g., a fractured midshaft femur with overlap.

Remodeling will not help:
- the child near the end of growth;
- rotational deformity;
- angulation in the anteroposterior (sagittal) plane at the midshaft, e.g., fracture of both bones of the forearm;
- angulation in the coronal plane at right angles to the plane of movement of the adjacent joint causing valgus or varus deformity;
- gross shortening of more than 4 cm;
- displaced fracture across a growth plate, whether the fracture is intra-articular or not.

REHABILITATION
- muscle atrophy and joint stiffness after immobilization in a cast are normally
- not a problem in children;
- rapid mobilization is, therefore, unnecessary in a child and should
- not be used as an excuse for open reduction and internal fixation.
- physiotherapy is
  —rarely indicated after a fracture has healed because the
  —high activity level of the child will soon
  —regain joint mobility and muscle strength.

BIRTH INJURIES

Etiology

Single fracture
- difficult delivery, especially breech, or
- hurried delivery to avoid hypoxia;
- often unavoidable;
- better to have a normal baby with a broken arm than a decerebrate baby with a normal arm.

Multiple fractures

- usually pathological, e.g., osteogenesis imperfecta.

Clinical features

- fractures of the clavicle, humeral shaft (proximal fragment pulled into abduction by deltoid) and femoral shaft (proximal fragment in abduction and flexion) are the commonest;
- epiphyseal separations are less common;
- dislocations are rare;
- the obstetrician or midwife usually hears and feels the bone break, but epiphyseal separation is silent and diagnosis is often missed until callus appears, especially in the distal humerus, because secondary centers of ossification appear after birth;
- a baby with a fractured clavicle will not move the arm (pseudoparalysis). Differentiate this from brachial plexus injury (which may coexist) by neurological examination and x-ray.

Treatment

- these fractures heal quickly and well with nonoperative treatment, and remodeling can be remarkable. A fracture of the
- clavicle needs only gentle handling. For the
- humerus, strap the arm to the chest over padding to keep the arm abducted;
- treat a femoral fracture by vertical (Byrant's) skin traction to both lower limbs for 3 weeks (avoid ischemia);
- treat epiphyseal injuries about the elbow or knee with the joint slightly flexed. Do not attempt reduction.

PATHOLOGICAL FRACTURES

- common causes are
  —osteomyelitis and septic arthritis,
  —metabolic disease such as rickets,
  —bone cyst,
  —primary malignant bone tumor, and
  —osteoporosis in neurogenic disease or after prolonged immobilization.

BATTERED CHILD SYNDROME

- most common in the first 2 years of the child's life;
- if a child presents with
  —multiple bruises, fractures or other injuries, or is seen on
  —consecutive occasions with new injuries, or has
  —several fractures and bruises in different stages of healing,
- think of this possibility.

- osteogenesis imperfecta may mimic this syndrome, but helpful differential points in this disease may be
  - —family history,
  - —minimal trauma,
  - —blue sclerae and
  - —hypotrophic shafts of bones.

chapter 4

Treatment of Recent Fractures: General Principles

First Aid

Treatment of an injured patient is urgent and should be started at the place of the accident by

- removal of the accident victim to a safe place, e.g., from the middle of the road to the side of the road,
- establishment of an airway,
- arrest of external hemorrhage by manual compression (tourniquet can be dangerous),
- careful and gentle treatment of the patient to diminish pain and shock, and
- temporary immobilization of the injured limb(s) to avoid further damage to soft tissues (vessels and nerves) and to bone and to avoid the aggravation of shock. Then
- rapid transport to a treatment center should be provided.

Treatment in Emergency Department

- initial examination of the vital systems and institution of appropriate life-saving measures, the seven Bs (see Chapter 2);
- once the airway is established and shock has been treated, a
  —fractured limb should be
  —splinted BEFORE sending the patient to the x-ray department. The splint may be of ready-made metal or plastic, plaster backslab, or anything suitable that is available; it must be well padded. All previous
- bandages should be removed, wounds should be inspected and then cleaned with soap and water and an antiseptic, and then clean dressings should be applied before splinting.

Principles of Definitive Treatment

GENERAL COMMENTS

- treatment of a patient with a fracture is urgent, so do not delay.
- particularly urgent problems are

—fracture with signs of ischemia,
—fracture with bleeding and shock,
—supracondylar humeral fracture, especially in a child,
—wrist and ankle fractures, and
—any dislocation.
- open fracture is a special case (see below), and
- vascular injuries are considered elsewhere (Chapter 32).
- this chapter deals with general principles; exceptions are dealt with in the relevant chapters.

AIMS OF TREATMENT
- promote healing of the fracture by
  —reduction and
  —maintenance of reduction of the fracture. But remember:
  —treat the patient, not the x-ray!
- restore normal function to the limb;
- rehabilitate the patient in his society.

PROTECTION OR IMMOBILIZATION ALONE WITHOUT REDUCTION
Protection
- certain stable fractures, e.g., a fibula shaft fracture with intact tibia, may require only crutches and non-weight-bearing (NWB) on the injured side until the pain subsides;
- certain stable impacted fractures need only a minimum of protection; e.g., an impacted fracture of surgical neck of the humerus in the aged patient requires a sling and Velpeau bandage for 5 days, then active shoulder exercises with the sling only.

Immobilization
- certain fractures do not require reduction but must be immobilized, e.g.,
  —undisplaced fracture of the tibial shaft,
  —displaced fracture with good alignment of the humerus or femur,
  —any undisplaced fracture in a child because he will surely fall again and displace the fracture if he has no cast.

REDUCTION AND IMMOBILIZATION
- most fractures can be reduced by closed means, but
- a few require open reduction.
- all fractures which have been reduced must be adequately immobilized afterward. If the
- limb is very swollen, elevate it first, then reduce the fracture when the swelling has disappeared.

Indications for reduction

- rotational deformity;
- angulation in the coronal plane
  —varus or valgus deformity;
- marked angulation in the sagittal plane, i.e.,
  —angulation in the anteroposterior (AP) plane, the same plane as that of the movement of the nearest joint;
- intra-articular fracture which is
  —displaced;
- overlap of
  —forearm or
  —tibia fracture, especially with
- shortening of
  —more than 2 cm in the lower limb;

Technique of closed reduction

- be gentle
  —to avoid further injury to the limb;
- anesthesia
  —local (into the fracture hematoma),
  —regional, spinal or
  —general, depending upon the circumstances and the patient's general condition;
- manipulation
  —accentuate the deformity to disimpact the fracture, then apply
  —traction and
  —re-engage the fragments in the anatomical position.
- traction
  —pull in the direction of the long axis of the proximal fragment;
  —the periosteal sleeve and adjacent soft tissues help the reduction by guiding the fragments into alignment;
- x-ray control is
  —important to confirm reduction and apposition of the fragments and
  —should be done while the patient is still anesthetized.
- special tricks
  —fractures, like patients and doctors, have their idiosyncracies, and every surgeon has his own tricks for reducing them. Although these tricks will be described in the relevant chapters, they are best learned by demonstration and experience. You cannot learn everything from books!

Immobilization by plaster cast

General indications

- protection and to
- maintain reduction.

General rules

Joint immobilization

- joints immediately proximal and distal to the fracture should be immobilized in the following positions according to the injury unless the nature of the injury requires otherwise:

—shoulder:	against the trunk or 70° of abduction;
—elbow:	90° flexion;
—forearm:	neutral rotation;
—wrist:	15° dorsiflexion or palmar flexion;
—metacarpophalangeal (MP):	90° flexion;
—interphalangeal (IP):	25° flexion, less for the index finger and more for the little finger;
—thumb:	in opposition;
—hip:	20° flexion and neutral rotation, with no abduction or adduction;
—knee:	20° flexion
—ankle:	neutral;
—subtalar:	neutral.

- do not immobilize joints unnecessarily;
- do not use a plaster cast on a limb with burned skin because ischemia will follow!

Padding

- put padding between the skin and the cast to allow for swelling; an
- unpadded cast is DANGEROUS!
- subcutaneous bony prominences such as those that follow may need extra padding:
    - —scapula, acromion and clavicle,
    - —elbow and wrist,
    - —patella and the head and neck of the fibula,
    - —tibial tuberosity and anterior tibial border,
    - —heel, malleoli and instep (dorsum of foot),

—spinous vertebral processes and the sacrum, and
—iliac crest and spines.

Circular versus backslab cast

- always split a circular plaster cast to the skin after reduction, unless the patient is in a hospital bed and can be observed regularly;
- if the patient goes home immediately after reduction, maintain the reduction by a backslab or split cast and complete this the next day at the fracture clinic if neurovascular status is normal.

Molding (Fig. 4.1)

- cast should be molded around the limb to prevent rotation through the fracture. Limbs are seldom circular, so
  —mold the cast to follow the natural contours of the limb, e.g.,

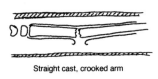

Before reduction

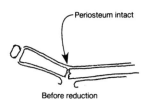

Straight cast, crooked arm

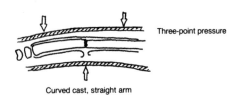

Curved cast, straight arm

Figure 4.1. Use of the periosteal hinge to maintain reduction. (Modified from Charnley J: *The Closed Treatment of Common Fractures*, ed 3. Edinburgh, Churchill Livingstone, 1961, p 54.)

—oval in the distal forearm and distal thigh;
- molding uses the three-point fixation principle to prevent redisplacement of the fracture. Slightly curve the cast in a direction opposite the original angular displacement;
- intact periosteum on the concave side of the fracture acts as a hinge and prevents overcorrection;
- remember: "curved plaster, straight limb; straight plaster, curved limb!"

Additional fixation with Kirschner wires
- intramedullary K wire introduced percutaneously without necessarily opening the fracture will prevent angulation of an unstable fracture in the cast, e.g., for
  —oblique fracture of ulnar shaft (unstable) with dislocation of the radial head (Monteggia lesion) in a child, use intramedullary wire in the ulna;
- transverse K wires (in forearm) or Steinmann pins (in tibia) through the proximal and distal fragments, with the ends held in the plaster cast, will
  —help reduction and prevent shortening of unstable radial or tibial fractures;
- remove wires at 4 weeks or less.

Postplaster x-rays
- confirm that reduction is maintained in the cast, by two radiographs through the cast. If
- fracture has a moderate angulation, correct this by
  —cutting the padded cast three quarters of the way around at the fracture when the cast is dry,
  —opening the wedge until the bones are straight, and then plastering the wedge (see Chapter 23). But
  —do not wedge an unpadded cast. If a
- cast is unpadded or
- reduction is totally lost,
- start all over again.

Postreduction care
- the patient should be seen the next day to check the neurovascular status of the limb;
- the patient should keep the limb elevated for 4 to 6 days after fracture reduction;
- draw the fracture and write the date on the cast to make your task easier in the fracture clinic;
- x-ray through plaster at regular intervals, usually 1, 2 and 3 weeks

after reduction, to be sure that the fracture does not redisplace. Remanipulate if necessary.

Physiotherapy

- important in the treatment of adults. Encourage
- isometric muscle contractions of the injured limb in plaster several times a day;
- all joints not immobilized, including normal limbs, must be exercised with full range of motion (FROM) daily;
- start the day after reduction;
- particularly important for
  —shoulder,
  —elbow and
  —all finger (MP and IP) joints because these stiffen quickly if not actively exercised;
- remember that
  —malunion with mobile fingers is
  —better than
  —anatomic reduction and sound union with stiff fingers, and that a
  —normal hand provides a good incentive for the patient to use the limb and mobilize the proximal joints after the cast is removed.

Plaster disease

- immobilization in plaster cast causes
  —muscle atrophy,
  —joint stiffness,
  —local, disuse osteoporosis,
  —dystrophic skin changes, and
  —plaster sores in skin;
- avoid plaster disease by
  —careful application of the cast,
  —padding the plaster well over bony prominences, and by
  —physiotherapy from Day 1. Remember that
- immobilization by hip spica may cause all the complications of prolonged bed rest (recumbency) (see Chapter 6) as well as these local problems.

Immobilization by continuous traction

- treatment of a fracture by traction is long and difficult and
- requires daily careful evaluation of pin sites, cords, pulleys, weights, direction of pull, position of patient and fracture, skin pressure areas, joint mobility, and muscle activity;
- main indications are supracondylar fracture of the humerus, fracture of the femoral shaft, or fracture of the distal femur.

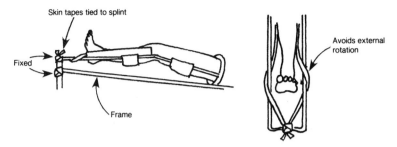

Figure 4.2.   Fixed skin traction.

Skin traction

- vertical traction (Bryant's or gallows) to both lower limbs of a child weighing less than 15 kg with a fractured femur,
    - —but ischemia of either distal extremity is a great danger, particularly if the child is heavier than this;
- fixed, horizontal traction for a child with a femoral fracture who is under 8 years old;
- use skin traction only on healthy skin;
- do not use with a pull of more than 5 kg (11 lb);
- protect the skin with Friars balsam or tincture of benzoate;
- protect the Achilles tendon, malleoli, and the front of the ankle from pressure sores and the peroneal nerve at the fibula neck from compression.
- correct malrotation by
    - —winding traction straps
    - —clockwise or
    - —counterclockwise around bars of the Thomas splint (Fig. 4.2).

Skeletal traction

Position of transverse pin (Fig. 4.3)

- olecranon, start on the
    - —medial side to avoid the ulnar nerve, at the level of the coronoid process;
- distal femur
    - —immediately proximal to the femoral condyles at the level of the adductor tubercle midway between the anterior and posterior surfaces of the femur in an adult and more proximal in a child to avoid the growth plate. Start on the
    - —lateral side anterior to the biceps tendon to avoid the common

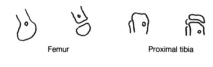

Femur   Proximal tibia

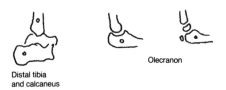

Olecranon

Distal tibia
and calcaneus

Figure 4.3. Pin placement for skeletal traction.

peroneal nerve. The pin must not enter the suprapatellar synovial
pouch;
- proximal tibia
  —2 cm posterior and distal to the tuberosity in the adult, just distal
  to it in the child (to avoid the growth plate of the tuberosity).
  Start
  —laterally to avoid the anterior tibial nerve and artery;
- distal tibia
  —2 cm proximal to the ankle joint in an adult (3 cm proximal to
  the tip of the medial malleolus) or 4 cm proximal to the ankle
  joint in a child and from the lateral side to avoid vessels;
- calcaneus
  —3 cm distal and posterior to the tip of the lateral malleolus, to
  counteract the pull of the Achilles tendon and prevent fixed
  plantar flexion. A Steinmann pin is preferred because a K wire
  will cut through the cancellous bone like a cheese cutter cuts
  cheese.

Fixed traction for fractured femur (Fig. 4.4)
- first, reduce the fracture under anesthesia, then
- fix the traction cord to the end of a Thomas splint, with the
  countertraction being pressure by the ring on the perineum and
  buttock;
- keep the end of the splint elevated and tied to the end of bed (in
  the child) or suspended to facilitate movement of the patient, skin
  care, and use of a bedpan (in the adult);
- a major indication is the child between 4 and 12 years old with a
  fractured femur;

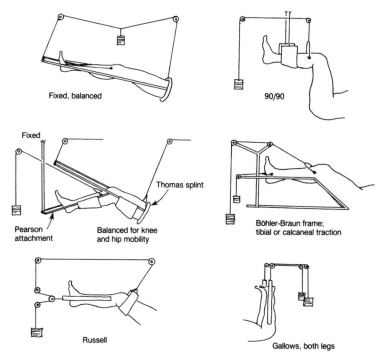

Fixed, balanced

90/90

Fixed

Thomas splint

Pearson attachment

Balanced for knee and hip mobility

Böhler-Braun frame; tibial or calcaneal traction

Russell

Gallows, both legs

Figure 4.4. Sliding traction techniques for femoral fractures. (Modified from Charnley J: *The Closed Treatment of Common Fractures*, ed 3. Edinburgh, Churchill Livingstone, 1961, p 170.)

- a disadvantage is that the patient cannot bend the knee.

Balanced traction (Figs. 4.4 and 4.5)

- reduction and maintenance of reduction by balanced traction for femoral shaft fracture;
- spiral, oblique or comminuted fractures can be reduced in the first 2 or 3 days and then held in place by continuous balanced traction;
- direction of traction is in line with the axis of the proximal fragment;
- countertraction is applied by use of the patient's weight (with the foot of the bed elevated);
- suspend a Thomas splint from an overhead beam by cords and weights over pulleys;
- do not use a frayed cord!
- cords should run over well-oiled pulleys;
- weights must be clear of the bed and floor (check this twice a day)

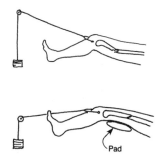

Figure 4.5. Padding and realignment of traction reduces angulation. (Modified from Charnley J: *The Closed Treatment of Common Fractures*, ed 3. Edinburgh, Churchill Livingstone, 1961, p 172.)

and should not be touched by anyone but yourself. (Instruct floor cleaners not to lift the weights if they sweep under the bed!) Do not remove weights to get the bed into the elevator for x-ray control. Ask for

- regular x-rays in two planes with a portable machine, with the patient held in traction, to confirm the position of the fracture and the correct alignment. For the
- AP x-ray, the tube must be at right angles to the long axis of the femur, not perpendicular to the bed, to avoid distortion;
- if x-rays are unavailable, check clinically the position of the fracture by
  —comparing visually alignment and rotation of the fractured limb with that of the normal limb and by
  —measuring the length of the limb with a tape measure or string and comparing it with that of the other limb. If the fractured limb is
  —shorter than the normal one, traction should be increased; if it is
  —longer, traction should be reduced.
- a Pearson knee attachment allows knee movement;
- suspension of the apparatus allows freedom of movement in bed.

Sliding traction for humeral fractures (Fig. 4.6)

- arm overhead with patient on his back,
  —edema subsides quicker;
- suitable for comminuted elbow fractures, an elbow injury with gross swelling, and a supracondylar fracture in a child.

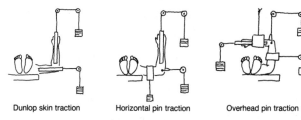

Dunlop skin traction   Horizontal pin traction   Overhead pin traction

Figure 4.6.   Traction for humeral shaft and supracondylar fractures.

Cast after traction
- when callus is sufficiently strong to prevent redisplacement of fracture, traction can be replaced with a cast and the patient can be sent home.

Physiotherapy
- isometric muscle exercises (contraction of muscle without moving the joint) whould be started within a few days;
- isotonic exercises (moving the joints) immediately for normal limbs and as soon as the fracture becomes "sticky" for the injured limb;
- respiratory exercises immediately, especially for the aged patient;
- physiotherapy will help to prevent complications of recumbency (traction disease), e.g.,
  —hypostatic pneumonia,
  —venous stasis and thrombosis with danger of embolism,
  —osteoporosis and renal stones,
  —decubitus skin ulcers,
  —muscle atrophy and joint stiffness, and
  —boredom!

Immobilization by external fixation
- Roger Anderson and Hoffman type systems are best because
  —fixation is firm and
  —plaster unnecessary; the
- pins and plaster method described already is simple and relatively cheap but is more cumbersome, and pins should be
  —removed at 3 or 4 weeks to avoid distraction and delayed union.
- indications for external fixation:
- open fracture with
  —damaged skin, loss of skin, or a large skin flap of doubtful viability (Type III wound) because this method

—allows easy skin care and dressing changes and because debridement and skin grafting can be done without removing the apparatus and disturbing the fracture. It also
—prevents plaster disease and allows movement of adjacent joints;
- closed fracture with skin damaged by
  —abrasions, ulcers or other skin lesions requiring daily care;
- bone loss. When a segment of bone is missing, the apparatus
  —maintains the length, and the bone defect can be
  —grafted without removing the apparatus.

Open reduction and internal fixation

- have many attendant risks and should not be undertaken if a good closed method can be used;
- fractures treated by open reduction should have internal fixation as well, which
- must be excellent. If it is not, you will gain nothing with your operation.

Indications

- vascular injury requiring exploration and vascular suture;
- displaced intra-articular fracture which cannot be treated well by other methods;
- displaced fracture crossing the growth plate in a child in whom other methods are inadequate;
- failure of closed methods, e.g., interposition of muscle;
- to maintain position after closed reduction of an unstable fracture, e.g., subcapital fracture of the hip;
- to accelerate rehabilitation and reintegration into the work force, e.g., intramedullary nailing of a fractured femoral shaft in a young adult;
- to decrease morbidity and mortality (intertochanteric fracture in the aged patient);
- pathological fracture, for excision biopsy and bone grafting.

Contraindications

- concurrent infection in any site;
- inadequate equipment and/or inadequate operating facilities;
- inexperienced surgical team;
- fracture which can be managed equally well or better by closed methods.

Advantages

- anatomical reduction;
- rigid fixation;
- prevention of traction and plaster disease;

- permits early physiotherapy of all muscles and joints but not weight-bearing (fracture usually must still be protected);
- promotion of early functional and social rehabilitation.

Disadvantages

- risk of infection with pseudarthosis, a disaster! When this occurs,
  —years of surgery and antibiotics
  —(blood, sweat and pus) lie ahead. Eventual
  —amputation may be the consequence;
- increased damage to muscles and periosteum, with risk of delayed union or pseudarthrosis. Almost the only way to obtain a pseudarthrosis in certain bones is to operate, e.g., the clavicle in the adult and femur in the child;
- failure of material,
  —screws loosen, pull out or break or a plate or nail breaks. This signifies a
  —pseudarthrosis;
- screw holes weaken bone, and a new fracture may occur here;
- material should be removed after 1 or 2 years, especially a compression plate because the bone underneath it remains relatively weak and osteoporotic as long as the plate is present.

Implants

- usually made of
  —stainless steel (bendable),
  —vitallium, a nonferrous, cobalt-chrome-molybdenum alloy (very hard to bend or cut),
  —titanium, or
  —high-density polyethylene;
- metals should never be mixed, e.g., a plate of stainless steel and screws of vitallium, because electrolysis with corrosion around the contact sites will occur.

Intramedullary femoral nail

- reaming destroys the intramedullary blood supply, a major disadvantage;
- closed reduction and percutaneous nailing are best but require a special table and intraoperative x-ray control;
- major indication is transverse fracture of the midshaft of the femur;
- contraindication is comminution or fracture of metaphysis (the canal is too large for nail).

Plate and screws

- adequate for most long bone fractures when open reduction is indicated;
- further damage to muscles and periosteum is unavoidable and is a disadvantage;
- should not be used on segmental fracture (the intramedullary blood supply of the middle fragment is already destroyed).

Screws

- used as an adjunct with other forms of fixation, e.g., two screws in a butterfly fragment plus a long plate;
- displaced fracture of the scaphoid, tibial condyle, medial malleolus, and neck of the talus are the only relative indications for use of screws by themselves (spiral fractures of the humeral, femoral or tibial shaft cannot be held securely by screws alone and are best treated by closed methods).

Bolt

- used with washers and a nut for displaced condylar fractures of
  —distal humerus,
  —distal femur or
  —proximal tibia.

Nail plate

- used for fractures of the hip
  —subcapital, transcervical or intertrochanteric, and
- supracondylar T fracture of the femur.

T plates

- used for fracture dislocation of the humeral head,
- Smith's fracture of the distal radius (Ellis plate), and
- comminuted fracture of the proximal or distal tibia.

Vertebral plates

- various designs are available for fixation of fracture dislocations of the spinal column;
- should be used only in conjunction with posterior vertebral fusion and have really been superseded by
- Harrington instrumentation.

Wire

- is weak and does not provide firm fixation, so it
  —should not be used by itself
  —except posteriorly in the cervical spine with a bone graft;
- two Kirschner wires and a figure-of-8 or cerclage wire are useful

for displaced fracture of the olecranon and patella and comminuted fracture of the medial malleolus;
- cerclage wire round an oblique or spiral shaft fracture should not be used because
  —it kills the periosteum and
  —destroys the blood supply of underlying bone with consequent osteolysis and pseudarthrosis.

Kirschner wires
- one wire alone is not sufficient because it does not prevent rotation at the fracture site;
- two crossed wires are useful for small fractures, e.g., fracture of the lateral humeral condyle in a child or an oblique, unstable fracture of the phalanx.

Bone
- cortical bone from the tibia, as onlay or inlay and held with screws, is best used in combination with a plate and cancellous bone graft to bridge a long bone defect;
- cortical bone alone is too weak to immobilize a fracture.

Care after reduction and immobilization
- elevate the limb on pillows, or by suspension from an intravenous pole or overhead beam, for 24 to 48 hours to reduce edema;
- observe carefully the neurovascular status of the limb;
- start physiotherapy for normal muscles and joints the day after injury;
- when the plaster cast is removed, wrap the limb in an elastic bandage for 10 days to support soft tissues and prevent edema.

OTHER TREATMENT METHODS
- prosthetic replacement, e.g.,
  —recent, displaced subcapital fracture of the hip in an older patient treated by Moore arthroplasty, to
  —avoid complications of long convalescence, delayed union or nonunion and avascular necrosis of the femoral head;
- excision arthroplasty, e.g.,
  —comminuted fracture of the radial head or patella in an adult, to
  —avoid articular incongruity and posttraumatic osteoarthritis.

PHYSIOTHERAPY
- 50% of the patient's treatment;
- twin objectives of physiotherapy are to
  —mobilize joints and
  —strengthen muscles.

- a perfectly reduced and well-united fracture is of little value to the patient if his
  —hand and fingers are stiff or his
  —foot is painful, swollen and fixed in equinus. He will not use his hand, nor can he walk on his foot; in effect he will have a
  —functional amputation.
- to avoid this, the patient must
  —actively exercise daily every muscle and joint which is not immobilized, and the
  —muscles crossing immobilized joints should have isometric exercises every day.
- active physiotherapy for uninjured structures must start the day after injury. But
- do not mobilize injured joints and soft tissues before the end of the inflammatory phase because
  —mobilization too early causes repeated serofibrinous exudation in and around the joint and increases fibrous adhesions and stiffness;
  —wait 2 to 3 weeks, then start active mobilization of the injured structures;
- activities of daily living provide excellent motivation for use of muscles and joints, so wherever possible
  —encourage the patient to continue household activities and light work while the fracture or injured joint is immobilized.
- teach the patient with a
  —lower limb injury the use of
  —crutches if weight-bearing on that limb is prohibited. Later, when weight-bearing is permitted, give the patient
  —gait training.
- physiotherapy helps prevent
  —edema, periarticular and intra-articular adhesions, and resulting
  —joint stiffness;
  —muscle atrophy and intramuscular adhesions;
  —disuse osteoporosis; and some of the
  —psychological problems which result from temporary or permanent disability.

Open Skeletal Injury—A Special Case

- you should assume that a skin wound near a skeletal injury communicates with it even if you cannot find the communication;
- your first concern must be to remove all contaminated material from the wound as soon as possible and to promote healing of the skin without infection.

- for classification of open wounds, see Chapter 2.
- all open fractures should be treated as follows:

EMERGENCY DEPARTMENT

- provide prophylaxis against tetanus if the patient is not already protected;
- take a swab of the wound for culture and sensitivity. If
- dirty bone protrudes through skin, do not reduce the fracture or dislocation unless the limb is ischemic;
- clean the skin and protruding bone thoroughly with soap and water.
- dress the wound, and
- do not remove the dressing until the patient is in the operating room;
- use a broad spectrum antibiotic for a large, dirty wound (but antibiotics are only of secondary importance to surgical debridement).

OPERATING ROOM

- take the patient to the operating room (not the emergency department operating room, this is not minor surgery);
- provide adequate anesthesia;
- the surgeon, assistant, and instrument nurse should scrub, gown and glove as for any elective orthopaedic procedure;
- elevate the limb and scrub it with soap and water for 10 minutes;
- then prepare the skin in a routine way (do not put alcohol or iodine on the wound as these chemicals kill cells);
- drape the limb as for a major surgical procedure. (There are no minor surgical procedures in orthopaedics and traumatology. Minor surgery is for minor surgeons!)

SURGICAL TECHNIQUE

- remove dirty bone spicules that had protruded through the skin,
- excise 2 to 3 mm of skin all around the edges of the defect with a scalpel (not scissors because these crush tissue) and
- reduce the bone beneath the skin;
- enlarge the defect by a lazy S incision if necessary (your skin incision should be sufficiently long to see inside the wound);
- do not undermine skin;
- wash out the wound with 500 ml of sterile saline;
- explore the wound carefully and lengthen the incision even more if necessary. (A skin incision heals from side to side, not from end to end! Do not be afraid of enlarging the wound.)
- remove all
  —dirt,
  —dead tissue (does not bleed, and dead muscle does not react to pinching by forceps),

—tissue of doubtful viability,
—contaminated tissue,
—dirty bone and
—loose bone fragments unattached to muscle or periosteum. Then
- irrigate again with 500 ml of sterile saline and
- reduce the fracture;
- close subcutaneous tissue over bare bone only if you can do so without tension. If bone has to be left exposed, petal the cortex to encourage granulations and cover with moist dressing;
- do not close the skin;
- apply bulky, occlusive dressing;
- immobilize the fracture with a
  —backslab cast or a cast with a window, or by
  —external fixation, or by
  —traction.

DELAYED PRIMARY CLOSURE

- 3 to 4 days after initial treatment; if the wound is clean and adjacent skin is viable, it should be closed under sterile conditions in the operating room, provided the skin is not under tension.

REPEATED DEBRIDEMENT

- if the wound is infected, dead tissue remains, or the viability of the skin is questionable, repeat the debridement as often as necessary and pack the wound open until it is clean and healthy.

SECONDARY CLOSURE

- when the wound is clean and no tissue or skin of doubtful viability remains,
  —close the skin if it is not under tension, or
  —cover the granulation tissue with split-thickness skin graft, or
  —let Nature close the wound by granulation, epithelialization and wound contracture;
- relaxing incisions to help close a skin defect can be dangerous, so use them with caution.

ANTIBIOTICS

- beware of antibiotics because
  —"covering the patient with antibiotics" may lull you into a false sense of security;
- use antibiotics but do so
  —intelligently and
  —not indiscriminately;
- give a broad-spectrum antibiotic, by injection when possible, for
  —a large dirty wound or

—an established infection while awaiting the results of the culture and sensitivity testing;

• remember that antibiotics are not a substitute for good and prompt surgery.

SUMMARY

The following are the cardinal rules in the treatment of an open fracture:

• do not wait;
• scrub the skin;
• provide a large exposure;
• copious irrigation;
• thorough debridement;
• leave the skin open; and give
• tetanus prophylaxis and
• antibiotics when necessary.

Communications

• talk to your patients and
• listen to them;
• give them the time that they need, and if you
• make a mistake,
• tell the patient. He has the right to know, and he will
• respect your honesty.

chapter 5

Sprains, Subluxations and Dislocations of Synovial Joints

Anatomy and Physiology

JOINT STABILITY (Fig. 5.1)

- three components

Structure

- bone and cartilage structure of some joints, e.g., the hip, provides great inherent stability, whereas
- other joints, e.g., the shoulder, have no inherent structural stability whatsoever.

Ligaments and capsule

- certain joints are almost entirely dependent on strong ligaments for stability, e.g., the knee;
- capsule is important in most joints.

Muscles

- good musculature is necessary for some joints which have weak ligaments and no structural stability, e.g., the shoulder

LIGAMENTS

Anatomy

Fibers

- collagen fibers arranged longitudinally in parallel bundles, which give great tensile strength in the direction of the fibers;
- few scattered elastic fibers;
- very few vessels, since collagen is a nonliving material.

Cells

- fibrocytes that lie between collagen bundles, with just enough
- vessels to nourish them.

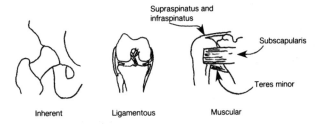

Figure 5.1. Joint stability.

Attachment to bone
- junction of collagen fibers and bone is mineralized fibrocartilage;
- collagen fibrils of the ligament intermingle with those of lamellar bone; these fibrils are called Sharpey's fibers.

Nerves in ligaments
- mediate
  —sensation, pain and
  —proprioception;
- proprioceptive fibers send information on
  —position of the joint surfaces,
  —change of speed of joint movement, and
  —ligament tension.

Healing in ligament
- repair occurs through collagen synthesis by fibroblasts which are
- recruited from surrounding areolar tissue;
- fibrocytes in ligament have little or no role in repair;
- if ends of the severed ligament are closely apposed,
  —repair is accelerated,
  —formation of mature, oriented collagen fibers is quicker, and the
  —scar is small.
- if ends of the severed ligament are *not* apposed,
  —they retract and surgical repair is not possible after 2 weeks;
  —the gap between the ends enlarges;
  —the scar is large, consists of immature fibrous tissue, and is
  —weak;
  —the ligament is longer than normal, with resultant instability of the joint;
- length of time for healing may be
  —3 weeks for ligaments in fingers and
  —3 months for ligaments in knee joint.

CAPSULE

Anatomy

- a thin sheet of collagen with
- fibers oriented in different directions but in one plane;
- capsule can resist stretching in the direction of the fibers;
- fibrocytes lie between collagen bundles;
- capsule contains few vessels,
- is usually attached to the edge of articular margin or to bone nearby in the same manner as the ligament (by fibrocartilage),
- is continuous with the periosteum of the bones forming the joint,
- is lined with synovium, and
- forms the boundary of synovial joints;
- in certain joints the collateral ligaments are attached to capsule (medial ligament of knee) or may even be a thickening in the capsule itself (shoulder);
- capsule is sometimes attached to structures within the joint (knee menisci).

Nerve endings

- capsule contains nerve endings similar to those in ligaments, for
  —sensation,
  —pain and
  —position sense.

Healing

- healing of capsule is similar to healing of ligaments.

Joint Injuries

SPRAINS

Definition

- sprain is a traumatic lesion of a ligament and sometimes the joint capsule, with no clinically evident displacement of the articular surfaces of the joint.

Etiology

- usually forced movement beyond the normal range or in an abnormal direction from an indirect force;
- particularly common in the ankle, especially during participation in a sport;
- young adults usually affected,

—children suffer growth plate injuries, whereas older adults sustain fractures;
- predisposing causes may be
  —muscle weakness or
  —congenital lax ligaments (e.g., Ehlers-Danlos syndrome).

Pathophysiology

- ligaments may be stretched or partially torn;
- capsule beneath and on both sides of the ligament and occasionally the synovium are stretched or torn too;
- capillaries and nerves in the ligament and capsule and also in the periarticular connective tissue are damaged or torn.

Clinical features

History

- is important for an understanding of the lesion, especially about the knee and ankle, and may indicate the diagnosis.

Physical examination

- relatively easy to perform just after the injury but becomes more difficult as time goes by because of pain, swelling and muscle spasm; its chief signs are
- localized pain and tenderness over the ligament and/or its insertions,
- swelling and ecchymosis around the lesion,
- immediate effusion of blood into the joint if the synovium is torn,
- serous effusion gradually developing after a few hours if the synovium is irritated by injury but not torn, and
- minimal or no instability (compare with the other side);
- request standard x-rays to eliminate the possibility of fracture, and
- if the diagnosis is still in doubt, perform a stress x-ray.

Treatment

Mild sprain (ligament stretched)

- for a mild sprain, the following are sufficient:
  —rest with the limb elevated,
  —ice, and a supportive bandage or
  —strapping and crutches or a cane (if injury is in the lower limb) for a few days;
- the objective must be to protect the ligament from further injury during the healing process;
- physiotherapy may help once pain has disappeared.

Severe sprain (partial tear)

- degree of damage to ligaments, capsule and synovium is worse and the
- treatment is longer with severe sprain than with mild sprain; if some
- instability is detected on examination or the injury involves the
- knee or ankle, a plaster cast should be applied for 5 weeks, followed by a supportive bandage and physiotherapy;
- if there is no instability, a supportive bandage or plaster cast should be applied, followed by physiotherapy after soft tissues have healed. If
- tense effusion is present in the joint, aspiration will relieve some of the discomfort. (But never put a needle in any joint if you are not sure of the sterility of your procedure. A sprain is one condition; iatrogenic septic arthritis is quite another!)

Sequelae

usually none if the injury is treated correctly from the start. If treatment is inadequate, the following complications may occur:

- instability of the joint (especially a weight-bearing joint) with recurrent sprains, due to
  —stretching of the ligament and
  —disruption of the proprioceptive system;
- recurrent posttraumatic synovitis;
- Sudeck's atrophy;
- posttraumatic osteoarthritis.

SUBLUXATION AND COMPLETE LIGAMENT TEARS

Definition

- subluxation is a partial separation of the articular surfaces of a joint.

Etiology

- similar to that for a sprain, but the force is sufficiently great to rupture completely the ligament and capsule.

Pathophysiology

- subluxation and complete tear of a ligament usually coexist;
- the collateral ligament may be torn through its substance or may be
- torn from its origin or insertion with or without a flake of bone;
- underlying capsule and synovium are torn for varying distances;
- articular surface damage usually occurs;
- at the time of injury the joint surfaces separate to a considerable degree but may return spontaneously to their normal relationship. Failure to do this, with resultant
- persistent subluxation, may be caused by an

—intra-articular fracture or

—invagination and interposition of the ligament and capsule.

- blood vessels and nerves are disrupted to a greater degree with a complete tear than with a partial tear, resulting in more swelling;
- articular cartilage or meniscal damage may be present.

Clinical features

History

- is very important, as it is with sprains;
- the patient may have heard or felt something snap in the joint or
- may have seen the joint in an abnormal position (subluxed or even dislocated) before it returned to normal.

Physical examination

- pain, tenderness, swelling and
- instability;

—with a complete ligament tear, instability is always present;

—if the lesion is recent, instability may be demonstrated without use of anesthesia, but you must gain the confidence of the patient, get him to relax as much as possible, and examine the joint gently;

—if the lesion is more than 2 or 3 hours old, reflex muscle spasm may prevent demonstration of instability, and anesthesia (local or general) will be needed.

Radiographic examination

Standard films

- anteroposterior (AP) and lateral views are mandatory;
- look for small, osteochondral fractures (Fig. 5.2).

Rotational views

- radiographs with the joint in different degrees of rotation may help, especially for the shoulder.

Stress x-rays

- are made during the clinical examination for instability;

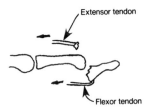

Figure 5.2. Fracture subluxation of the distal interphalangeal joint of the finger.

- you should perform the clinical examination yourself. The x-ray technician cannot do it for you;
- you must wear a lead apron and lead gloves;
- you must make comparison x-rays of the normal side because different people have a different degree of joint laxity which is normal for them;
- stress views will show whether there is any
  —abnormal joint laxity or instability and its
  —degree, by demonstrating subluxation of the articular surfaces.

Arthrography

- arthrograms are difficult to interpret. Ask for one if the radiologist is experienced with arthrography.

Treatment

- reduction of the subluxation and coaptation of the torn ends of the ligament are mandatory.

Closed treatment

- satisfactory for most joints;
- once the subluxation is reduced, the position can be held by a plaster cast for 4 to 8 weeks, depending on the circumstances (the joint and the age of the patient);
- upper limbs require shorter immobilization than do lower limbs;
- space between the ligament ends or between the ligament and the bone is usually large and eventually fills with fibrous scar tissue;
- this scar is not as strong as the original ligament, and the ligament is usually elongated;
- the consequence may be some weakness and instability, especially in the knee. This may also be due to
- interruption of proprioceptive nerves in the ligament.

Open treatment

- surgery has the following advantages:
- articular surfaces can be inspected and the
- extent of synovial, capsular, ligamentous and meniscal injury can be assessed;
- meniscus can be removed if necessary,
- synovium and capsule can be accurately repaired and
- ligament can be tightened and repaired anatomically, whether its substance is torn or it is pulled off its origin or its insertion, with or without a bone flake;
- repair can be reinforced if necessary;

- after accurate suture the structures will heal with minimum scar tissue and maximum strength;
- indications for surgery include
  —irreducible subluxation,
  —associated meniscal tear,
  —displaced, intra-articular fracture, even if the fracture fragment is small (if it is left as a loose body in the joint, it will cause instability, locking and osteoarthritis), and
  —complete tear of collateral or posterior cruciate ligament of knee.

Old untreated injury

- instability is the problem;
- ligaments have usually retracted too much for direct repair, so they must be
- reconstructed with use of tendon or fascia;
- persistent subluxation may be difficult to reduce because of shortening of soft tissues and malunion of an associated fracture;
- certain parts of the articular cartilage may degenerate for lack of nourishment by synovial fluid, which will compromise the final result.

DISLOCATION

Recent

Definition

- dislocation is complete separation of the articular surfaces of a joint.

Etiology

- similar to that of ligament tears;
- differs in the degree of force required to produce the injury;
- this force is usually indirect, with the limb acting as a lever.

Pathophysiology

- degree of damage to ligaments, capsule and synovium is usually worse with a dislocation than with a subluxation but varies with circumstances; e.g.,
  —anterior dislocation of the shoulder may produce a rent (tear) only in the front of the capsule, whereas
  —dislocation of the knee may completely tear capsule and ligaments all the way around;
- osteochondral fracture or meniscal tear (knee) may be associated;
- articular cartilage may be damaged without fracture through bone, causing osteoarthritis later;
- articular cartilage which is no longer bathed in synovial fluid is

deprived of nutrients. If dislocation is not reduced early, degenerative changes will start after about 10 days.

Clinical features

- 1 dislocation for every 10 fractures is the norm;
- 77% of dislocations occur in the upper limb; 20% occur in the lower limb;
- more common in young adults than in other persons and are found 3 to 4 times more often in men than in women;
- symptoms and signs include pain, swelling, deformity, tenderness and loss of function.

Complications

all the complications of a fracture and of its treatment apply to dislocations, but the following should be noted:

- vessels, peripheral nerves and spinal cord are particularly vulnerable around joints;
- articular fracture may be associated and may prevent reduction;
- avascular necrosis is common in the
  —femoral head and
  —talus;
- late complications include:
  —persistent instability,
  —recurrent dislocation,
  —joint stiffness,
  —degenerative arthritis and
  —myositis ossificans (in the elbow and hip).

Treatment

- dislocation is an emergency and should be reduced as soon as possible;
- reduction must be perfect to restore normal congruity of articular surfaces;
- imperfect reduction will always remain imperfect, even in children (unlike fracture alignment which may be improved by remodeling);

  Closed reduction

  - closed reduction without anesthesia may be possible for a short period after injury;
  - after a few hours, muscle spasm will be too strong and anesthesia will be necessary;
  - dislocation usually reduces with an obvious "clunk," and a full passive range of motion is restored;
  - x-ray the joint to confirm reduction;
  - if passive movement is still restricted after reduction, either

—the joint is still subluxed due to soft tissue interposition, e.g., the capsule, or

—there is an associated fracture;

• if closed reduction fails, open reduction is indicated.

Open reduction

indications include

• failed closed reduction due to the following:

—hole in capsule may be too small to allow epiphysis to return through it (bouttonière or buttonhole), e.g., the hip;

—capsule and ligaments may trap the epiphysis, e.g., the second metacarpophalangeal joint of the hand;

—interposition of collateral ligament, e.g., the ankle;

—osteochondral fracture fragment in the joint; some

• fracture dislocations require open reduction; e.g.,

—dislocation of the head and fracture of the neck of the humerus or femur is an indication for open reduction.

Treatment after reduction

• stability versus mobility is the problem;

• certain joints, e.g., the knee, should be immobilized until the ligaments heal (because stability is important);

• other joints, e.g., the interphalangeal (IP) joint of the finger, should be protected for a few days only, then mobilized (by strapping the injured finger to the adjacent normal finger, which is called buddy taping) because mobility is important;

• certain joints, e.g., the shoulder, should be immobilized for 3 to 5 weeks in a young person but should be immobilized for only a few days in an older patient;

• start immediate active mobilization of all joints of the limb which are not immobilized;

• active physiotherapy for the injured joint is important once the joint is stabilized and the soft tissues have healed;

• passive manipulation should not be ordered because it

—stiffens the joint by increasing fibrous reaction around it and encourages

—myositis ossificans.

Results

• even when treated properly, the results of a dislocation are often not as good as those of a fracture. Sequelae include

—limitation of movement,

—instability and

—osteoarthritis.

Old untreated dislocations

Pathophysiology

- after 3 weeks the hematoma is organized into fibrous tissue, fills the space between the articular surfaces, and adheres to cartilage;
- articular cartilage is deprived of nutrients and degenerates;
- soft tissues shorten and
- muscles atrophy.

Clinical features

- similar to those of an acute dislocation except that
  —pain is diminished or may be absent,
  —muscle atrophy is marked, and
  —movement in the joint is reduced or absent. But
- function of the limb may be surprisingly good.

Treatment

- if function of the limb is satisfactory to the patient, do not reduce the dislocation;
- if function of the limb is unsatisfactory, you must answer this question:
  —"Can I improve the function of this limb by surgery?"
  —if the answer is "yes," you have following alternatives:

Closed reduction

- usually impossible and may cause fracture through osteoporotic bone;

Open reduction

- difficult!
- all fibrous tissue must be removed from the articular surfaces. But it is
- difficult to distinguish between fibrous tissue and degenerated articular cartilage, so in removing fibrous tissue you may unwittingly remove some cartilage too;
- shortened, contracted soft tissues have to be released and
- muscles and tendons may have to be lengthened;
- the result may improve the position of the limb, but the limitation of movement is permanent and osteoarthritis will occur, especially in weight-bearing joints.

Arthroplasty

- dermis arthroplasty is sometimes satisfactory in the elbow when articular cartilage is destroyed;
- total joint replacement, e.g., for the hip, may work well but consider the patient's

—age, occupation and the

—risk of infection. Would the patient be better off with a Girdle-stone resection than with the hip in the dislocated position?

Arthrodesis after reduction

- may be indicated in weight-bearing joints when articular cartilage is destroyed, particularly for a manual worker;
- provides a painless stable limb, corrects malposition of the limb, and improves the shortening;
- there are fewer indications in the upper limb where mobility is more desirable.

OPEN JOINT INJURY

- an emergency! So
- treat the injury as soon as possible, following the principles outlined for open fractures in Chapter 4; i.e.,
- antibiotics;
- wide arthrotomy, copious irrigation and debridement, and removal of small bone spicules;
- reduction and stabilization of intra-articular fractures;
- closure of the wound primarily over a drain without skin tension. This latter step differs from treatment of an open fracture, which should be left open, because

—joint tissues are less resistant to infection than is muscle and

—articular cartilage deteriorates when it is exposed to air and is no longer bathed by synovial fluid. If

- skin is under tension, perform

—delayed primary closure (do not let the wound close by secondary intention!) and

- immobilize the limb.

chapter 6
Nonbacterial Complications of Skeletal Injuries

General Complications

HYPOVOLEMIC SHOCK
- most likely to occur with multiple trauma, but the
- patient with fracture of the femoral shaft may lose one liter of blood into the thigh muscles, and the
- patient with a fractured pelvis may lose several liters of blood into the retroperitoneal space and may even die. So
- beware of occult hemorrhage from bone.

GASTROINTESTINAL
- paralytic ileus may be associated with injury to vertebral column or pelvis, due to the retroperitoneal hematoma which irritates the peritoneum;
- treat by intermittent aspiration through gastric tube.

FAT EMBOLISM SYNDROME

Definition
respiratory distress syndrome in which fat globules are found in the blood stream and in certain vital organs.

Pathogenesis
- several theories have been postulated for the origin of the fat emboli:

  Physical theory
  - the most plausible theory;
  - free fat is liberated from the bone marrow at the site of injury and
  - is forced into blood vessels by increased interstitial pressure;
  - the fat globules form emboli which block capillaries in certain organs, e.g., lung, where the fat is
    —hydrolyzed by lipase to form fatty acids, e.g., oleic acid. These fatty acids may then combine with calcium to produce a
    —calcium soap which
    —affects tissue cohesion and produces

    —hemorrhagic lung infarcts and

    —chemical pneumonitis. Or the

- emboli may pass through the lung and reach the systemic circulation, i.e.,

    —brain, kidney, and skin.

Chemical theory

- emboli leave the marrow and reach the lung, as discussed under physical theory;
- trauma and stress alter the stability of lipids already in the blood and, with changes in

    —blood coagulability, may cause

    —chylomicrons to coalesce and form larger fat droplets which then

    —block tissue capillaries with consequent

    —tissue hypoxia.

- breakdown of fat in the lung into fatty acids may cause a
- chemical pneumonitis (as discussed previously).

Clinical features

Associated factors

Fractures (most often)

- multiple (more than 11% mortality rate);
- femur and tibia in young adults and the
- hip in the aged.

Soft tissue trauma

- cranial, thoracic or abdominal or with
- major arterial injuries.

Surgery

- especially bone surgery.

Others

- osteomyelitis and
- diabetes mellitus.

Fat embolism without clinical manifestations

- incidence of fat emboli in the lungs is high after trauma, especially multiple trauma, but not all these patients develop the fat embolism syndrome. The
- clinical syndrome is rare in children.

Fat embolism with clinical manifestations

- there are two main clinical syndromes: The

- fulminant systemic syndrome may occur within a few hours of an accident, with rapid onset of
  —pulmonary edema and marked respiratory distress,
  —shock, coma and death. The
- classical systemic syndrome is the
- most common and may present
- any combination of the following features:

Latent period

- short latent period after trauma, 6 to 48 hours, then
- rapid development of symptoms and signs which may regress and then recur.

Cerebral symptoms

- may continually change; they include
- headache, restlessness and obstreperousness (patient becomes difficult to manage and does not cooperate);
- confusion, delirium and coma;
- may have localizing signs, long tract signs or decerebrate rigidity;
- retinal hemorrhages, exudates and infarcts;
- cerebral damage may be permanent.

Pulmonary symptoms

- dyspnea,
- cough,
- hemoptysis and
- rapid respiration, 30/minute or more.

Fever

- high, 103° to 104° F (39° to 40° C).

Cardiovascular system

- pulse very rapid, 140/minute or more;
- blood pressure low; patient may go into shock.

Anemia

- low hemoglobin, continually falling in spite of transfusions.

Skin

- petechiae across chest, axilla, root of neck, and conjunctiva, which may fade rapidly, then recur.

Laboratory studies

Blood

Anemia

- decrease in red blood cells and

- decrease in platelets (important diagnostic sign);
- hematocrit drops, sometimes precipitously.

Blood gases

- pO_2 of less than 60 mm Hg;
- serial tests useful as index of effectiveness of treatment;
- pCO_2 elevated more than 50 mm Hg.

Serum lipase

- elevated in half the patients but a late sign.

Urine

- free fat (triglycerides) occurs in half the patients and, when present, always indicates systemic fat embolism to the kidney;
- occurs between the first and the third day and is
- present in 50% of severe cases.

Radiography

- serial chest x-rays show progressive "snow storm" infiltrations. But these changes are
- not specific for fat embolism syndrome, often
- occur late, and
- disappear within 1 or 2 days.

Summary of major clinical problems

- shock,
- pulmonary insufficiency,
- anemia,
- hypoxemia (major clinical importance), progressive
- confusion and coma.

Differential diagnosis

Posttraumatic pulmonary insufficiency

- shock lung (adult respiratory distress syndrome), especially aspiration (chemical) pneumonitis,
- pulmonary contusion, and
- diffuse intravascular coagulation.

Coma

- coma due to cerebral trauma may be difficult to differentiate from that due to fat embolism syndrome (see Table 6.1).

Treatment

General measures

Cardiorespiratory support

- the most important aspect of treatment;

Table 6.1
Comparison of Clinical Features of Cerebral Fat Embolism and Craniocerebral Trauma

Clinical Features	Cerebral Fat Embolism	Cerebral Trauma
Lucid interval	12 to 48 hours	6 to 10 hours
Confusion	Marked	Moderate
Heart rate	Increased	Decreased
Blood pressure	Low	High
Respiration rate	Rapid	Slow
Localizing signs	Usually absent	Usually present

- maintain an open airway;
- give oxygen immediately and maintain a pO_2 higher than 70 mm Hg (give less than 40% oxygen; higher percentages cause toxicity);
- endotracheal tube or tracheostomy if necessary; e.g., when adequate pO_2 (more than 70 mm Hg) cannot be maintained on the safe inspired oxygen content (less than 40%). Tube or tracheostomy
  —allows suctioning,
  —prevents aspiration into lungs, and
  —increases oxygenation of alveolar air by decreasing the dead space;
- mechanical ventilator;
- digitalization if acute right heart failure is present.

Shock

- restore blood volume,
- restore fluid and electrolyte balance, and
- monitor fluid replacement with a central venous pressure (CVP) line to avoid overload;
- fluid replacement more with colloid than crystalloid solution because the latter leaks into pulmonary interstitial tissue and increases pulmonary edema.

Coma

- general care of the unconscious patient.

Treatment of fractures

- is important;
- fractures must be immobilized to avoid further emboli;
- transport the patient gently and only when absolutely necessary;
- keep manipulations of injured parts to a minimum.

Specific measures

Steroids

- improve gas exchange by decreasing inflammation in alveolar membranes;

- IV Solu-Cortef
  - —125 mg stat, then
  - —80 mg q6h (every 6 hours) for 3 days or
- IV methylprednisolone sodium succinate
  - —100 to 200 mg q6h.

Heparin
- lypolytic agent which
- prevents platelet aggregation but
- is not recommended.

Alcohol
- IV alcohol is not recommended.

Summary of treatment
- airway and oxygen,
- blood and
- steroids.

Prevention
- impossible at present, except for
  - —moving the patient as little as possible and
  - —stabilizing the fractured limbs.

Prognosis

Severe syndrome
- prognosis is poor with marked pulmonary insufficiency and coma (50% mortality);
- the earlier the diagnosis is made and treatment started, the better the prognosis.

Mild syndrome
- good prognosis

Overall prognosis
- if the diagnosis is made, the overall mortality rate is 10% to 15%.

IMMOBILIZATION

Hypostatic pneumonia
- due to
  - —pain preventing deep breathing and coughing or due to
  - —recumbent position, with intra-abdominal viscera limiting full excursion of diaphragmatic movement.

Decubitus ulcers (pressure sores)
- due to immobilization in bed, especially if the patient's skin is insensitive (e.g., in paraplegia) or macerated;
- cachexia (loss of protein and fat) predisposes to pressure sores;

- for prevention and treatment, see Chapter 30.

Osteoporosis
- may increase serum calcium and
- cause renal and bladder stones, especially when it is associated with
- urinary stasis in the bladder.

Vascular
- venous stasis, thrombosis and embolism in pelvis or lower limb.

Muscle atrophy
- especially of the injured limb.

Local Complications
- for complications involving the
  —skin, see Chapter 4,
  —viscera, see Chapters 15 and 30;
  —spinal cord, see Chapters 27, 29 and 30;
  —peripheral nerves, see Chapter 31; and
  —blood vessels, see Chapter 32.

ARTICULAR
Stiffness
- likely when fracture is
  —near the joint or is
  —intra-articular, causing serofibrinous exudate and adhesions;
- local edema due to dependency (gravity) or disuse (circulatory and lymphatic stasis) and
- infection near the joint, e.g., pin track infection in the distal femur, produce periarticular adhesions and joint stiffness;
- muscles may stick to fracture callus, and these adhesions prevent gliding of muscles, thereby limiting motion of the joint distal to the fracture, e.g., quadriceps in supracondylar femoral fracture;
- treatment of joint stiffness by active functional physiotherapy usually succeeds, but soft tissue release is occasionally necessary.

Posttraumatic degenerative osteoarthritis
- when intra-articular fracture leaves incongrous joint surface or when
- malunion of fracture alters the axis of the joint, with resultant unequal wear, degenerative arthritis may occur;
- common in weight-bearing joints, especially the hip and knee, and
- uncommon in the upper limb joints.

PROBLEMS RELATED TO UNION OF FRACTURE

Malunion (Fig. 6.1)

- often is an iatrogenic complication and should be foreseen and prevented;
- minor deformity is usually not important, but major deformity is.

Shaft

- angulation in coronal plane,
- malrotation, and
- overlap with marked shortening are generally unacceptable.

Epiphysis and metaphysis

- cubitus valgus may cause tardy ulnar nerve palsy;
- cubitus varus is ugly but is not often a problem functionally.
- incongruity of joint surface causes osteoarthritis, as does
- malalignment; e.g.,
  — genu valgum causes osteoarthritis in the lateral compartment and
  — genu varum causes it in the medial compartment.

Delayed union

Definition

- union is slow or delayed when it has not occurred within the normal time for that particular fracture in that age group;
- unusual in children.

Predisposing factors

- infection is the single most frequent cause of delayed union and the most difficult to treat;
- open fracture causes
  —extensive periosteal stripping, and
  —tissue is devascularized;
  —bone loss may also cause delayed union or nonunion;
- comminuted and segmental fracture increases the amount of devascularized bone;

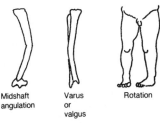

Midshaft angulation   Varus or valgus   Rotation

Figure 6.1. Unacceptable forms of malunion.

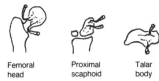

Femoral   Proximal   Talar
head   scaphoid   body

Figure 6.2. Bones with precarious blood supply.

- pathological fractures usually do not heal unless underlying pathology is treated too;
- soft tissue interposition by
  —periosteum (medial malleolus),
  —muscle (femur),
  —tendon (phalanx) or
  —nerve (supracondylar fracture of humerus);
- bones with vulnerable blood supply (Fig. 6.2), e.g.,
  —scaphoid,
  —femoral head,
  —talus and
  —segmental fracture,
- bones known to heal slowly, e.g.,
  —subtrochanteric femoral fracture,
  —ulna shaft and
  —distal tibia;
- iatrogenic, often due to
  —distraction of femoral fragments in traction,
  —inadequate immobilization,
  —excessive periosteal stripping during open reduction, or
  —infection!

Treatment

- with patience and plaster cast immobilization, most fractures will unite without surgery. If the fracture does not, immobilization and
- bone grafting and/or electrical stimulation are justified.

Nonunion

- exists when fracture fails to heal, which is usually evident within 12 months of fracture in an adult. It is
- uncommon in children.

Etiology

- inadequate immobilization in either method or duration, especially that allowing rotation or sliding movement at the fracture site, is the major cause of nonunion;
- predisposing factors of delayed union, which are cited previously, combined with inadequate immobilization, may cause nonunion.

General features (Fig. 6.3)

- clinical symptoms and signs may include
  —pain and tenderness at the fracture site on weight-bearing or stressing of the fracture,
  —movement at the fracture site, and
  —redness and swelling of skin over the fracture.
- fibrous union or
- pseudarthrosis forms, and the fracture ends are
  —enlarged, sclerotic and smooth in the hypertrophic ("elephant foot") type and
  —tapered and osteoporotic in the atrophic type;
- cellular activity has ceased and will not start up again without intervention;
- implant failure or a broken plate or screw is a sign of nonunion; as the metal is stressed beyond its limits, the molecular structure is rearranged and the metal breaks.

Treatment

- stabilization of the fracture and
- bone grafting to stimulate osteogenesis are usually necessary;
- autogenous bone is always best;
- free, vascularized bone graft can bridge a gap, but this technique is
  —long and difficult and requires a
  —specialized team and equipment.
- for grafting, consider the following:
- skin is often of
  —poor quality, so
  —plan to make the surgical approach through the best skin possible, to avoid infection. It may be necessary to
  —graft skin before grafting bone;
- preoperative physiotherapy with
  —active muscle exercises and mobilization of joints is important and will also
  —improve blood flow and nourishment of the limb,
  —reverse trophic changes in skin and bone, and

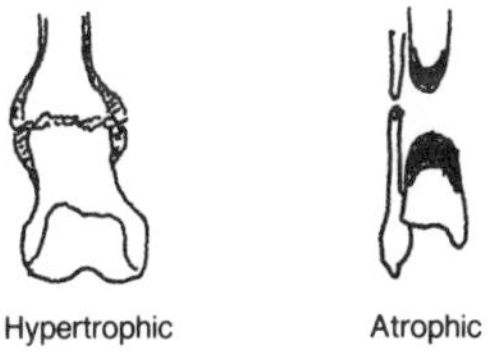

Hypertrophic   Atrophic

Figure 6.3. Types of pseudarthrosis.

—improve chances of successful rehabilitation afterward;

—ends of ununited bone usually are embedded in fibrous tissue, and physiotherapy is neither painful nor harmful. The limb can be protected with a brace if necessary;

- if there is infection, it must be treated with
  —antibiotics and
  —stabilization of the fracture because the infection will persist as long as movement occurs at the fracture site;
- cure of infection is not a prerequisite for bone grafting, but infection should be controlled as much as possible.
- electrostimulation augments the normal bioelectrical potential of bone, whereas electronegativity encourages osteogenesis. Electrostimulation may become an alternative to bone grafting, but its value is still being assessed.

PREMATURE FUSION OF GROWTH PLATE

- occurs in children and adolescents after an epiphyseal growth plate injury.

Complete fusion of plate

- causes shortening but is usually only
- significant in the lower limbs; estimate the final discrepancy with Green-Anderson or Moseley's growth charts and
- treat by epiphyseal closure of the opposite growth plate at the appropriate time if predicted shortening will be more than 2 cm. Do not operate for an upper limb discrepancy.

Incomplete fusion

- causes progressive angular deformity but is usually only
- significant in a lower limb.
- correct by osteotomy, repeated if need be until the end of growth, or by
- completion of epiphysiodesis if angulation is insignificant, then
- arrest growth of the opposite side if predicted shortening is more than 2 cm.

AVASCULAR NECROSIS (Fig. 6.2)

- occurs in the femoral head, the body of the talus, and the proximal third of the scaphoid when a fracture disrupts the blood supply;
- on x-ray the dead bone appears to be denser than does the adjacent osteoporotic bone, but
- this may not become radiologically evident for a year or more.

OSTEOPOROSIS

Local osteoporosis

- of disuse (immobilization);

- confined to injured limb;
- disappears once the fracture is healed and the patient starts using the limb;
- active, isometric muscle exercises during the period of immobilization help prevent this complication.

Sudeck's atrophy

Etiology

- neglected trauma, most frequently
- minimal soft tissue trauma, or a small fracture which is treated usually
- without immobilization and
- without exercises.

Pathology

- muscle inactivity causing
- hyperemia of the limb,
- swelling in soft tissues, and
- decalcification of bones of the limb. The bone has a characteristic spotty appearance;
- vasomotor (sympathetic) reaction may also be involved.

Clinical features

- more common in the hand than in the foot;
- very tender and painful limb, out of proportion to the injury;
- edema of the distal part of the limb;
- stiff joints;
- trophic lesions of the skin
  —smooth, glossy,
  —hairless, warm and
  —dry;
- patient terrified to move or even to touch the hand and fingers or the foot;
- functional (psychological) problems soon develop.

POSTTRAUMATIC MYOSITIS OSSIFICANS

Etiopathology

- fibroblasts, collagenoblasts and osteoblasts from torn or raised periosteum invade the hematoma around the fracture or differentiate from multipotential cells in the region;
- hematoma ossifies;
- delayed reduction and passive stretching exercises increase the likelihood of periarticular and intramuscular ossification;
- intramuscular ossification after injury may be due to cellular metaplasia in the muscle;

- associated particularly with head injuries;
- ectopic bone matures 6 to 12 months after injury.

Clinical features

- elbow (brachial muscle) and thigh are common sites;
- region is warm, tender and swollen;
- if new bone is near the joint, movement is diminished or may be abolished;
- may simulate an osteosarcoma on x-ray;
- appears 15 to 30 days after injury.

Treatment

- passive physiotherapy will make it worse;
- hematoma and ectopic bone usually diminish in size or are even resorbed spontaneously, but
- surgical removal, once the bone is mature (not before 6 months), may be necessary. If bone is excised before it is mature, the condition will recur.

TENDON RUPTURE

- tendon sliding over sharp edge of fracture will rupture;
- most often an extensor tendon at wrist ruptures after a Colles fracture, causing a drop finger;
- treatment
  —remove cause and
  —repair or graft the tendon.

Complications of Treatment

- the complications of treatment are
  —iatrogenic, caused by the medical personnel treating the patient, and the
- best treatment is
- prevention, by
  —educating the medical and paramedical personnel and by
  —anticipating the problems.

NONOPERATIVE TREATMENT

Plaster cast

Vascular

Ischemia

- due to increased swelling of limb inside encircling plaster. Volkmann's contracture is the end result;
- circular cast and padding should be split to the skin immediately after reduction;

- safest method of cast immobilization immediately after reduction is to use
  —backslab (posterior splint) and
  —complete the cast the next day.

Venous thrombosis

- especially in the lower limb, due to venous stasis.

Neurological

- radial nerve compression in the midarm by a long arm plaster made too short. This cast should end just below the axillary folds, not in the middle of the arm;
- common peroneal nerve compression at fibula neck by below-knee or long leg cast. This cast should be well padded over the fibula head and neck.

Gastrointestinal

- hip spica or thoracolumbar jacket, with immobilization of the patient in bed, may cause
  —paralytic ileus or
  —duodenal obstruction at the ligament of Treitz through compression by the superior mesenteric artery.

Plaster disease

- joint stiffness in the adult. Joints that are especially susceptible are the
  —shoulder and elbow (forearm rotation),
  —wrist and fingers in the upper limb, and the
  —knee and
  —subtalar joints in the lower limb;
- disuse,
  —muscle atrophy and
  —osteoporosis;
- dermatitis and dystrophic skin changes;
- pressure (plaster) sores over bony prominences, especially the
  —elbow,
  —malleoli and heel, and
  —sacrum and iliac spines;
  —if the patient complains of pain beneath the cast, do not wait; make a window and inspect the skin. Always replace plaster window afterward to avoid window edema;
- venous stasis and thrombosis;
- hip spica causes problems of prolonged recumbency (see previous discussion).

Traction

- treatment of the patient in traction is more exacting than a plaster cast because the patient, the fracture and the traction equipment have to be carefully checked daily.

Skin traction

- dermatitis under the traction band;
- skin ulcers at the edge of the traction band;
- compression of the common peroneal nerve.

Skeletal traction

Pin

- subcutaneous, with skin necrosis;
- piercing ulnar nerve (olecranon traction) or common peroneal nerve (tibial traction) or vessels;
- infection, with ring sequestrum, or even acute osteomyelitis or septic arthritis;
- pin driven through a growth plate with growth disturbance later.

Thomas splint or Braun frame

- common peroneal nerve compression when the leg lies in external rotation, with the bar of the splint compressing the nerve against the fibula;
- skin ulcers by pressure from a Thomas splint ring or Braun frame or from the supporting bands.

General

- nonunion due to distraction,
  —traction too strong;
- malunion due to malalignment or too little traction;
- equinus deformity,
  —ankle should be maintained in neutral position by board or bandage and regular exercises;
- all the complications of recumbency, called "traction" or "hip spica disease" (see previous discussion).

OPERATIVE TREATMENT

Early (within 48 hours) local complications

Skin

- a closed fracture is converted to an open fracture, with all the complications that may ensue!

Vascular

Tourniquet

- must be

- at least 6 cm wide because a narrow band may cause arterial spasm or compression of nerves with neuropraxia;
- placed around the most muscular part of the limb, to avoid vessel or nerve damage, e.g., at the
  —midarm,
  —proximal forearm,
  —proximal thigh and
  —midcalf;
- inflated after stripping the limb, by emptying the veins with an Esmarch bandage (but not in the case of infection or tumor!);
- removed after 90 minutes maximum. If surgery is not finished, release the tourniquet after bandaging the wound, confirm that blood is circulating by the color of the finger tips or toes, then 10 minutes later reapply the tourniquet for no longer than an hour.

Vascular wounds

- accident while dissecting;
- drill bit or screw too long;
- too much distraction at the fracture site.

Peripheral nerves

- poor position of the patient on the table, e.g.,
  —radial nerve compression, when the arm is allowed to fall sideways and rests on the table edge, or
  —brachial plexus or ulnar nerve paralysis, when the patient is positioned prone with the arms above the head;
- accident while dissecting, particularly of the
  —radial nerve during internal fixation of a fractured humeral shaft, or
  —deep motor branch (posterior interosseous) of radial nerve during exposure of proximal thirds of the radius and ulna;
- these accidents are avoidable by
  —thorough knowledge of anatomy,
  —careful dissection,
  —exposure of the nerve, and gentle retraction with a Penrose drain or folded gauze, at the beginning of the operation.

Surgical technique

- possible errors of surgical technique are legion! A
- good surgeon knows not only how to
  —stay out of trouble but how to
  —get out of trouble too. This generally comes with experience!

Late (after 48 hours) local complications

Skin

- necrosis due to
  - —incision through skin of poor quality;
  - —skin sutured under tension;
  - —subcutaneous dissection over too large an area; or
  - —subcutaneous hematoma under tension.

Vascular

- arteriovenous fistula,
- aneurysm or
- thrombus after damaging the vessels.

Muscular

- myositis ossificans;
- adhesions, especially between the quadriceps and femur, with use of an anterior incision (which is therefore not a good approach).

Osteoarticular

- avascular necrosis of bone;
- malunion, due to
  - —poor reduction or
  - —poor fixation;
- nonunion, due to
  - —infection,
  - —inadequate fixation,
  - —destruction of blood supply to the fracture area by subperiosteal dissection over too wide an area, or
  - —distraction of fragments.

Surgical implant failure

- heralds nonunion.

Refracture

- removal of external support too early;
- screw holes act as stress risers and weaken the bone.

General complications

Anesthesia

- hypoxia or anoxia;
- aspiration pneumonia;
- allergy and hypersensitivity;
- atelectasis and pneumonia.

Fat embolism

- see previously.

chapter 7

Bacterial Complications of Skeletal Injuries

Posttraumatic and Postoperative Osteitis

DEFINITION

- this is an infection of bone introduced by direct inoculation of bacteria at the time of injury or surgery or, more rarely and usually in children, by hematogenous spread to the injured area from an infected focus elsewhere.

ETIOLOGY

Origin of bacteria

- dirty wound or skin,
- contaminated surgical instruments,
- poor surgical technique,
- concurrent infection elsewhere in the patient's body, or
- concurrent infection on surgical staff.

Bacteria

Initial infecting organisms

- *Staphylococcus aureus* alone: 85% to 90%
- *S. aureus* and others (mixed): 5% to 10%

Secondarily infecting organisms usually

- *Escherichia coli*,
- *Pseudomonas* or
- *Proteus vulgaris*.

PATHOLOGY

Local factors favoring infection

- in a wound, whether surgical or traumatic, establishment of infection is different from hematogenous osteomyelitis because
- tissue planes are opened,
- tissues are devitalized, and
- vessels bleed and form a hematoma;
- ends of the fracture are necrotic;

- internal fixation devices change the blood supply and may cause ischemia;
- dead spaces always form, no matter how carefully a wound is sutured and drained, and usually fill with
- hematoma which is an ideal culture medium for bacteria because it is
  —warm,
  —filled with nutrients, and
  —well protected from the host's defense mechanisms;
- all these factors decrease the local blood supply and favor the establishment and spread of infection.

Spread of infection

- infection usually involves bone and soft tissue from the start;
- pus is generally not under pressure and does not spread up and down the shaft, along the marrow cavity and under the periosteum, as it does in acute hematogenous osteomyelitis, but it does
- spread along the planes already opened for it by the injury or surgery.

CLINICAL FEATURES

Acute infection

Early, acute phase

Local signs

- the four classical signs of inflammation,
  —rubor (redness),
  —tumor (swelling),
  —calor (heat) and
  —dolor (pain,) were
- described by Celsus, a Roman physician who lived in the first century A.D.;
- any combination of these signs may be present, but the
- symptoms and signs are generally not as acute as with hematogenous osteomyelitis.

Systemic signs

- malaise,
- persistent fever, and
- white blood cells (WBC) and erythrocyte sedimentation rate (ESR) raised.

Abscess and pus formation

- if the infection is left untreated, it progresses and
- a fluctuant abscess forms;
- needle aspiration is of doubtful value in making the diagnosis because you may

—miss the pus or the pus may be

—too thick to enter the needle.

If you do aspirate, do it under rigorously aseptic conditions. If the wound remains untreated, it will start to drain, usually frank pus, and if the diagnosis was not obvious before, it surely is now!

- the wound fills with infected necrotic debris and pus.

Chronic phase

- draining sinuses;
- surrounding skin red, dystrophic, possibly edematous, and adherent to underlying muscle or bone;
- fracture usually ununited;
- sequestra;
- exploration of the sinus with a probe may tell you
  —the direction of the sinus and
  —whether there is a mobile sequestrum.

Subacute infection

Nature of bacteria

- may be due to organisms which do not produce acute, pyogenic infection (unusual) or
- may be an infection modified and masked by previously administered antibiotics (more likely).

Clinical features

- may not be clinically evident for many weeks with
- little pain,
- minimal edema,
- no redness or heat; there may be
- drainage of thin, serous fluid.

RADIOGRAPHIC EXAMINATION

Standard radiographs

- early, no changes;
- after 1 week
  —localized osteoporosis;
- at 2 weeks
  —superiosteal reaction and
  —streaky, lytic areas in bone, only visible when 40% of bone substance has been destroyed. In the
- chronic stage bone shows
  —lytic and
  —sclerotic areas with marked
  —subperiosteal new bone formation. The
- fracture is

—slow to heal or remains ununited, with margins becoming more sclerotic with time and closing the medullary canal, or

—may be united with large, osteoporotic callus looking like a sponge with areas of sclerosis and lysis and sometimes multiple small sequestra.

Special radiographs

Tomography

- when standard radiographs are inconclusive, a tomogram can show the
  —existence
  —number, and
  —location of
  —sequestra, as well as the
  —extent of bone infection and the
  —state of adjacent bone.

Sinogram (fistulogram)

- inject radiopaque liquid, under sterile conditions, into the sinus and make
- two radiographs at right angles (90°) to each other, the anteroposterior (AP) and the lateral.
- sinogram will show the
  —direction of the sinus and
  —with what it communicates,
  —size, shape and extent of the abscess cavity, and
  —presence of sequestra in the cavity.

Computerized axial tomography (CAT scan)

- CAT scan may show clearly the sequestra lying in bony lacunae.

SCINTIGRAPHY

- bone scanning with the radioactive isotope
- gallium-67 citrate aids in the detection of
  —infection in the bone or joint as early as 24 hours after injury because the isotope is taken up by
  —leukocytes. Uptake is
  —less strongly positive in other inflammatory conditions and has a
  —more localized uptake pattern with malignant bone tumors.
- technetium-99m phosphate is less specific and may be positive in any condition associated with increased bone turnover because this isotope is
  —absorbed onto hydroxyapatite crystals.

COMPLICATIONS

Local

- pseudarthrosis is a
  —catastrophe because an infected pseudarthrosis is very difficult to treat, adjacent joints will be stiff, and the
  —patient may be handicapped the rest of his life;
  —if the pseudarthrosis persists, with florid chronic infection in spite of treatment, amputation may be the only practical solution.
- pathological fracture occurs through adjacent, osteoporotic or infected bone.
- growth arrest may occur when the adjacent growth plate is damaged, and part or all of it may close prematurely, causing shortening or deformity.
- stiff joints due to
  —prolonged immobilization,
  —adherence or fibrosis of muscles in the infected area,
  —adherence or fibrosis of joint capsule, or
  —intra-articular adhesions from suppurative arthritis.
- muscle atrophy due to
  —prolonged immobilization or
  —infection.
- skin over infected bone becomes thin, scarred, fragile and easily damaged by minor trauma, developing sinuses and chronic edema.
- epithelioma may develop in the edge of the sinus in
  —1% to 2% of patients with chronic osteitis and a sinus.
- latent infection is always a possibility because
  —chronic osteitis is seldom permanently cured;
  —infection may recur 20 or more years after an apparent cure;
  —any procedure involving the infected bone, no matter how long after the last signs of infection, may rekindle the infection.

General

- nutritional state may deteriorate, with
  —weight loss,
  —anemia and
  —hypoproteinemia.
- secondary amyloidosis is a manifestation of
  —deranged reticuloendothelial system function and abnormalities of immunoglobulin synthesis;
  —deposition of amyloid substance (proteinpolysaccharide complexes) occurs in the liver, spleen, kidney and adrenals;
  —a rare complication.

TREATMENT

Acute phase

Drainage

- surgery should be performed as soon as possible, in the operating room, with the patient under anesthesia;
- the pus must be thoroughly drained, and
- all infected and doubtful tissue must be removed;
- copious irrigation is necessary;
- do not remove the internal fixation device if this immobilizes the fracture;
- the wound should be opened widely and either
- left open, packing the wound lightly to allow pus, blood and serous fluid to escape, or
- closed over irrigation and aspiration tubes. But this technique is
  —difficult because the tube system often malfunctions and
  —dangerous because the closed space is ideal for spread of infection from any bacteria remaining in the wound.
- dressing changes made too frequently increase the risk of secondary infection by resistant hospital flora. Resist the temptation to "peak at the wound to see how it looks!" Every dressing change removes fragile granulations. Always
- put the limb at rest.

Culture and sensitivity (C & S)

- is mandatory before starting antibiotic therapy.

Antibiotics

Interim therapy

- while waiting for the results of C & S, start a broad-spectrum antibiotic such as a cephalosporin.

Appropriate IV or IM antibiotics

- start these as soon as results of the C & S are available.

Inappropriate prescription of antibiotics

- antibiotics are prescribed indiscriminately all over the world. Recent figures from the United States show that
  —50% of all drugs prescribed in the United States are antibiotics,
  —90% of antibiotics are prescribed without proper indications, and
  —50% of patients receiving antibiotics in hospitals do not have infection.
- is the situation any different elsewhere?

Principles of antibacterial therapy

- select the

        —most effective drug with the
        —least side effects;
- give it by an
    —appropriate route for a
    —sufficient length of time to eradicate the infection;
- check the patient regularly for
    —bacterial response and
    —the patient's tolerance to antibiotic;
- modify dosage when circumstances indicate;
- discontinue drug when
    —infection is cured, or
    —bacteria become resistant, or
    —intolerable side effects develop;
- operate when necessary;
- follow up with cultures after an apparent cure.

Skin coverage
- when the infection is cured and the wound is covered with healthy granulation tissue, apply a split-thickness skin graft;
- bare bone can be decorticated by fish scaling to encourage granulations, and then skin can be grafted.

Chronic phase
- C & S and
- appropriate antibiotics with
- surgery; the choice of
- surgical procedure depends on whether the fracture is united or not.

United fracture
- remove all implants;
- remove all infected, necrotic and doubtful soft tissue and bone;
- saucerize the bone, if necessary, but leave the far cortex. Do not fracture the bone!
- remove dead and diseased bone until only healthy, bleeding bone remains;
- fill the cavity with muscle belly, if possible, or leave it open to granulate. But if the
- cavity is large, fill it with autogenous cancellous bone chips (Papineau technique);
- apply split-thickness skin graft when granulations are healthy.

Ununited fracture
- infection cannot be cured while the fracture is unstable and moves;
- treatment is initially directed toward immobilization of the fracture and to osteogenesis:

Antibiotherapy

- is used as described previously.

Immobilization

- traction on a Thomas splint for a femoral fracture or use of a
- plaster cast, with a window for dressing changes, for fractures of the arm or tibia is sufficient;
- external skeletal fixation e.g., with the Hoffmann or Roger Anderson apparatus is excellent and allows exposure of the whole limb.
- duration of protection for an infected fracture is much longer than that for a noninfected fracture.
- remove sequestra early if this does not leave a bone gap. If a
- gap would result,
    —leave sequestrum until
    —callus and involucrum are
    —sufficiently strong to immobilize the fracture, then
    —remove the sequestrum. If the
- internal fixation device immobilizes the fracture, leave it in;
- if it does not, remove it and either
    —replace a small intramedullary nail with a larger one or use
    —plaster or external skeletal fixation.

Bone grafting

- if callus formation stops in spite of adequate immobilization, and nonunion is established,
- freshen the bone ends and
- use a cancellous (not cortical) bone graft from the iliac crest, if infection is quiescent. Cancellous bone may survive in an infected area but not if it is bathed in pus! If there is a
- gap in continuity,
    —hold the bone out to length with an external fixation device. Callus may form and close the defect in a child, but this is less likely in the adult; so in this case
    —graft the defect with cancellous chips. In the
    —leg the graft may be placed away from infected pseudarthrosis, between the two bones, as a posterior intertibiofibular graft, with use of a posterolateral approach to avoid poor skin and bone anteriorly;
- always irrigate the wound.

After union

- if the callus is strong enough,
- treat the infection as a chronic osteitis (as described previously).

Definitive skin coverage
- split-thickness graft lying on bone and devascularized tissues is usually of
  —poor quality and
  —susceptible to ulceration. Once the fracture is united and the infection is controlled,
- replace the poor skin with a
  —full thickness skin graft, using whichever technique is best suited to the circumstances, e.g.,
  —cross leg flap,
  —pedicle flap with or without delayed transference,
  —turnover flap, de-epithelializing the flap first and applying the split-skin graft to the dermal surface, or a
  —vascularized free flap with microvascular anastomoses.

PREVENTION OF INFECTION
- in the long run, prevention of infection will save you and the patient a lot of
  —blood,
  —sweat and
  —tears!

The patient
Examination
- always reexamine the patient the day before elective surgery for sources of infection, e.g.,
  —skin,
  —ear, nose, teeth and throat, and
  —urine.

Skin preparation on the ward
- bath and scrub the patient the day before the surgery;
- shave the whole limb to be operated, and
- prepare the skin of the limb by
  —washing in antiseptic soap.

The operating room (OR)
Staff
- all operating room staff, including nonmedical personnel, must obey standard rules of behavior, and the
- operating team must pay meticulous attention to aseptic technique. Keep

- movement and talking in the OR to a minimum.

Equipment

- evaluate periodically the sterilization technique for drapes, instruments and sutures;
- prophylactic antibiotic coverage is not a solution for faulty sterilization techniques;
- in the long run, it is cheaper and less dangerous to sterilize material properly than to "cover" every surgical patient with prophylactic antibiotics!

Operative technique

- handle tissues gently and
- operate reasonably fast,
  —the longer the wound is open, the more likely it is to become infected, but
  —do not operate so fast that you make a mistake. Surgery
  —is not a race!
- pay attention to hemostasis at the end of surgery (release the tourniquet) to prevent formation of hematoma;
- drain the wound whenever necessary, especially if you leave a dead space.

Posttraumatic and Postoperative Septic Arthritis

CLINICAL FEATURES

- similar to those of osteitis with general signs of
  —fever, raised ESR and leukocytosis and with local signs of
  —swelling with warm, red skin and pain. The patient will not move the joint;
- infected discharge drains from the wound;
- radiographs may show
  —soft tissue swelling, expanded capsular outline and, later, osteoporosis.

TREATMENT

- C & S, then
- broad-spectrum antibiotic, e.g., a cephalosporin;
- wide arthrotomy with
- copious irrigation and debridement, then
- closure of the wound, if skin is not under tension, over multiple
- irrigation and aspiration tubes, and
- immobilization of the limb;
- remove tubes when serial cultures are negative, and start
- protected, progressive mobilization of the joint.

Gas Gangrene

Etiology

- gas gangrene is caused by several organisms working in concert. These organisms are
- gram-positive, anaerobic, nonmotile rods.

Saccharolytic bacteria

- ferment sugars, e.g.,
  - *Clostridium welchii* (*perfringens*),
  - *Clostridium septicum* and
  - *Clostridium oedematiens.*
- these bacteria produce exotoxins, e.g., *C. welchii* produces at least 12, among which are
  - alphatoxin (hemolytic and necrotizing),
  - hyaluronidase (spreading factor) and
  - lecithinase alphatoxin. This latter exotoxin attacks the lecithin and cell walls and destroys them. It also causes hemolysis, jaundice, fever, hemoglobinuria, renal failure and death on IV injection.

Proteolytic saprophytic bacteria

- these bacteria break down dead tissue to putrid products and form foul-smelling gas, e.g.,
  - *Clostridium sporogenes* and
  - *Clostridium histolyticum.*

Origin of bacteria

- present in wet, heavy clay soils,
- less frequent in light sandy soils and deserts;
- *C. welchii* and *C. sporogenes* are normally present in the intestine of man, on the skin (20%), and in house and hospital dust;
- may be quiescent in an old war or farm wound.

PHYSIOPATHOLOGY

- clostridia are present in a high percentage of wounds, but development of gas gangrene is uncommon.

Prerequisite conditions

- essential factor for germination of clostridial spores is low oxygen tension (lowered oxidation-reduction potential);
- this occurs in large wounds with grossly devitalized tissue, in which blood supply is poor or absent, especially in muscle, in tissue under compression, or with an associated vascular injury, such as
  - war wounds,
  - high-speed motor accidents,
  - agricultural accidents and

—wounds containing contaminated foreign bodies;
- primary suture of traumatic wounds is an invitation to gas gangrene.

Pathology

Superficial wound

- clostridial organisms may cause
  —anaerobic cellulitis with
  —serous exudate and
  —foul-smelling gas. This is
- not gas gangrene.

Deep wound

- necrotizing myositis is the signature of gas gangrene.

Progressive muscle necrosis

- saccharolytic bacteria ferment carbohydrates and
- form lactic acid, hydrogen and carbon dioxide gases;
- gas is odorless;
- local, acute inflammatory response is poor, with little polymorpho-nuclear infiltration (which differentiates this from streptococcal myositis which has many polymorphs).

Rapid local spread

- destruction of tissue barriers, e.g., endomysium and perimysium, by exotoxins, hyaluronidase (spreading factor) and collagenase.

Tissue necrosis

- tissue is killed by exotoxins, and ischemia increases due to the pressure of gas;
- area is tense and edematous, with crepitation occurring due to gas in the tissue;
- muscle is odorless and brick-red.

Saprophytic activity

- proteolytic saprophytes break down dead tissue and cause
- putrefaction (now called gas gangrene, since this term means tissue death with putrefaction);
- muscles turn greenish black and have a
- foul odor.

Systemic toxemia

- caused by exotoxins;
- starts with beginning of infection and increases, and is associated with
- intense shock,
- hemolytic anemia, and

- cardiotoxicity (lecithinase);
- at death, the blood stream may be invaded by bacteria.

CLINICAL FEATURES

Contamination

- 20% to 50% of traumatic war wounds are contaminated with clostridial spores which may
- proliferate in dead tissue, e.g., clots, without invading viable tissue, causing a
- thin, brown, foul-smelling discharge, with deeper parts of the wound turning greenish black;
- clostridia usually disappear without specific therapy.

Anaerobic cellulitis

- develops in 5% of war wounds contaminated by clostridia;
- incubation period is from 3 to 4 days;
- onset is gradual;
- bacteria multiply in superficial connective tissue spaces around the wound but with
- no muscle invasion; there is a
- moderate quantity of brown, foul-smelling seropurulent discharge, but there is
- little pain, edema or discoloration of skin; there
- may be a lot of gas but only in the superficial, fascial planes;
- systemic reaction is minimal.

Gas gangrene (anaerobic myonecrosis)

- endangers life;
- developed in 1.5% of World War II wounds contaminated by clostridia;
- is 6 times more frequent in a wound treated 4 days after the injury than in a wound treated the same day as the injury;
- is 5 times more frequent in wounds of the thigh and buttock than in wounds of the leg or arm.

Diagnosis

- should be made clinically, not bacteriologically nor radiologically, because you do not have time to wait for these examinations;
- incubation period is from 6 hours to 4 days with *C. welchii* and up to 6 weeks with *C. oedematiens*, but the average is from 12 to 24 hours;
- success of treatment depends on early diagnosis.

Early symptoms and signs (in first few hours)

- local
  —tight, shiny skin, whitish in color, and
  —pain.

- systemic
  —toxemia,
  —mental confusion and
  —fever;
  —pulse rate rises faster than the patient's temperature. Normally, pulse rate rises 10 beats/minute for every degree Fahrenheit (half a degree centigrade) rise in temperature.

Later signs (after several hours)

- local
  —edema and pain increase,
  —skin reddens, and
  —blisters appear containing reddish brown serous fluid;
  —skin sloughs with
  —seropurulent, brown, foul-smelling discharge;
  —crepitus appears (gas bubbles) and the
  —wound bursts open (if it was closed);
  —muscles are red and swollen at first, then become
  —greenish black and no longer bleed; there is a
  —foul smell (hydrogen sulfide) with gas in muscles.
- systemic
  —hemolytic anemia,
  —shock with high pulse rate (hypovolemia),
  —oliguria,
  —hemoglobinuria,
  —jaundice and
  —metabolic acidosis;
  —death may occur within 24 hours of onset of systems.

Predisposing factors

- ischemic vascular disease,
- diabetes mellitus,
- delay in treatment,
- site of wound or
- primary closure of wound.

Differential diagnosis

Other gas-producing bacteria

- gram-negative bacteria can produce gas in patients with lowered resistance, e.g., in a patient who is
  —cachexic or who has
  —diabetes mellitus or
  —leukemia, but the
- clinical syndrome of gas gangrene is not present.

- *Klebsiella* brings about an
  —insidious onset of pain and has a
  —slow course,
  —gas in superficial fascial planes only, and
  —no necrotizing myositis.

Streptococcal myonecrosis

- anaerobic streptococcus plus either aerobic streptococcus or staphylococcus may produce
- clinical features similar to those of gas gangrene, but
  —symptoms and signs are less marked,
  —the course is slower and less fulminant,
  —odor and gas are less, and
  —exudate has few bacteria but many polymorphonuclear leukocytes.

TREATMENT

Anaerobic cellulitis

- surgery with
  —local debridement,
  —leaving the wound open;
- immobilization of the limb;
- antibiotics.

Gas gangrene

- if in doubt as to diagnosis, treat the patient as though he has gas gangrene.

Surgery

- the cornerstone of prevention and treatment.
- immediate surgery is essential, the single most important therapeutic act;
- open the wound widely and perform
- fasciotomy on all fascial compartments;
- remove all dead, dying and doubtful tissue (the entire muscle mass if necessary)
  —*Clostridium* is anaerobic and does not like oxygen;
- irrigate the wound thoroughly with hydrogen peroxide and/or Dakin's solution;
- leave the wound open and
- immobilize the limb;
- if amputation is necessary, do not hesitate to amputate high because the
  —patient may die if you wait too long.

Antibiotics

- adjunct to surgery;
- massive IV doses of betalactamine antibiotics
  —penicillin, 24 million units daily, or
  —ampicillin or
  —cephalosporin,
- with either a wide spectrum antibiotic of the aminoside group
  —streptomycin,
  —kanamycin,
- or tetracycline, 500 mg IV q6h

Antitoxin

- anti-gas gangrene serum is of doubtful value and should not be given prophylactically at the time of injury;
- if antitoxin is available, treat established infection with 40,000 to 60,000 units q4h, the first three doses IV, the rest IM, for 24 to 48 hours;
- antitetanus serum is mandatory.

Supportive measures

- blood transfusion;
- correct electrolyte imbalance;
- rehydrate the patient.

Hyperbaric oxygen (O_2)

- oxygen delivered in a pressure chamber at 3 times the pressure of air at sea level;
- no action on toxins already released but
- may prevent extension of the infection by inhibiting the growth of organisms;
- four to six periods in a chamber at 6-hour intervals, each period lasting 60 to 90 minutes;
- hazards are considerable:
  —decompression sickness (N_2 bubbles in blood vessels),
  —convulsions,
  —otitis media and
  —claustrophobia.

Summary of treatment

- as soon as a diagnosis is made, proceed with treatment in this order:
  —fluid and electrolyte replacement to prepare patient for surgery,
  —antibiotics,
  —surgery, and
  —hyperbaric O_2.

PREVENTION

Traumatic wound

- wide exposure;
- clean it thoroughly;
- excise dead and doubtful tissue, especially muscle;
- remove all foreign bodies, if possible, and
- always leave the wound open, even Type I punctiform wounds.
- incidence of gas gangrene among wounded American troops was
  —2% in World War I and
  —0.5% in World War II, when primary closure was common practice;
  —0.2% in the Korean Conflict in which delayed primary closure was introduced toward the end, and
  —0.016% in the Vietnamese War in which no wounds were closed primarily. In
- civilian practice reported from Miami,
  —all 27 patients with gas gangrene had
  —primary closure. The
- moral is clear: Treat traumatic wounds by
  —adequate debridement and
  —delayed closure.

Circular casts

- are dangerous, so
- split a cast along its entire length down to skin or bivalve it and hold it on with a bandage and
- remove completely all tight dressings.

Antibiotics

- of secondary importance to surgery.

Tetanus

ETIOLOGY

Bacteria

- *Clostridium tetani* is a gram-positive, anaerobic, motile rod that
- produces exotoxins such as
  —tetanospasmin, which is a very toxic neurotoxin, and
  —tetanolysin, a hemolysin and cardiotoxin. *C. tetani* has
  —no saccharolytic or proteolytic activity.

Epidemiology

- spores exist in the superficial layer of soil where
  —the population of people is dense,

—climate is warm and humid, and
—the soil is rich in organic matter, e.g., clay;
- in towns and densely populated countryside, spores are found
  —in the gastrointestinal tract of inhabitants,
  —on the skin of outdoor workers,
  —on clothes and
  —in house dust.
- patients who walk barefoot, and all children, should be immunized before surgery is performed on the feet.

PHYSIOPATHOLOGY

Entry wound
- may be very small and seemingly insignificant and is therefore
- most dangerous because the surgeon tends to ignore it;
- large wounds are generally better cared for and therefore less likely to be associated with tetanus;
- in 20% of cases, no entry wound is evident.

Local conditions
- for exotoxin production the bacterium requires
  —a low oxygen tension and
  —tissue necrosis;
- other factors favoring exotoxin production are a
  —foreign body in the tissues or
  —associated infection of the wound with other organisms;
- infection with *C. tetani* always remains localized. The bacterium is not invasive.

Exotoxin
- travels to the spinal cord via
  —lymphatics,
  —blood vessels and
  —perineuronal space, between neurones.
- tetanospasmin acts at the
  —interneuronal synapse to prevent inhibitory impulses at the
  —neuromuscular junction, and it also acts
  —directly on the muscles;
- once the toxin is fixed to the tissue, it is invulnerable to antitoxin.

CLINICAL FEATURES
- diagnosis is made clinically, not bacteriologically, because the bacteria are often no longer present in the wound when the first tetanic spasms appear.

Incubation period

- 2 to 60 days;
- the shorter the incubation period, the worse the prognosis.

Signs

Trismus

- spasm of the masseter muscles which clench the jaw.

Generalized muscle contractions

- occur 24 to 72 hours after onset of trismus and
- appear
  —on the face (risus sardonicus),
  —neck (hyperextension) and spine (opisthotonos which is hyperlordosis),
  —arms (rigid in flexion),
  —legs (rigid in extension) and
  —larynx and pharynx (spasm of the glottis and dysphagia);
  —these contractions are persistant and painful.

Paroxysms

- paroxysmal muscle spasms occur at intervals superimposed on persistent muscle contraction, and their
- frequency, duration and intensity add to the severity of the disease.

COMPLICATIONS

- death from
  —asphyxia,
  —cardiac arrhythmias and arrest.
- atelectasis and pneumonia,
- urinary obstruction,
- fractures and muscle ruptures,
- fecal impaction and
- decubitus ulcers.

PROPHYLAXIS

Types of immunization

Active

- vaccination by antitetanus toxoid
- is so effective that no tetanus occured in the United States Army from 1956 to 1971;
- three injections of 1 to 2 ml of antitetanus toxoid IM according to age, the second and third at 6 weeks and 6 months after the initial injection;

- a booster injection 1 year later;
- effective for 10 years;
- in patients vaccinated many years previously, one booster dose will produce a rapid rise in antibody production;
- modern vaccine is usually associated with poliomyelitis and whooping cough vaccines.

Passive

Antitetanus horse serum

- give a test dose to elicit allergy, and
- if there is no reaction within 20 minutes, give 1500 units IM;
- effective for 15 days; give a
- second injection of 1500 units at 2 weeks if the wound is still infected. But
- if patient has already received horse serum, he has antibodies against the horse proteins; consequently, the serum will be increasingly less effective and may cause an allergic response. For this reason, this vaccine is
- no longer used in North America.

Human hyperimmune gammaglobulin

- 250 international units IM;
- no allergic reaction;
- eliminated more slowly than horse serum but is
- expensive.

Programs of prophylaxis

Patient already properly vaccinated

- recently
  —give booster injection of toxoid, 0.5 ml;
- more than 5 years ago give
  —one booster dose of toxoid and
  —one injection of serum or immune globulin.

Patient not vaccinated or vaccinated more than 10 years ago

- give antitetanus serum, then a
- few hours later, with a different syringe and into a different muscle (to avoid precipitation), give the first dose of the toxoid;
- complete the vaccination with toxoid in the normal way.

Surgery

- in all cases the wound must be
  —cleaned,
  —debrided (all dead and doubtful tissue and foreign bodies, when possible, must be removed),

—irrigated and

—left open;

—pay attention to the smallest wounds as well as the big ones.

Antibiotics

- effectiveness is doubtful.

TREATMENT

Surgery

- explore, clean and debride the wound even if it has since closed, and
- leave it open.

Passive immunity

- give 50,000 to 200,000 units IM of horse serum, after a test dose to elicit allergy is administered; better still, give

  —3,000 to 6,000 units of immunoglobulin (less for a child).

Tracheotomy

- end-assisted ventilation by a respirator at the earliest sign of pharyngeal or laryngeal spasm. But if

  —tracheotomy becomes infected, the patient may die, so in uncertain circumstances it is

  —better to intubate the patient and perform tracheotomy only as a last resort.

Sedation

- quiet, dark room;
- Valium in high doses or
- 1% sodium pentothal IV with 5% glucose and water;
- curarization to control spasms. This treatment must be supervised by an anesthetist.

Antibiotics

- penicillin, 20,000 units IV q6h, and
- steptomycin, 0.5 gm IM q12h.
- doubtful effectiveness.

Supportive therapy

- fluid and electrolytes.

Prognosis

- treatment may last 4 to 6 weeks;
- mortality rate is about 50% and increases with the age of the patient!
- prophylaxis is more effective and less expensive than treatment;
- there is no substitute for immunization.

chapter 8

Injuries of the Scapula, Clavicle and Shoulder Joint

Fractures of the Clavicle (Fig. 8.1)

MIDDLE THIRD (Fig. 8.2)

Etiopathology

- 80% of fractures of the clavicle occur in the middle third; these fractures are
- especially common in children and often are caused by a
- fall on the point of the shoulder with a
- shearing force transmitted to the middle third (the clavicle is shaped like a lazy S);
- fracture may be displaced by the
  —sternocleidomastoid muscle pulling the proximal fragment up and back and by the
  —weight of the arm, pectoralis major and deltoid pulling the distal fragment down and forward.

Clinical features

- the patient usually supports the injured arm with the other arm;
- symptoms and signs are the same as those of most fractures, i.e., pain, swelling, tenderness and functional impotence of the limb;
- the injured shoulder is lower and more medial than the noninjured shoulder if the fracture is displaced, but if there is no displacement,
- no deformity other than swelling should be found;
- gently examine the scapulohumeral joint also to exclude injury to it.

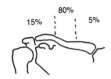

Figure 8.1.   Frequency ratio of clavicular fractures.

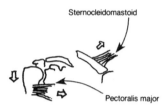

Figure 8.2.   Mechanical forces on a middle third fracture of the clavicle.

Radiological examination

- anteroposterior (AP) view and
- 45° oblique view upward and backward (upshot view).

Complications (Fig. 8.3)

- as for any fracture. In particular, the
- clavicle is subcutaneous and a fracture fragment may threaten to perforate the skin, although open fracture is rare;
- the subclavian vessels and brachial plexus are immediately posterior and may be injured by the fracture or may be compressed on the rib later by exuberant callus;
- pleural perforation with subcutaneous emphysema;
- pseudarthrosis is rare and may be of little functional consequence. Treat by internal fixation and grafting if it is symptomatic. Do not confuse pseudarthrosis caused by fracture with congenital pseudarthrosis.
- malunion with an ugly bump may concern a young woman. Treat by osteotomy and realignment if necessary, but beware because this exchanges a
  —bump for a scar, and you may exchange a
  —malunion for a nonunion!

Treatment

Closed

- closed reduction by pulling the shoulders up and back and
- holding the position by a figure-of-8 bandage

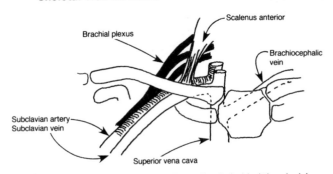

Figure 8.3. Important structures immediately behind the clavicle.

—well padded over the clavicle and under the axilla and
—tightened every few days.

Open

- indications include
  —open fracture or associated
  —vascular injury. But
- beware of surgery on this bone; the
  —hard, cortical bone and
  —subcutaneous position increase the risk of
  —skin necrosis,
  —pseudarthrosis and
  —infection, and
  —behind it lie the subclavian vessels and brachial plexus.
- if you must operate, do so
  —cautiously and use a
  —plate or threaded pins;
  —never use smooth pins unless they are bent outside the bone to prevent migration.

Results

- for closed treatment, results are
  —almost always good;
  —nonunion is rare if closed treatment is employed.

MEDIAL THIRD

- 5% of all clavicle fractures. Caused by
- direct trauma and may involve
- articular surface of sternoclavicular joint.
- treatment is nonoperative with a sling or figure-of-8 bandage.

LATERAL THIRD (Fig. 8.4)

- stable fracture has
  —intact coracoclavicular ligaments. Fracture is unstable when
  —coracoclavicular ligaments are ruptured; the proximal fragment displaces upward. In this instance,
  —delayed union is common because the distal fragment moves constantly with the scapula.
- treatment for a stable fracture is with a sling; for an
- unstable fracture, treatment consists of application of a
  —bandage or cast which pulls the shoulder itself backward. A
  —figure-of-8 bandage should
  —not be used because this pulls the medial fragment backward and exaggerates the deformity.
  —open reduction and internal fixation may be necessary for failure of closed treatment.

Sternoclavicular Lesions

RECENT LESIONS

Etiopathology

- rare. Caused by
- direct or indirect force, with the shoulder acting as the lever;
- injury may be
  —mild or
  —moderate sprain with tearing of part of the ligaments or may be
  —complete anterior (more common) or posterior dislocation, depending on the direction of the force;
- posterior dislocation may be associated with
  —venous engorgement in the neck by compression of the innominate (brachiocephalic) veins (Fig. 8.3), or with
  —pneumothorax, or with

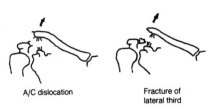

A/C dislocation   Fracture of
                         lateral third

Figure 8.4. Acromioclavicular (A/C) dislocation versus unstable lateral third fracture. The ligaments are torn.

—dyspnea by pressure on the trachea, or with

—dysphagia by compression of the pharynx.

Diagnosis

- is clinical;
- radiographs are difficult to interpret.

Treatment

Mild and moderate sprains

- symptomatic treatment

Dislocation

Anterior

- closed reduction by
  —traction on the arm in abduction and extension;
  —push the bone back and
  —hold with a figure-of-8 sling;
- may be stable after reduction. If it is
- unstable but
  —asymptomatic, accept this. Otherwise, perform
  —open reduction and internal fixation, repairing or reconstructing capsule and ligaments.

Posterior

- closed reduction under anesthesia by
  —traction on the arm in abduction and extension. If it is
- still dislocated, grasp the clavicle with fingers or a sterile towel clip and pull forward.
- after reduction, the joint is nearly always stable.
- do not put pins or K wires across this joint because they may migrate into vessels, lungs or heart!

OLD UNREDUCED DISLOCATIONS

Anterior dislocation

- is usually asymptomatic and requires no treatment. If it is
- symptomatic, treat by
  —open reduction and ligamentoplasty, with fascial strips used to replace the sternoclavicular ligament;
  —if the costoclavicular ligament is torn, replace it by transfer of subclavian muscle tendon, and detach the clavicular head of the sternocleidomastoid muscle to protect the ligamentoplasty.

Posterior dislocation

- whether symptomatic or not, this can produce complications and should be treated by

—open reduction and ligamentoplasty or by

—excision of medial end of clavicle proximal to costoclavicular ligament.

Acromioclavicular Lesions

RECENT LESIONS

Etiopathology

- 12% of all dislocations about the shoulder girdle. commonly caused by a
- direct force such as a fall on the point of the shoulder;
- indirect force, with the arm acting as a lever, is uncommon.

Classification

Type I

—mild sprain with pain and local tenderness,

—no deformity, and

—stable.

Type II

—subluxation with rupture of acromioclavicular capsule and ligaments but with coracoclavicular ligaments intact;

—mild deformity in comparison with the other side;

—stress x-ray of the patient standing and holding 5 kg in each hand with the arms by the side will show the displacement.

Type III (Fig. 8.4)

—dislocation with rupture of all ligaments;

—deltoid and pectoralis major muscles or periosteum torn off the clavicle; the

—clavicle rides up high, above the acromion, and is clinically obvious;

—unstable in both sagittal and coronal planes.

Treatment

Type I

- treatment is symptomatic;
- protect from injury for 6 weeks;
- results are excellent.

Type II

- treatment is symptomatic, e.g.,
  —analgesics and a
  —sling for a few days until the pain disappears, followed by
- pendulum exercises.
- no sport or heavy work for 8 weeks, to avoid further injury.

Type III

Nonoperative

- closed treatment is unlikely to maintain reduction of the joint; with
- symptomatic treatment the
- functional result is satisfactory but the
- aesthetic result is not.

Operative

- open reduction and internal fixation is not necessary unless the patient is a sportsperson or is someone who depends on looks for a livelihood and prefers a thin scar to an unsightly bump.
- at surgery
  —repair the coracoclavicular ligaments, the periosteum and attachments of the deltoid and pectoralis major muscles, and the capsule and ligaments of the joint;
  —excise the meniscus and
  —stabilize the joint with threaded pins crossing from the acromion to the clavicle. These pins must be removed later;
  —limit abduction for 6 weeks after surgery, until the pins are removed.

Results

- 80% regain normal function with either method;
- degenerative arthritis and meniscal problems developing in Types II or III may require excision of the distal end of the clavicle later.

OLD UNREDUCED DISLOCATIONS

- usually asymptomatic and require no treatment. But if they are
- symptomatic with no degenerative changes in the joint, for Types II and III lesions perform
  —open reduction and transfer of the coracoid process, with attached muscles, to the undersurface of the clavicle in the locality of the coracoclavicular ligaments (Dewar-Barrington procedure) and
  —fix the coracoid with a screw;
  —transferred muscles act as dynamic ligament. Or
- transfer with a piece of bone the acromial end of the coracoacromial ligament, and stabilize it with a Bosworth screw for 10 weeks. When
- degenerative changes are present,
  —excise the distal end of the clavicle and meniscus;
- for Type III lesions, perform ligamentoplasty also, as described previously.

Scapula Fractures

- the scapula is embedded in muscle and is
- mobile;

- fractures are uncommon and are generally undisplaced. They may be caused by
- severe trauma, so look for other injuries in the patient.
- x-rays should include an
  —AP view of the chest and shoulder and a
  —30° tangential view, to see the scapula in profile;
- treatment is symptomatic;
- results are good and
- complications are rare.

Glenohumeral Joint Lesions

- common in adults because
  —structural stability of the joint is nil,
  —ligamentous stability is poor, and the
  —joint is very mobile. In
- children, the humeral growth plate is weaker than the ligaments, so the plate is injured instead.

RECENT INJURIES

Sprain

- no instability;
- treatment is symptomatic, but no sports are allowed for 6 weeks.

Anterior subluxation

- an athlete's injury

Diagnosis

- history is very important and usually involves an
  —external rotation injury of the shoulder which patient can often describe. On
- examination, look for the
  —"sign of apprehension"; i.e., ask the patient to hold both arms in 90° abduction. He does not allow external rotation and extension of the injured arm to the same extent as the uninjured arm because this would recreate the displacement.
- x-rays usually show nothing.

Treatment

- anterior subluxation is usually a chronic, recurrent problem, so surgical repair, using one of the methods described for recurrent anterior dislocation, is necessary (see below).

Anterior dislocation

Etiopathology

- the humeral head is levered out of the glenoid by an abduction, extension and external rotation force on the arm, with the acromion acting as a fulcrum. The
- capsule is
  —torn through its substance, especially in older patients, or is
  —avulsed from the glenoid labrum or
  —avulsed with part of the glenoid labrum or even with a flake of bone from the glenoid. The
- humeral head may have a
  —compression fracture on the posterolateral surface, the Hill-Sachs lesion. The
- position of the head may be
  —subcoracoid (most common), with the head distal to coracoid process, or may be
  —subglenoid, with the head below and in front of the glenoid, or may be
  —subclavicular (rare), with the head medial to the coracoid and distal to the clavicle.

Clinical features

- complete loss of function of the shoulder;
- the injured arm is in slight abduction and external rotation and is supported by the normal arm;
- shoulder contour is flat and squared-off; the acromion is prominent;
- the head is usually palpated below the coracoid and medial to the acromion; and the
- glenoid fossa is empty;
- exception is subglenoid dislocation in which the arm is in the "forward pass" position.

Radiography

- confirm clinical diagnosis and
- look for associated fractures;
- an axillary view, with the arm in 90° of abduction, will show the dislocation clearly.

Complications

- compression of the axillary artery, nerves of the brachial plexus, or the axillary nerve. These may equally be iatrogenic, i.e., compressed during reduction, so examine the neurovascular status carefully before and after reduction and write down your findings;
- associated fractures may occur of the

—greater tuberosity, with the fragment pulled upward, medially and posteriorly by the supraspinatus (the rotator cuff inserts into this fragment which usually returns to its place after reduction of the dislocation, but if it does not, open reduction and internal fixation may be indicated);

—glenoid, especially of the anterior margin;

—surgical neck of humerus (closed reduction under anesthesia may be possible if the fracture is impacted; otherwise, open reduction is necessary); and

—anatomical neck, which is rare; avascular necrosis may result;

• recurrent dislocations.

Treatment

Closed reduction

- do not delay. Closed reduction is usually
- possible without anesthesia within a few hours of injury by
  —gaining the patient's confidence,
  —making no sudden painful movements, and
  —talking your way through the procedure to encourage the patient to relax his muscles;
- if muscle spasm is too great, reduction is easy with general anesthesia or a narcoleptic;
- traction (hippocratic) method:
  —patient supine,
  —gentle traction in the direction of the arm as it lies,
  —countertraction in the axilla or laterally on the arm;
  —technique described by
  —Hippocrates 2400 years ago.
- external rotation (Kocher's) method:
  —patient supine;
  —flex elbow to 90°;
  —adduct the elbow at the same time as gentle
  —lateral traction is applied on the arm by an assistant; then
  —rotate the arm externally until the shoulder reduces
  —or the arm is in more than 90° of external rotation; then
  —rotate the arm internally until the forearm is across the chest, with the hand on the opposite shoulder. The humeral head is reduced by this maneuver.
  —this technique may be more traumatic to capsule and humeral head than are straight traction methods;
  —technique described by Kocher in the nineteenth century A.D. but demonstrated on Egyptian tomb paintings 3000 years ago.

Open reduction
- indications include
  - —failed closed reduction (the usual cause is soft tissue interposition, e.g., long head of biceps tendon or buttonholing of capsule);
  - —unstable fracture of surgical neck when closed reduction obviously is impossible;
  - —fracture of greater tuberosity which remains displaced after reduction of humeral head (this requires open reduction and fixation).

Care after reduction
- aim for stability in the younger patient and mobility in the older patient, as the older shoulder very quickly stiffens;
- allow the anterior capsule to heal, and prevent abduction and external rotation by a
  - —Velpeau or a
  - —sling and swathe bandage around the arm and chest, with the arm in nearly full internal rotation. For the
- young adult
  - —5 weeks immobilization, followed by
  - —graduated exercises, with both abduction and external rotation avoided, for 5 more weeks. Return to sport when there is a full range of movement, no muscle atrophy or weakness, and no pain. For the
- patient over 35 years old
  - —5 days immobilization, followed by sling protection and pendulum exercises. No sport for 5 weeks.
- the older the patient, the greater the risk of stiffness of the shoulder, so the sooner the joint should be mobilized.

Posterior dislocation

Etiopathology
- usually caused by leverage on the arm during an epileptic fit or electroconvulsive treatment;
- pathology is the reverse of that for anterior dislocation and may include a
  - —stretched or torn posterior capsule or avulsion or fracture of the posterior glenoid rim, or a
  - —stretched or avulsed subscapularis muscle or avulsion fracture of the lesser tuberosity, or a
  - —compression fracture of the anteromedial part of the head.
- position of humeral head is usually
  - —beneath the acromion with the

—articular surface facing posteriorly (90° internal rotation) and the
—lesser tuberosity in the glenoid fossa. Less common positions of the
head are
—subglenoid or subspinous.

Clinical features

- rare; occurs in only about 2% of all shoulder dislocations;
- diagnosis is clinical more than the radiological,
- the arm is held in adduction and internal rotation and the forearm is held against the chest;
- abduction and external rotation are impossible, which is the key to the clinical diagnosis;
- on palpation, a mass is felt posteriorly and emptiness is felt anterolaterally (where the humeral head should be).

Radiological features (Fig. 8.5)

- subacromial dislocation
  —the AP film gives a lateral view of the head of the humerus. The head, neck and shaft then resemble an upside-down onion;
  —there may be no overlap of the head and glenoid that is normally seen on the routine AP x-ray;
  —the head is not obviously dislocated;
  —axillary and true lateral views (not transthoracic, since the scapula lies obliquely on the chest wall) are helpful in showing displacement between the head and the glenoid;
- subglenoid and subspinous dislocations are more obvious both clinically and radiographically.

Treatment

- closed reduction as soon as possible, with the patient under general anesthesia, by
  —traction in the line of the humeral shaft with direct pressure over the humeral head to push it forward or with

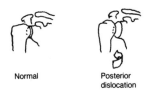

Normal   Posterior
                      dislocation

Figure 8.5. In posterior dislocation of the shoulder, the anterior two thirds of the glenoid are empty, and the humeral head is more symmetrical because the arm is internally rotated.

—gentle internal rotation to dislodge the head from the glenoid rim, followed by

—gentle external rotation and traction;

- closed reduction usually succeeds, and open reduction is seldom necessary;
- once the dislocation is reduced, the joint is usually stable and recurrence is rare;
- care after reduction is similar to that for anterior dislocation unless the joint is
- unstable, in which case apply a

—shoulder spica with the arm in 30° of external rotation for 5 weeks.

OLD UNREDUCED DISLOCATIONS

Anterior

Etiopathology

- may occur in
  —old people because weak muscles and capsule allow dislocation with minimal trauma and mental status may prevent the patient from going to the doctor;
  —younger people who live far from medical facilities;
  —developing countries where medical facilities are insufficient;
  —patients with epilepsy; or may be
  —iatrogenic, with the injuries unrecognized by the doctor, especially in patients with multiple injuries. Often
- associated with
  —fractures of humerus and scapula and
  —neurological injuries.
- capsule and muscles contracted;
- adhesions involve
  —articular surfaces and
  —neurovascular bundle.

Clinical features

- in the young patient,
  —pain and stiffness usually persist because capsule and muscles are strong and tight. But in the
- older patient,
  —pain decreases and mobility increases with time, and there may be no symptoms when you see the patient;
  —scapulothoracic joint allows 60° of abduction, which may be sufficient for the patient's needs.

Treatment

Asymptomatic

- no treatment

Symptomatic

- in the old patient, leave well enough alone.
- in the younger patient with dislocation less than 3 weeks old,
  —perform gentle closed reduction by traction (not leverage) with the patient under general anesthesia;
  —if you lever the head, you will fracture the osteoporotic bone;
  —if closed reduction fails, do not pull harder; perform an open reduction.
- in the younger patient with dislocation more than 4 weeks old,
  —perform open reduction with use of a wide anterior approach;
  —protect brachial plexus and axillary vessels;
  —release subscapularis and contracted capsule, if necessary, and
  —remove fibrous tissue from the glenoid fossa;
  —suture anterior structures neither too tight (stiff joint) nor too loose (redislocation). Start the patient on
  —active movements at 3 weeks.
- in the younger patient with a dislocation more than 9 months old,
  —no treatment.

Posterior

Clinical features

- usually a subacromial dislocation because this is not obvious clinically or radiographically, and the diagnosis is often missed;
- no external rotation is the key to diagnosis;
- abduction to a maximum of 60° (for the scapulothoracic joint);
- muscle atrophy;
- often treated for many weeks as a "frozen shoulder" (adhesive capsulitis).

Treatment

- if the dislocation is asymptomatic, leave well enough alone and encourage mobility. If it is
- symptomatic but

Less than 3 weeks old

- perform gentle closed reduction by traction with the patient under anesthesia, as is used for treatment of acute posterior dislocation;
- if closed reduction fails, perform open reduction.

3 weeks to 6 months old

- with small or no humeral head defect (compression fracture),
  —perform open reduction through an anterior approach, followed by a
  —shoulder spica for 5 weeks in 30° external rotation; then start the patient on
  —graduated exercises; the prognosis is poor.
- with large head defect but
  —good cartilage and muscle control,
  —perform open reduction and
  —transfer the lesser tuberosity with the subscapularis muscle into the defect to stabilize the joint and prevent recurrent dislocation. But with
- damaged cartilage and poor muscles, though with good scapulo-thoracic movement and control,
  —perform replacement arthroplasty or
  —arthrodesis.

More than 6 months old

- encourage mobilization.

RECURRENT DISLOCATION

Anterior

Etiopathology (Fig. 8.6)

- recurrent dislocation is the most common complication of acute, traumatic, anterior dislocation of the shoulder;
- 80% to 90% of acute dislocations in young patients (under 20 years old) recur,
- 60% recur in patients under 30 years old and
- 15% to 20% recur in patients over 40 years old;
- most recurrences happen in the first 2 years after acute dislocation;
- when acute dislocation is associated with
  —fracture of the glenoid rim, the recurrence rate is more than 95%; when it is associated with
  —fracture of the greater tuberosity of the humerus, the rate is less than 30%;
- 4 to 6 times more common in men than in women;
- the incidence of recurrence is affected more by the age of the patient and initial damage than by the initial treatment;
- one or a combination of the following anatomical factors may be associated with recurrence:
  —fracture of glenoid margin, avulsion of glenoid labrum or of capsule from the scapula neck anteriorly (Bankart lesion),

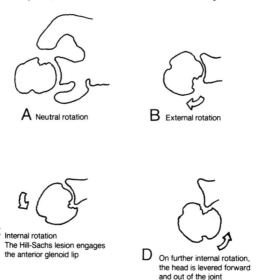

A Neutral rotation

B External rotation

C Internal rotation
The Hill-Sachs lesion engages
the anterior glenoid lip

D On further internal rotation,
the head is levered forward
and out of the joint

Figure 8.6. Mechanism of recurrent anterior dislocation due to a Hill-Sachs lesion.

 —stretched anterior capsule,
 —weak and partly torn subscapularis muscle, and
 —depressed fracture of posterior humeral head (Hill-Sachs lesion).
- mechanism (abduction and external rotation) is similar to that in acute dislocation, but much less force is usually required to redislocate the humerus.

Clinical features

- dislocation may recur during swimming, from throwing, or even from turning in bed during sleep;
- the patient often is able to reduce it himself;
- little pain and some anterior tenderness;
- the sign of apprehension, discussed previously, may be evident. On the
- axillary lateral x-ray, look for the "hatchet" deformity of the Hill-Sachs lesion.

Treatment

Bankart's repair of anterior capsular lesion

- indications are
  —lesion of capsule at its insertion on the anterior neck of the scapula or

—avulsion of glenoid labrum, with or without a flake of bone.
- technique is performed through
  —anterior approach,
  —osteotomy of coracoid,
  —division of subscapularis and capsule, then
  —reattachment of glenoid labrum by sutures through bone or by staple;
  —capsule is sutured with overlap;
  —subscapularis is sutured without overlap.

Putti-Platt subscapularis muscle shortening

- indications are
  —elongated capsule and muscle without tear, or
  —central tear of capsule, or
  —compression fracture of humeral head (Hill Sachs lesion);
- technique is performed through
  —anterior approach,
  —division of subscapularis 3 cm medial to the lesser tuberosity,
  —division of capsule in the same line, and
  —overlap of capsule and muscle anteriorly, so that external rotation is limited. Verify this on the operating table before closing the wound.

Watson-Jones

- combines Putti-Platt with Bankart when there is both
- anterior capsular lesion at the glenoid insertion and
- stretched subscapularis muscle.

Postoperative care

- 6 weeks in a Velpeau type dressing before starting young athletes on graduated range of movement (ROM) exercises;
- 2 to 4 weeks for patients over 40. The
- recurrence rate for these three pocedures is between 1% and 8%.
- like all operations, what works well with one surgeon does not always work well with another. When several different operations give similar results, the technique that a surgeon chooses is usually the one that he knows best and that gives him the best results.

Posterior

- an uncommon problem. Few acute posterior dislocations recur when treated promptly and properly.

Surgical repair

- treatment is through posterior approach;
- in any of the following procedures, the humeral head can be stabilized by two K wires through it and the glenoid.

Reverse Bankart

- for capsular lesion at the glenoid without a large humeral head defect;
- reattach capsule to scapula.

Reverse Putti-Platt

- for capsular tear and laxity of infraspinatus and teres minor muscles without a large humeral head defect;
- overlap these two muscles or overlap the first by itself.

Bone block

- wedge of bone from posterior lip of acromion or from ilium is
- screwed onto the back of the glenoid to deepen the cavity and prevent the head from slipping posteriorly.

Combination bone block and reverse Putti-Platt

- "belt and braces" operation which has
- better results than soft tissue reconstruction alone.

McLaughlin-Neer subscapularis transfer

- for a large anterior defect (compression fracture) of more than 40% in the anterior head. Through an
- anterior incision,
- screw the lesser tuberosity, with attached subscapularis tendon, into the defect;
- tuberosity helps to fill the defect, and
- muscle prevents posterior dislocation.

Postoperative care

- 4 to 6 weeks in a shoulder spica with the arm in neutral rotation;
- the older the patient, the shorter the time of immobilization;
- then graduated ROM exercises.

Prognosis

- is good with most techniques, but
- the larger the head defect, the worse the prognosis.

chapter 9

Fractures of the Proximal End and Shaft of the Humerus

Fracture of the Proximal Humerus

ETIOPATHOLOGY

- 4% to 5% of all fractures;
- usually results from a fall on an outstretched, abducted arm;
- common in the elderly with osteoporotic bone;
- fracture line nearly always through the surgical neck;
- may have associated fractures of greater and lesser tuberosities.

CLASSIFICATION

Stable fractures

- no major fragment is displaced more than 1 cm and
- angulation is less than 30°;
- fracture is stable and will not displace without further trauma;
- rarely associated with dislocation of the humeral head.

Unstable fractures (Fig. 9.1)

- four major segments (Neer's classification); these are the
  —head (articular fragment);
  —shaft (usually fractured from the head through the surgical neck), with the pectoralis major acting as the main displacing force;
  —greater tuberosity (may be comminuted) with rotator cuff; and
  —lesser tuberosity with subscapularis muscle attached;
- other fragments are not important.
- regardless of the number of fracture lines and the number of fragments, the classification is based on these four major fragments, as follows:

Two-part fracture

- one major fragment is displaced more than 1 cm. The
- two parts are the
  —displaced fragment and the
  —remaining fragment or fragments (these latter, being undisplaced and therefore stable, are considered as one fragment).

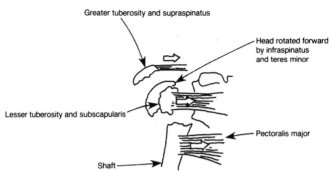

Figure 9.1. Four-part proximal humerus fracture and the forces acting on the fragments. (Modified from Neer CS II: Displaced proximal humeral fractures. *J Bone Joint Surg* 52A:1077–1089, 1970.)

Three-part fracture
- two major fragments are displaced. The
  —other fragments are undisplaced and therefore
  —stable and for practical purposes are considered as one fragment.

Four-part fracture
- all four major fragments are displaced.

Fracture dislocations
- unstable, two-, three- or four-part fractures may be associated with
  —anterior or
  —posterior dislocation of the humeral head.

CLINICAL AND RADIOLOGICAL FEATURES
- clinical features often are not obvious in shoulder fracture, but in a patient
- with pain and tenderness and a hematoma which may extend to the chest and elbow, you should suspect an injury and order
- good x-rays in two planes;
- the shoulder joint does not lie in the coronal plane but lies at 35° to it, facing backward. For
- good anteroposterior (AP) and lateral (scapular) views, have the patient
  —lie on his back, tilt him 35° toward the injured side, and take the
  —AP view in an axis vertical to the floor and the
  —lateral view in an axis horizontal to the floor;
  —the patient may sit or stand for these views, but the principle remains the same;
- an axillary view may be necessary for classification but should not be performed routinely because abduction of the shoulder to 90° is painful. This is the best view for diagnosing posterior dislocation and glenoid fractures.

TREATMENT

- these fractures heal well and rapidly if displacement is not too great;
- the shoulder joint stiffens rapidly in the adult and poses a much greater problem than the fracture;
- the maxim for fracture in adults is early motion.

Stable fractures

- 80% of all proximal humeral fractures. Treat with a
- sling for days 1 to 5; then
- pendulum exercises, with a sling, for days 6 to 10; then
- pendulum exercises, without a sling, for days 11 to 15; then
- no sling but continued graduated active range of movement (ROM) exercises; from the day of injury
- do not forget to mobilize the
  —elbow,
  —wrist and
  —fingers.

Unstable fractures

Two-part fracture (10% of proximal humoral fractures)

Before end of growth

- is an epiphyseal plate injury, usually a Salter-Harris Type II fracture, although Type I is more common in children under 5 years old. If it is
  —displaced more than 2 cm or
  —angulated or rotated more than 30°, perform
- closed reduction, then shoulder spica for 2 weeks with the arm in
  —any position in which reduction is stable (monitor with an image intensifier).

Adult

- shaft displaced, perform
  —closed reduction and immobilize with a
  —sling and swathe for 2 weeks. Then start the patient on
  —pendulum and graduated ROM exercises, with a sling. If
  —closed reduction fails, perform open reduction and fix with a Rush nail.
- shaft displaced and comminuted, treat with
  —overhead traction with neutral rotation until fracture is "sticky," then start the patient on
  —graduated ROM exercises.
- greater tuberosity displaced by
  —more than 1 cm, a tear in the rotator cuff is implied. Perform

—open reduction through a transacromial approach,
—repair torn cuff, and
—fix the bony fragment with wire or strong suture material. If
—repair is stable, use a sling and swathe for 2 weeks postoperatively. If it is
—unstable, use an airplane splint or shoulder spica for 2 weeks with the shoulder in 70° abduction.
- lesser tuberosity displacement requires
  —open reduction and a screw, through the anterior approach.

Three-part fracture (3%)

- consists of
  —displaced surgical neck fracture and either
  —displaced greater tuberosity (and head is rotated posteriorly by the subscapularis) or
  —displaced lesser tuberosity (and head is rotated anteriorly by the infraspinatus and teres minor);
- anatomical distortion is greater with this fracture than with the two-part fracture.
- treat by open reduction through the
  —anterior approach,
  —derotate the head,
  —reattach the tuberosity with wire, then
  —reattach the head to the shaft with wire or a Rush nail;
  —do not disturb soft tissue attachments of the head. The ascending branch of the anterior circumflex humeral artery is the main blood supply to the head in this injury;
  —repair the tear in the rotator cuff;
- postoperatively, treat with a sling and swathe for 3 weeks, then start the patient on
- graduated ROM exercises.

Four-part fracture (4%)

- called "Humpty Dumpty" fracture of the shoulder. Attempt
- open reduction and internal fixation. If this fails, replace the head with a prosthesis and attach muscle groups to it.

Fracture dislocation

Anterior dislocation

- two-part
  —nearly always the greater tuberosity is fractured and displaced. Perform
  —closed reduction; the greater tuberosity usually falls into place. If there is

—more than 1 cm of displacement after closed reduction, perform open reduction and fixation of the tuberosity, with repair of the rent in the rotator cuff.
- three-part
  —usually the greater tuberosity and shaft are displaced; perform
  —open reduction and wiring and repair of the rotator cuff.
- four-part
  —very difficult to repair because the shell of the head is avascular;
  —replace head with prosthesis.

Posterior dislocation

- two-part
  —usually the lesser tuberosity is displaced; perform
  —closed reduction. If the
  —tuberosity is still displaced, reduce it surgically and fix it.
- three-part
  —lesser tuberosity and shaft are displaced; perform
  —open reduction with a wire loop and Rush pin fixation.
- four-part
  —rare;
  —replace head with prosthesis.

Fracture of anatomical neck

- rare;
- incidence of avascular necrosis is high whatever the treatment; perform
- open reduction, with wire loop fixation for the displaced head, followed by a
- sling and swathe for 2 weeks; then start the patient on graduated ROM exercises.

COMPLICATIONS

- vessel injury;
- axillary nerve injury is rare with fractures alone;
- soft tissue interposition preventing reduction, e.g., biceps tendon.
- malunion
  —but great mobility of shoulder can compensate for 45° of angulation;
- nonunion is unusual;
- avascular necrosis of head with
  —pain,
  —limited movement and subsequent
  —degenerative arthritis.
- stiffness of
  —shoulder,

—elbow,

—wrist and

—fingers. Prevent this by early, active physiotherapy.

PROGNOSIS

- for one- and two-part fractures, prognosis is good if motion is started early;
- for three- and four-part fractures, results are often poor whatever the treatment;
- for dislocation with three- or four-part fracture, prognosis is generally poor; and
- for anatomical neck fractures, prognosis is poor because of avascular necrosis.

Fractures of Humeral Shaft

ETIOPATHOLOGY

- direct violence causes
  —transverse, butterfly or comminuted fracture;
- indirect violence causes an
  —oblique or spiral fracture;
- uncommon in children.

CLINICAL AND RADIOLOGICAL FEATURES

Diagnosis

- classical triad of pain, tenderness and swelling;
- displacement and
- abnormal mobility may not be evident.

Displacement (Fig. 9.2)

- related to
  —site of fracture,
  —fracturing force and
  —consequent muscle pull.

Fracture of proximal half

- when fracture lies between pectoralis major insertion (above) and deltoid insertion (below), the
- proximal fragment is pulled forward and medially by the pectoralis major while the
- distal fragment hangs straight.

Fracture of distal half (Fig. 9.3)

- if fracture is below the deltoid insertion, the
- proximal fragment is pulled into abduction by the deltoid and the

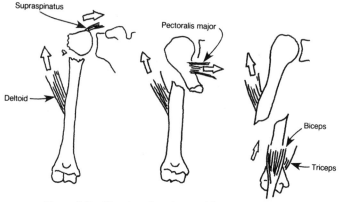

Figure 9.2.   Muscle pull on humeral fractures.

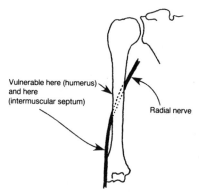

Figure 9.3.   Radial nerve winds around the humerus.

- distal fragment is pulled proximally by the biceps and triceps, especially if fracture is oblique or spiral;
- radial nerve is particularly vulnerable because the nerve lies on bone, then passes through lateral intermuscular septum. So
  —evaluate nerve function before and after treatment.

Radiological features

- x-ray in two planes to see the
- whole length of bone plus shoulder and elbow joints.

TREATMENT

Closed treatment

- treat a closed shaft fracture not associated with arterial injury by
  —closed reduction, with the patient sitting or standing,
  —molded sugar tong (U-shaped) plaster splint, and a sling; and
- start the patient on active elbow, wrist and finger exercises as soon as the pain has subsided. The adult may also start gentle
- pendular exercises for the shoulder.
- remove splint at 6 weeks and
- test union clinically. Radiologically, the callus around the humeral shaft does not show well. If the
  —fracture is "sticky," protect it with a sling, then start the adult patient on active graduated ROM exercises for the shoulder and elbow and
  —remove the sling 20 days later. If it is
  —not "sticky," protect it with plaster backslab for 4 more weeks, then reevaluate healing. In an active child,
- robust plaster shoulder spica may be preferable to a sugar tong cast.

Operative treatment

- for open reduction, Henry's anterolateral approach is the safest. Beware of the radial nerve, especially in the distal part of the incision.
- major indications include:
- open fracture
  —debridement and external fixation;
- arterial injury
  —usually associated with an open wound;
  —repair the fracture with external fixation preferably, or a six-hole plate and screws or intramedullary nail, then
  —repair the artery;
- nerve injury. If
  —radial nerve paralysis is a result of manipulation or develops late,
  —explore the nerve (see below);
- associated injuries, e.g.,
  —fractures elsewhere in the limb or
  —prolonged recumbency for multiple injuries may
  —require humeral stability without a cast to facilitate nursing, treatment and mobilization;
- double segmental fracture of the shaft may be better aligned by use of an intramedullary nail because of the difficulties of closed reduction.

Prognosis

- closed treatment produces
  —good results;

—malunion with mild residual angulation, rotation or shortening can be accepted because mobility of the shoulder joint compensates for this;

—nonunion is rare. In

- operative treatment for
  —open fracture, prognosis depends on success in preventing infection; for
  —arterial injury, prognosis depends on successful repair;
  —nonunion and infection are more likely after surgery. So operate only for proper indications.

COMPLICATIONS

Radial nerve injury (Fig. 9.3)

Neurapraxia and axonotmesis

- requires no special treatment other than a
  —cock-up lively banjo splint with the thumb in opposition and the metacarpophalangeal and interphalangeal joints in extension. Elastic bands to fingers and thumb allow active flexion and grasp, but return the fingers and thumb to a position of extension. This
  —splint protects long extensors and abductors and prevents stretching of paralyzed muscles.
- prognosis of
  —neurapraxia is excellent,
  —axonotmesis is good (70% recovery).
- if activity in the brachioradialis muscle does not begin within 3 months of injury, explore the nerve. If it is
  —cut, repair it; and if it is
  —trapped in callus or fibrous tissue, release it and perform neurolysis;
- if fracture of the distal third remains separated by soft tissue or if radial nerve palsy appears after closed reduction, explore the radial nerve immediately. It may be in the fracture!

Neurotmesis

- usually associated with open fracture;
- should be explored at the time of initial debridement, with the ends identified and tacked together to prevent retraction;
- later, when the wound is closed and dry, reexplore, excise the neurofibroma (proximal nerve end) and fibroma (distal nerve end), and suture the nerve, or graft it if necessary (see Chapter 31). In the meantime,
- protect paralyzed extensors with a banjo splint.

Delayed union and nonunion

Etiology

- there is
  —delayed union if healing takes 2 to 4 months, and there is
  —nonunion if the fracture is not healed at 4 months;
- union is likely to be slow, or to stop altogether, with
  —open fracture,
  —comminuted or transverse fracture,
  —soft tissue interposition,
  —inappropriate open reduction or
  —inadequate internal or external fixation.

Treatment

- for delayed union, continue with plaster immobilization. For
- nonunion,
  —identify and carefully dissect the radial nerve which may be stuck in fibrous tissue at the fracture site; then
  —freshen the fracture fragments and use
  —cancellous graft and
  —firm internal fixation supplemented by a cast if necessary.

chapter 10
Elbow Injuries in Children

General Observations

DIAGNOSIS (Fig. 10.1)
- is sometimes difficult. To make it easier, order
  —good anteroposterior (AP) and lateral radiographs centered on the joint, and
  —AP and lateral radiographs of the noninjured side for comparison, if necessary; and look at all the ossification centers. Order
  —oblique x-rays if you think there is a lesion (pain and swelling), even though the AP and lateral views appear to be normal.
- occasionally, an
  —air arthrogram and
  —stress films may help.

TREATMENT
- to avoid vascular complications
  —do not split an unreduced fracture in flexion,
  —always remove or splint immediately a cast or bandage of any child when you suspect vascular insufficiency, and
  —admit a child overnight for observation after closed reduction, especially of a supracondylar fracture;
- always make a careful neurovascular examination of the hand
  —before and
  —after reduction and write down your findings.
- malunion is often iatrogenic, seldom the result of a growth disturbance; do not blame Nature for your mistakes.

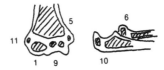

Figure 10.1. Appearance (in years) of ossification centers about the elbow.

Supracondylar Fracture of Humerus

ETIOPATHOLOGY (Fig. 10.2)

- commonest elbow injury in children (60% of all elbow injuries);
- a fall on the hand with hyperextension of the elbow results in extension fracture, with the distal fragment being displaced posteriorly;
- a fall on a flexed elbow results in flexion fracture (2% to 10% of all supracondylar fractures);
- displacement is usually a blend of angulation and rotation;
- periosteum is intact but lifted off the humeral metaphysis on the
  —medial side with medial displacement,
  —lateral side with lateral displacement,
  —posterior surface with extension fracture, and
  —anterior surface with flexion fracture (Fig. 10.5);
- periosteum is torn on the opposite side.
- fracture is in the
  —distal metaphysis of the humerus and crosses the olecranon fossa proximal to the epicondyles. It
  —may tear the synovium. Thus the fracture may be intrasynovial, though articular cartilage itself is never damaged.

CLASSIFICATION (Fig. 10.3)

- both extension and flexion fractures can be classified as follows (Lagrange and Rigault):
  —Type I: greenstick fracture with or without anteroposterior angulation;
  —Type II: complete fracture with minimal or no displacement;

Figure 10.2. Supracondylar fracture in a 10-year old. The fracture line crosses the olecranon and coronoid fossae.

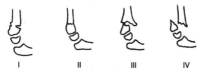

Figure 10.3. Classification of supracondylar fractures. (Modified from Lagrange J, Rigault P: Fractures supra-condyliennes. *Rev Chir Orthop* 48:337–414, 1962.)

—Type III: complete fracture with rotation of the distal fragment and only one remaining point of contact;
—Type IV: complete displacement with total loss of contact between the fragments.

DIAGNOSIS

Clinical

- examine blood supply to the hand first, next
- examine neurological function of the hand, and lastly
- examine the elbow. Features are
  —pain,
  —increasing swelling, and
  —inability to move the elbow.
- splint the limb in the position in which it lies and send the patient to the x-ray department.

Radiological

Technique

- AP and
- lateral
  —a good lateral x-ray is only possible if the techician moves the tube through 90° rather than the arm through the fracture site. Splint the limb first and educate your technicians.

Interpretation

- undisplaced fracture is difficult to see. Look for the
  —anterior and posterior fat pads displaced by hemarthrosis;
- anteroposterior displacement is
  —obvious on a good lateral x-ray, but
  —rotation and tilting are not. Suspect
- rotation on a lateral x-ray when you see an
  —oblique view of one fragment and a
  —lateral view of the other; it helps to
  —know the radiological appearance of a normal elbow;
- angulation (varus or valgus) of distal fragment can be seen on an
  —AP x-ray; look for
  —unilateral overlap of the two fragments, usually on the medial side of the fracture line (because angulation of this fracture is almost always in varus). On a good
  —lateral x-ray centered on the joint, look for the sign of the crescent moon (Fig. 10.4). This shows an
  —overlap of the capitellum by the sigmoid notch of the olecranon when the fracture is angulated. The overlap has the shape of the

Figure 10.4. Sign of the crescent moon.

—moon in its first quarter. If there is a

—clear space between the capitellum and the sigmoid notch, the fragment is not tilted. If the

—lateral x-ray is not accurately centered, the crescent moon sign may be falsely positive or falsely negative.

TREATMENT

Extension and flexion fractures: Types I and II

- long arm backslab with the
  —elbow at 90° of flexion for an extension fracture, less for a flexion fracture, and the
  —forearm in pronation. No tight bandages.
- complete the cast the next day if there is no vascular impairment. This is a safe way to treat the child.

Extension fractures only: Types III and IV

Closed reduction

Technique (Figs. 3.2 and 10.5)

- with the patient under general anesthesia,
- disengage the fracture fragments by
  —traction on the forearm, with the elbow in extension and with countertraction applied to the arm by the assistant;
- correct lateral displacement first by manipulating the distal fragment between the finger and thumb and
- reproduce the normal angle of valgus (compare with normal arm). Then
- manipulate the distal fragment forward with the thumb on the olecranon. The posterior periosteal hinge will prevent overcorrection and anterior displacement. Once the elbow is
- reduced, flex it to 120° while maintaining pressure on the olecranon. Then
- pronate the forearm if the distal fragment was displaced medially (common);
  —pronation will close the gap on the lateral side, with intact medial periosteum used as a hinge. Or

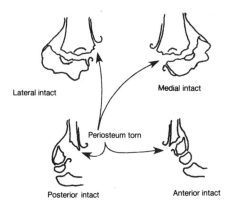

Lateral intact

Medial intact

Periosteum torn

Posterior intact

Anterior intact

Figure 10.5.   Periosteal hinge prevents overreduction.

- supinate the forearm if the distal fragment was displaced laterally,
  —using intact lateral periosteal hinge to close the gap on the medial side.

Confirmation

- AP, shooting through the flexed elbow, and lateral x-rays to confirm reduction;
- on AP x-rays, look again for
  —residual displacement in the coronal (lateral) plane and
  —unilateral overlap of the fracture surfaces (rotation and angulation).
- on lateral x-rays, look for
  —rotation (lateral view of one fragment, oblique of the other) and
  —angulation (crescent moon).

Immobilization

- hold the elbow at 100° with the forearm in pronation or supination;
- the assistant applies backslab and holds it on with gauze or flannel bandage, using figure-of-8 technique at the elbow to allow for swelling and to prevent compression in the antecubital fossa;
- collar and cuff sling is attached firmly to backslab at the wrist to avoid displacement in the cast. The child should not be able to remove the sling;
- x-ray again the next day, and if
  —reduction is maintained and the
  —vascular status is normal, complete the cast (loosely in front of elbow) and maintain the sling. If

- reduction is lost,
    - —attempt closed reduction once more, with the patient under general anesthesia;
    - —if the second attempt fails, treat the child in traction.

Vascular impairment

- if
    - —flexion of the elbow to stabilize the fracture stops the radial pulse and the fingers are white, and
    - —extension of the elbow until the radial pulse reappears and the fingers are pink causes displacement of the fracture,
    - —treat the child in traction. If the
- pulse disappears but the fingers are pink and warm, maintain flexion. The radial pulse usually reappears after a few minutes.

Traction (Fig. 4.6)

- indications are
    - —failed closed reduction or
    - —gross edema about the elbow;
- technique may be
    - —overhead traction with olecranon pin (beware of the ulnar nerve) or
    - —Dunlop's horizontal method with skin traction or an olecranon pin. This technique is
- safe but requires daily attention. At
- 14 days the fracture is
    - —"sticky" and will not displace. Put the arm in a
    - —cast for 2 more weeks.

Percutaneous pins (Fig. 10.6)

- indications are for
    - —open fracture,
    - —associated vascular injury,
    - —associated fractures of both bones of the same forearm, or an

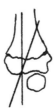

Figure 10.6. Two percutaneous pins.

—unstable fracture;
- with the patient under general anesthesia and with rigidly sterile conditions,
  —reduce the fracture and
  —immobilize it with
  —two pins, either one pin through
  —each epicondyle (careful of the ulnar nerve) or
  —both just lateral to the olecranon, one vertically in the humeral medullary canal and the other obliquely into the far cortex. Then apply plaster backslab. But if you
- fail with two attempts, do not try again. The elbow is not a dart board! Treat the child in traction.

Open reduction

- indications are
  —vascular injury if vessels are to be explored,
  —open fracture of Type II or III skin wound, or
  —failure of all closed methods to reduce the fracture and maintain the reduction.
- approach the fracture through an
  —anterior S-shaped incision if vessels are to be explored, or
  —through the skin wound if fracture is open, or
  —through the Campbell posteror approach if fracture is closed or the wound is dirty or poorly placed for surgery;
- reduce the fracture and stabilize under direct vision with two K wires (as discussed previously), and
- apply plaster backslab with the elbow at 90° flexion and with the forearm in neutral rotation.

Postoperative care

- if the fracture has been pinned, remove the
  —pins at 3 weeks and the
  —cast at 4 weeks;
- the child will mobilize his own elbow and does not need physiotherapy. Full range of movement may take 2 years or more to return, so warn the parents.

Flexion Fracture: Types III and IV

- closed reduction is
  —more difficult with flexion fractures than with extension fractures;
  —disimpact the fracture and
  —correct lateral displacement and the carrying angle as is done for extension fracture, then

—push the distal fragment backward and

—apply a long arm cast with the elbow in 30° of flexion and the forearm in supination;

- percutaneous pins can be used for
  —unstable or
  —open fractures or for associated
  —forearm fractures of the same side;
  —technique and postoperative management are the same as for extension fractures;
- open reduction is indicated for similar reasons as with extension fractures, but the incidence of failed closed reduction is higher with flexion fractures.

COMPLICATIONS

- complications of the fracture and of its treatment are common. The following could be secondary to either the fracture or its treatment.

Vascular (Fig. 10.7)

Pathology

- in an extension fracture the brachial artery may be
  —speared by the sharp edge of the proximal fragment,
  —compressed by the proximal fragment,
  —caught and squeezed in the fracture, especially if the elbow is flexed before the fracture is reduced, or
  —angulated posteriorly over the proximal fragment so that the lumen is occluded;
- in flexion and extension fractures, the vessels may be
  —compressed by hematoma and edema.

Treatment

- if the
  —radial pulse is absent but the
  —fingertips are pink and warm, and

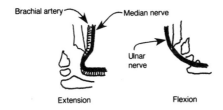

Figure 10.7. Structures endangered in supracondylar fractures.

—capillary filling of the finger pulp is normal, even after the fracture is reduced,

—elevate the arm and wait. If the fingers remain pink and warm and extension of the fingers is painless, exploration is unnecessary;

- if the fingers are
  —pale and cool, even after reduction,
  —remove all constricting bandages,
  —extend the elbow to 80° or 60°,
  —elevate the arm, and wait for 30 minutes. If the
- circulation does not return,
  —explore vessels as soon as possible and perform a complete
  —fasciotomy at the same time. Do not wait. It is better to
  —operate too soon than to operate too late.

Neurological (Fig. 10.7)

- median nerve in an extension fracture may be
  —speared by a proximal fragment or
  —caught and compressed in the fracture site;
- radial nerve in extension fractures, with the distal fragment displaced medially, may be pulled backward over the proximal fragment and speared;
- ulnar nerve is vulnerable in flexion fractures.
- almost all nerve injuries recover spontaneously over several days or months once the fracture is reduced.

Others

- less than 5% are open fractures, and these are almost always from within without.
- elbow injury may be accompanied by forearm or humeral shaft fracture of same side, so
  —order radiographs of the full length of the humerus and forearm bones.
- cubitus varus (10%) is due to
  —poor reduction with uncorrected angulation or rotation or to
  —loss of reduction. This causes
  —no functional problems but is an ugly deformity.

PROGNOSIS

- generally good;
- anteroposterior displacement may remodel, especially in the young child, but
- rotation and varus or valgus will not remodel;
- most elbows regain a full range of motion with time.

UNTREATED DISPLACED FRACTURES

Pathology (Fig. 3.5)

- fracture always unites but usually with
  - —varus (gunstock) and
  - —rotation deformity and either
  - —posterior or
  - —anterior (rare) displacement of the distal fragment;
- coronoid and olecranon fossae may be filled with callus and limit movement;
- varus and rotation in a child will not remodel, but continued
- growth of the elbow away from the fracture site and
- remodeling of the fracture deformity will allow increased flexion and extension.

Clinical features

- limitation of flexion and extension, less marked in children than in adults;
- forearm rotation is normal;
- varus (rarely valgus) deformity;
- no pain; and
- no osteoarthritis.

Treatment

- closed reduction is not possible in the child after 10 days and in adult after 14 days;
- surgery to correct varus and rotation is difficult, and the results are not always good due to
  - —insufficient correction of varus,
  - —failure to correct rotation,
  - —difficulty with internal fixation,
  - —nonunion,
  - —stiffness of the elbow,
  - —myositis ossificans and
  - —an unsightly bump on the lateral side of the arm.
- if you must treat the elbow,
  - —wait until the child has regained as much movement as he can, then perform
- closing wedge osteotomy through a lateral incision and
  - —fix the bone with a plate and screws or K wires; during surgery
- compare the correction with the normal side;
- this is

—cosmetic surgery and will
—not improve function. So
—warn the parents!

Fracture of Lateral Condyle of Humerus

ETIOPATHOLOGY (Fig. 10.8)

- 10% of elbow injuries in children. The injury
- occurs when the fully extended elbow is forced into varus. The ulnar trochlear ridge acts as a fulcrum and the
- lateral condyle is avulsed by the lateral collateral ligament and the common extensor muscle. This is a
- Salter-Harris Type IV growth plate injury. The
- fracture line
  —crosses the lateral corner of the distal
  —metaphysis, the
  —growth plate and the distal
  —epiphysis. Then, either the fracture line
  —enters the joint in the trochlear sulcus, and the fracture fragment then includes the capitellum and lateral third of the trochlea, or the fracture
  —passes through the ossific nucleus of the capitellum and enters the joint lateral to the trochlea; the fracture fragment then includes only the capitellum, and the trochlea is intact. If the fracture is
- incomplete, leaving a hinge of epiphyseal cartilage at the medial end of the fracture line, the fragment will be undisplaced. If the fracture is
- complete, displacement may occur, and the fragment may be rotated in 3 planes by the extensor muscle pull. The
- injury may be accompanied by a
  —varus fracture of the olecranon (transverse greenstick fracture open laterally) and by

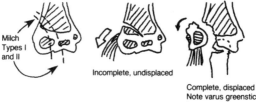

Milch
Types I
and II

Incomplete, undisplaced

Complete, displaced
Note varus greenstick
fracture of olecranon

Figure 10.8. Fractures of the lateral humeral condyle.

—subluxation and even dislocation of the ulna when the fragment includes the lateral third of the trochlea.

RADIOLOGICAL FEATURES
- displaced fracture is usually
- easy to diagnose if the capitellar ossific nucleus is visible because the
- capitellum is in the
  —wrong place, has a
  —strange shape (because of rotation), and has a
  —metaphyseal fragment attached (compare x-ray of the injured elbow with x-ray of the normal elbow). If the child is
- under 4 years of age, and the capitellum is still cartillaginous, a varus
  —stress film will prove the instability, and an
  —air arthrogram will show the fracture and the displaced fragment;
- hematoma on the lateral side distinguishes this from a Type II injury in which hematoma is medial and instability is in valgus. An
- undisplaced fracture may also be
- difficult to diagnose. Look for a
  —hairline fracture along the corner of the metaphysis and pay particular attention to the
  —alignment of the humerus, capitellum and radius when comparing the injured side with the normal side;
  —oblique x-rays,
  —stress film
  —and air arthrogram may be useful.

TREATMENT
Undisplaced fracture
- immobilization in long arm cast for 4 weeks with the elbow at 90° and the forearm in neutral rotation;
- x-ray every 4 days for the first 2 weeks because the fragment may displace in the cast; open reduction is then required.

Displaced fracture
- if displacement is more than 2 mm, treat by
  —open reduction through a lateral approach and
- immobilize the condyle with two fine Kirschner wires;
  —confirm reduction by x-rays before closing; apply a
- long arm cast for 4 weeks, then remove the pins and plaster;
- no vigorous activity is allowed for 4 more weeks;
- prognosis is good.

COMPLICATIONS

- malunion,
- nonunion,
- cubitus valgus,
- growth deformity and
- tardy ulnar nerve palsy.

UNTREATED DISPLACED FRACTURES

Pathology

- fracture is usually
  —ununited, the
  —condylar fragment and humeral fracture surface are covered with fibrous tissue. There is
  —retraction of the soft tissue attachments of the condyle and a
  —valgus deformity which generally does not increase with growth;
- no avascular necrosis, but
- osteoarthritis is common, and this together with valgus may cause
- tardy ulnar nerve palsy.

Clinical features

- cubitus valgus with
- bump on lateral side of elbow;
- flexion and extension are limited, about 70% of normal, but
- forearm rotation is normal;
- patient may have
  —pain occasionally with
  —weakness of the arm and a feeling of instability;
- tardy ulnar nerve palsy is the most disabling complication.

Treatment

Fracture less than 6 weeks old

- open reduction through lateral approach;
- carefully clean fibrous tissue and callus from all fracture surfaces and from the joint;
- do not damage articular cartilage. It is difficult to differentiate between this and the white fibrous tissue;
- orient the fragment and reduce it, but respect its soft tissue attachments in order to avoid necrosis. Then
- fix the fragment with two K wires.
- AP and lateral x-rays before closure are mandatory because the reduction is never as good as you think! If it is
- unsatisfactory, do it again. Then apply a

- long arm cast with the elbow at 90° and the forearm in neutral rotation,
- remove pins at 4 weeks and the cast at 6 weeks, and
- allow the child to mobilize the elbow himself.

Fracture more than 6 weeks old

- the poor results of open reduction of a fracture older than 6 weeks are due to the
- difficulties of reduction and resulting complications, which may include
  —malunion
  —nonunion,
  —premature growth plate closure,
  —avascular necrosis and
  —elbow stiffness, and
- do not justify this surgery. It is better to
- leave the lateral condyle alone and accept the deformity and limitation of movement, and
- advise the patient and parents to return at the first sign of hypoesthesia in the ulnar nerve territory. Then you can transpose the nerve.

Capitellum (Fig. 11.1)

- occurs usually in older adolescents;
- fragment comprises anterior, articular half of the lateral condyle. If the fracture is
- undisplaced, treat with a cast for 3 weeks. If it is
- displaced and the patient is still
  —growing, perform open reduction through a lateral approach and fix the fragment with a posteroanterior screw into subchondral bone. If the patient is
  —near the end of growth, excise the fragment (see Chapter 11).

Fracture of Medial Condyle of Humerus

ETIOPATHOLOGY AND RADIOLOGICAL FEATURES (Fig. 10.9)

- less than 2% of elbow injuries;
- pathology is similar to that of fractures of the lateral condyle, a
  —Salter-Harris Type IV growth plate injury;
- fragment includes the
  —medial epicondyle and the

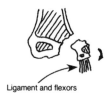

Ligament and flexors

Figure 10.9. Medial condyle fracture before ossification of trochlear center.

—medial third or half of the distal humeral epiphysis (the trochlea). Fragment is
- frequently displaced and rotated by the flexor muscles attached to it.
- because ossific nuclei of the trochlea appear in children at 8 years of age, the injury in a younger child is very
    —difficult to diagnose and is often
    —mistaken for avulsion of the medial epicondyle. In this case, the
    —clue is the metaphyseal fragment. If in doubt, order
    —stress x-rays or an
    —air arthrogram.

TREATMENT
- undisplaced, treat with a
    —long arm cast for 4 weeks;
- watch for displacement in the cast in the first 10 days. For
- displaced fracture, treat by
    —open reduction through a medial approach, taking care to protect the ulnar nerve, and by
    —fixation with two K wires;
    —verify accurate reduction both visually and radiographically before closure;
- remove pins and cast at 4 weeks, but forbid vigorous activity for 4 weeks more;
- complications and prognosis are similar to those for fracture of the lateral condyle.

UNTREATED DISPLACED FRACTURES
Pathology
- fragment usually includes the whole trochlea;
- fracture surfaces and medial joint space are filled with fibrous tissue, and the
- soft tissue attachments of the condylar fragment are retracted.

Clinical features

- occasionally, varus deformity and
- ulnar nerve neuritis;
- limitation of flexion and extension but
- normal forearm rotation;
- elbow may be unstable.

Treatment

- should have open reduction to stabilize the elbow regardless of the age of the fracture;
- protect the ulnar nerve;
- orientation of fragment is difficult due to
  —rotation and
  —fibrous tissue which fills the cavities and covers the fracture surfaces;
- fix the condyle with two K wires, and take
- AP and lateral x-rays before closure to verify the reduction. Then apply a
- long arm cast;
- remove pins at 4 weeks and the cast at 6 weeks, and
- allow the child to mobilize the elbow himself;
- results are better than those for late reduction of fractures of the lateral condyle.

Avulsion of Medial Epicondyle

ETIOPATHOLOGY AND RADIOLOGICAL FEATURES (Figs. 10.10 and 10.11)

- 8% of elbow injuries in children. Due to
- valgus injury of the elbow. The
- medial epicondyle is avulsed from the humerus, through the apophyseal line, and may be
- sucked into the joint while this is open medially at the time of injury;
- frequently associated with
  —dislocation of elbow or
  —fracture of radial neck.
- always compare x-rays of the injured elbow with those of the noninjured elbow, and check to see whether medial epicondyle is
  —in the joint!
- diagnosis is difficult before the epicondyle ossifies, at age 5. Medial painful swelling should arouse suspicion.

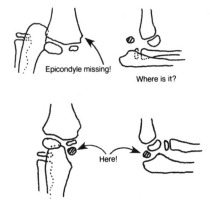

Figure 10.10. Intra-articular entrapment of the medial epicondyle after reduction of dislocation.

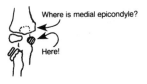

Figure 10.11. Valgus injury with radial neck fracture.

TREATMENT

Nonoperative treatment

- the majority of patients can be treated by
- protective plaster backslab for 10 days and then by
- mobilization. The fragment need not be reduced unless it is in the elbow joint;
- healing is often by fibrous union and is nearly always asymptomatic.

Operative treatment

- indications include the
  —epicondyle in the joint, an associated
  —ulnar nerve lesion or an
  —open skin wound;
- approach the lesion through a
  —medial incision,
  —extract the fragment from the joint (will have its flexor muscle

attachment intact) and suture it in place or fix it with two K wires. If there is an

—ulnar nerve lesion, transpose the nerve anteriorly and resuture the epicondyle and flexor muscles. After wound closure, apply a

- long arm cast, with the elbow at 90°, with the forearm pronated to relax the pronator teres, and with the wrist flexed 15° to relax the flexors, and remove after 3 weeks;
- then active mobilization;
- prognosis is good.

COMPLICATIONS

- ulnar nerve neuritis;
- late instability of the elbow is seldom seen;
- if the diagnosis is missed and the fragment remains in the elbow joint, pain, limitation of movement, and later osteoarthritis (see below) will result.

UNTREATED AVULSION

Pathology

- if the epicondyle is intra-articular, the elbow is
  —subluxed, since the fragment is interposed between the sigmoid (ole-cranon) notch of the ulna and the trochlea of the humerus. The injury may be
- associated with
  —impacted fracture of the radial neck or
  —reduced or unreduced dislocation of the elbow.

Clinical features

Extra-articular epicondyle

- usually no pain,
- no instability,
- no limitation of movement, a
- small bump on the medial side of the elbow and
- rarely ulnar nerve neuritis.

Intra-articular epicondyle

- pain and
- crepitus on movement of the elbow with
- marked limitation of flexion and extension. Rarely the patient may have reasonable pain-free function.

Untreated dislocation with avulsion of medial epicondyle

- the elbow is usually stiff in a few degrees of flexion, but
- occasionally the patient has surprisingly good painless function.

Treatment

Extra-articular fragment

- if you suspect instability, take
  —stress x-rays. If the elbow is unstable,
- reduce and fix the fragment with its muscular and ligamentous attachments.

Intra-articular fragment

- if the patient has a range of painless movement from 60° to 110°,
- do not operate. If
- function is poor and the elbow is painful,
- extract the fragment and its attached flexor muscles through a medial approach, taking care to
- protect the ulnar nerve;
- excise the fragment and suture the flexor muscle group to periosteum of the humerus. Put the arm in a
- cast for 2 weeks, then
- start the patient on early active movements;
- results may be surprisingly good.

Dislocation associated

- see below.

Arthroplasty

- if the articular cartilage of the elbow joint is badly damaged and
- function is severely limited, the older patient may require a
- dermis or fascial arthropalsty. This may
- convert a painful elbow to a relatively painless one.

Dislocation of Elbow

ETIOPATHOLOGY AND RADIOLOGICAL FEATURES (Fig. 10.10)

- direction of dislocation is usually posterior, sometimes with medial or lateral displacement, and is rarely anterior;
- often associated with avulsion of medial epicondyle, so look for this (visible on x-ray in a patient after the age of 5 years);
- occasionally accompanied by fracture of the radial neck when the
  —radial head may be angulated and impacted or may be
  —completely displaced;
- rarely associated with fracture of the coronoid (posterior dislocation) or epiphysis of the olecranon (anterior);

- subluxation or even dislocation may also accompany
  —fracture of the lateral condyle.

TREATMENT

- closed reduction of a simple dislocation under anesthesia is usually easy;
- correct the collateral (coronal) displacement first, then the
- anteroposterior displacement;
- once the dislocation is reduced, full flexion of the elbow is possible without effort; however, you must take
- postreduction x-rays and look for the
  —medial epicondyle. If it is
  —trapped in the joint, extract it through a medial incision and suture it in place or fix it with two K wires;
- treat associated fractures as described elsewhere in this chapter. If the dislocation is
- properly treated, the prognosis is good.

COMPLICATIONS

- vascular compression is common;
- neurological injuries are
  —more frequent and usually involve the
  —ulnar nerve; generally,
  —recovery is spontaneous after reduction;
- myositis ossificans may occur, especially in the brachialis muscle. In children, this may be
  —resorbed within a few months. If it is not and it
  —interferes with function,
  —excise the ectopic bone mass once it is mature.

UNTREATED DISLOCATION

Pathology

- usually posterior;
- triceps muscle is shortened,
- collateral ligaments are contracted,
- joint space anterior to the humeral condyles and in the sigmoid notch of the ulna is filled with fibrous tissue, and this tissue and the capsule adhere to the articular surfaces;
- muscles are atrophied and there is
- local disuse osteoporosis;
- callus may form beneath stripped-up periosteum of the humeral shaft, and
- myositis ossificans occasionally occurs.

Clinical features

- irreducible by closed methods 3 weeks after injury;
- range of movement is usually 20° to 50° or may be fixed in a few degrees of flexion;
- occasionally the patient has a satisfactory range of painless movement of 50° to 110°, but
- muscle power in the arm is reduced;
- forearm rotation usually is little affected.

Treatment

Satisfactory function

- if the child has
  —50° or more movement around the right angle, he does
  —not require surgery.

Poor function

- if the elbow is fixed or has a
- small range of movement in a useless arc (e.g., 10° to 30°), perform
- open reduction through a Campbell posterior approach, taking care to
- protect the ulnar nerve;
- dissect soft tissues from around the elbow joint,
- remove new bone that blocks reduction, and
- lengthen the triceps tendon when necessary;
- do not damage articular cartilage;
- reduction of the elbow must be gentle;
- if the elbow is unstable in reduced position, stabilize it with a K wire through the olecranon into the humerus;
- suture the triceps in its lengthened position and apply
- long arm backslab, with the elbow at 90° for a child and at 60° for an adult;
- remove the pin and cast at 2 weeks and have the patient
- start active (never passive) mobilization. The
- results are better than one would expect with an increased range of movement in the useful range, 60° to 120°. Obviously, the
- younger the patient and the shorter the period since dislocation, the better the result.

Fracture of Radial Neck

ETIOPATHOLOGY AND RADIOLOGICAL FEATURES

- 4% of elbow injuries in children.
- usually a
  —fracture of the radial neck, just distal to the growth plate, or

—a Salter-Harris Type II growth plate injury (less common);
- fracture of the radial head itself is a Type III lesion and is rare.
- half of these fractures are associated with other injuries:
  —avulsion of medial epicondyle (valgus injury) (Fig. 10.11);
  —transverse or oblique fracture of the olecranon, open medially (valgus injury), which may occur when the elbow is fully extended at the time of the accident and the olecranon is "keyed" into the olecranon fossa of the humerus;
  —fracture of the ulnar shaft (a Monteggia-like lesion);
  —dislocation of the elbow, sometimes with a
  —coronoid fracture;
- valgus injury causes varying degrees of angulation and impaction of the radial head on the neck;
- posterior dislocation of the elbow may fracture the radial neck, and during closed reduction the lateral condyle may knock the radial head off the radius. The head remains behind and closed reduction is impossible;
- good AP and lateral x-rays of the proximal radius are necessary to appreciate angulation and displacement.

TREATMENT

Undisplaced fracture

- backslab for 3 weeks with elbow at 90°.

Angulation (Fig. 10.12)

Less than 30° to long axis of radius

- long arm cast for 3 weeks;
- radius will remodel.

More than 30°

- avoid open reduction if possible;
- try closed reduction under anesthesia
  —rotate the forearm until you feel the prominence of the radial head,
  —then push the head medially and the shaft laterally. Then

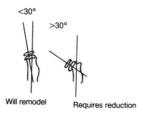

Figure 10.12. Radial neck fracture.

—x-ray to assess the new position and,

—if there is still more than 30° angulation,

—try again. If the second attempt fails, perform

- open reduction through a

    —lateral approach;

    —lever the radial head into position, rotating the forearm to help you, and

    —fix the head with one oblique Kirschner wire (this should not cross the capitellum and elbow joint as the wire usually breaks and is then difficult to remove).

Complete displacement

- never remove the radial head in a child because of subsequent growth disturbance;
- reduce the head through lateral incision and fix with K wire;
- avascular necrosis is not a problem because

    —fracture is usually distal to the entry of vessels, and even when these are damaged,

    —the small fragment is quickly revascularized.

Associated injuries

- avulsion of medial epicondyle,

    —leave it alone unless it is trapped in the elbow joint;

- olecranon fracture that is displaced,

    —half will reduce without operation simply by extension of the elbow and then by casting it in this position;

    —the other half may require open reduction, and half of these may need open reduction of the radial head too;

- ulnar shaft fracture is treated the same as a Monteggia lesion (see Chapter 12);
- dislocation of the elbow

    —reduce it;

- coronoid fracture

    —not usually a problem.

Postoperative care

- long arm cast for 3 weeks. Then
- remove the K wire and have the patient start
- active mobilization;
- prognosis is

    —excellent with nonoperative treatment and is

    —fair with operative treatment, with some residual loss of rotation.

COMPLICATIONS

- most frequent after open reduction;
- avascular necrosis of the head may occur, but necrosis of the whole head is rare;
- growth disturbance and early closure of growth plate;
- radioulnar synostosis.

UNTREATED FRACTURES

Pathology and clinical features

- head usually hypertrophies;
- molding usually improves displaced impacted fractures, but where there is
- no contact between the fracture surfaces, the result will be a nonunion. There may be
- some limitation of flexion and extension of the elbow and of
- rotation of the forearm;
- osteoarthritic changes may intervene much later.

Treatment

- do not remove the head before the end of growth because this may cause cubitus valgus and disturb the distal radioulnar joint. If the patient is a child and the head is
- angulated less than 30%, do not operate. If the
- angulation is more than 30°, use the
  - —lateral approach and perform
  - —osteotomy of the neck of the radius,
  - —push the head into position, and
  - —fix it with a K wire and a cast for 4 weeks. If the
  - —head is too large, shorten the neck.
- results are generally good. If the
- head is completely displaced,
  - —extract it (it has no soft tissue attachments),
  - —replace it on the neck, and fix it with a K wire and cast for 4 weeks;
  - —although the head has no blood supply, it is small and quickly revascularizes; and because the elbow is a
  - —non-weight-bearing joint, the head is unlikely to deform before revascularization is complete.
- if the patient has finished growing and the radial head limits movement and is painful, excise it.

Olecranon Fractures

ETIOPATHOLOGY AND RADIOLOGICAL FEATURES (Figs. 10.1, 10.8 and 11.4)

- the olecranon has a posterior epiphysis with a growth plate;
  —do not mistake this for a fracture (compare x-ray of injured side with x-ray of noninjured side);
- fracture line usually goes through the proximal metaphysis;
- varus or valgus force on the extended elbow, when the olecranon process is locked into the olecranon fossa, produces a
  —transverse greenstick fracture or
  —complete transverse fracture of olecranon and is often
- associated with
  —fracture of the lateral condyle (varus),
  —fracture of the radial neck (valgus) or
  —dislocation of the elbow (coronoid process fractures in posterior dislocation, olecranon epiphysis in anterior dislocation);
- complete fracture may be
  —undisplaced, with intact periosteum, or
  —displaced, with torn periosteum, either angulated or separated by the
  —pull of the triceps muscle.

TREATMENT

Undisplaced

- long arm cast for 3 weeks.

Displaced

Closed reduction

- by extension of the elbow the olecranon fossa may guide the fracture into position;
- minimal displacement can be accepted;
- 3 weeks in a long arm cast with the elbow in extension.

Open reduction (Fig. 11.5)

- indicated for failed closed reduction. The
- technique for children is similar to that for adults (see Chapter 11);
- two parallel or crossed K wires and a figure-of-8 tension wire through the posterior (Boyd) approach;
- protective long arm cast for 3 weeks, then
- active mobilization.

Pulled Elbow

ETIOPATHOLOGY

- occurs in a child 1 to 4 years of age;
- cause is a violent tug on the child's forearm in the axis of the arm;
- annular ligament is partially torn as the radial head subluxes distally and
- the ligament is interposed between the radial head and capitellum, preventing reduction.

DIAGNOSIS

- typical history
  —parent pulls child across the road;
- the child holds the elbow slightly flexed and will not move it;
- tenderness over the radial head and pain on attempted forearm rotation;
- no radiographical abnormality. The subluxation may be reduced by a technician positioning the elbow for the AP film!

TREATMENT

- no anesthesia;
- gently supinate the forearm with the elbow slightly flexed. You may feel or
- hear a click and no more screams!
- the child can use the elbow immediately,
  —no immobilization is needed;
- prognosis is excellent, provided the parents do not pull on the arm again!

chapter 11

Elbow Injuries in the Adult

General Remarks

- neurovascular lesions are common, so look for them;
- good anteroposterior (AP) and lateral x-rays are essential for the diagnosis, and oblique views may help too. Look for displacement of the anterior and posteror fat pads;
- differentiate those injuries which will do better with operative treatment from those which should be treated closed;
- many fractures about the elbow are unstable, with the fragments being displaced by the pull of various muscle groups. For these, open reduction and internal fixation are indicated;
- surgical treament should be prompt, but it may be technically difficult. If you do not have good x-rays, proper equipment, and an experienced team, it may be better to use closed methods because poor surgical treatment is worse than no treatment at all!
- the elbow joint is particularly prone to stiffness in the adult, so rehabilitation and physiotherapy should be prominent in your plan of treatment.

Supracondylar Fracture of Humerus

- rare in the adult;
- fracture line crosses the olecranon fossa (Fig. 10.2)

CLASSIFICATION (Fig. 10.7)

Extension

- the most common type. Generally caused by a
- fall on an outstretched hand;
- fracture line is transverse and oblique, downward and forward;
- distal fragment is displaced posteriorly with the elbow joint;
- radial and median nerves and the brachial artery are threatened by the proximal fragment anteriorly.

Flexion

- rare. Usually the result of a
- fall on the point of the elbow;
- fracture line is transverse and oblique, downward and backward;
- distal fragment is displaced anteriorly;
- ulnar nerve is threatened by the proximal fragment posteriorly.

Medial and lateral displacement

- may be associated with either type.

TREATMENT

- indication for reduction is malalignment with
  —rotation more than 5°,
  —angulation more than 20°, or
  —medial or lateral tilt.

Closed reduction

Manipulation and cast

- manipulation with the patient under anesthesia. Maintain reduction by
- posterior plaster slab, with the elbow at 100° of flexion if the radial pulse is not obliterated, and with the forearm in
  —pronation, if the distal fragment was displaced medially, or
  —supination, if the distal fragment was displaced laterally, with the intact periosteal hinge used to close the gap on the other side. If the
- radial pulse is obliterated, reduce flexion until it reappears;
- never apply a circular cast before the swelling starts to subside;
- support the cast with a collar and cuff sling;
- re-x-ray in the cast at 1 week to confirm the position;
- remove the cast at 4 weeks and reassess the fracture:
  —if it is united, start the patient on physiotherapy (adults need physiotherapy);
  —if it is not, apply a cast for 2 more weeks.

Skeletal traction

Indications

- elbow too swollen for manipulation,
- failed manipulation,
- recurrence of displacement in the cast,
- vascular insufficiency or
- open fracture Type I.

Technique (Figs. 4.3 and 4.6)

- pin through olecranon from medial side (to avoid ulnar nerve);
- overhead traction with the patient supine;
- pin suspended from beam with pulley and weight;
- forearm horizontal, supported by sling suspended from beam. Position
- requires daily clinical assessment and twice weekly assessment with x-rays.
- when fracture is "sticky," usually at 3 weeks, remove traction and put the elbow in a cast for 2 weeks; then start the patient on physiotherapy.

Manipulation and percutaneous pins (Fig. 10.6)

- indicated when closed reduction succeeds, but either the
  —fracture redisplaces in the cast or
  —extreme flexion is required to maintain reduction;
- pins should be placed as described in Chapter 10 and removed at 4 weeks, maintaining the cast for 1 or 2 more weeks.

Open reduction and fixation

Indications

- open fracture Types II and III,
- vascular injury or
- failed closed reduction.

Technique

- posterior approach (Campbell), but use the
- anterior approach if vessels are to be explored;
- fixation with
  —percutaneous pins or
  —screws or a
  —plate and screws.

COMPLICATIONS (Fig. 10.7)

- ischemia and
- nerve injuries are reasonably common with this fracture. So
  —always examine the neurovascular status of the hand before and after reduction,
  —write down your findings (negative ones are just as important as positive ones), and
  —monitor the status regularly;
- varus deformity,
- stiffness,
- myositis ossificans.

OLD UNTREATED FRACTURE

- may create a varus deformity with some loss of movement;
- osteotomy to correct angulation is
  —difficult and
  —does not improve motion. So
- think carefully before embarking on it!

Condylar Fractures

ETIOPATHOLOGY

- uncommon fracture in adult;
- usually intra-articular;
- size of fragment varies and may be
- displaced and rotated by attached muscles. Condylar fractures are often
- associated with other
  —fractures or
  —dislocation of the elbow.

CLASSIFICATION

Lateral condyle (Fig. 10.8)

- this fracture usually includes the
  —lateral half of the distal humeral epiphysis. This half has an articular surface, the capitellum (capitulum humeri), which articulates anteriorly and distally with the radial head, and a nonarticular surface posteriorly, to which is attached the common extensor origin. Also included with the fragment are the
  —lateral epicondyle and
  —usually a small corner of the distal metaphysis.

Capitellum (Fig. 11.1)

- uncommon;
- a coronal shear fracture of the articular eminence of the lateral condyle, leaving the posterior nonarticular part of the condyle intact;
- usually displaced upward and sometimes rotated.

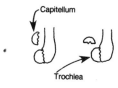

Figure 11.1. Fracture of the capitellum.

Medial condyle (Fig. 10.9)

- this fragment includes
  - —medial half of the distal humeral epiphysis, the trochlea (this half of the epiphysis is covered with articular cartilage except for the medial border which is in close contact with the ulnar nerve as it passes behind and below the medial epicondyle);
  - —medial epicondyle and
  - —corner of metaphysis.

TREATMENT

Lateral and Medial condylar fractures

Undisplaced

- cast, but watch for displacement in the cast. If this occurs, perform open reduction and fixation.

Displaced

- open reduction through medial (identify and protect the ulnar nerve) or lateral incision and
- internal fixation with screws (Kirschner wires in the adult are not strong enough). You should
- see the joint surfaces to ensure an accurate reduction before fixing the fragment. Incongruity of articular surface is unacceptable after open reduction. Ask for
- peroperative x-rays before closing, to confirm accurate reduction. If the
- reduction is poor, try again.
- motion should be started as early as possible without jeopardizing the fixation.

Old untreated fracture

- major problem is usually neurological, a
  - —tardy ulnar nerve palsy. To treat this, follow the principles described in Chapter 10.
- axial deformity is a
  - —cosmetic problem which can be treated by a varus or a valgus
  - —osteotomy. But this is
  - —difficult procedure technically and is not advised.
- mobility is usually adequate and seldom is an indication for treatment.

Capitellum fracture

- functionally this fracture is similar to a fracture of the radial head in the adult and can be treated the same way. If it is
- undisplaced (rare), treat with

    —backslab for 10 days, then
    —graduated active motion;
    —serial x-rays for 3 weeks are indicated to see that the fragment does not displace. If it is
- displaced,
    —excise the fragment through lateral incision, and start the patient on
    —active mobilization. Do not reduce and fix this fracture in the adult because the results are often poor due to stiffness, osteoarthritis and avascular necrosis. When the fracture is
- untreated, the fragment usually
    —unites with the anterior surface of the humerus and
    —limits flexion. Treat this by
    —osteotomy of the callus through a lateral approach,
    —excision of the capitellum and
    —early motion.

Intercondylar T or Y Fracture

ETIOPATHOLOGY

- uncommon; usually caused by
- direct injury to the elbow and consists of
- two fracture lines:
    —one crosses the supracondylar region transversely and may be straight or V shaped; the
    —other leaves this fracture line and descends vertically or obliquely into the joint, usually between the trochlea and capitellum.
- often associated with gross soft tissue damage, swelling and skin lesions.

CLASSIFICATION (Riseborough and Radin) (Fig. 11.2)

Type I

- no displacement.

Type II

- displaced but condyles have not rotated.

Type III

- displaced,
- condyles have rotated (by forearm extensor and flexor muscles groups), and
- distal humerus is thrust down between the condyles.

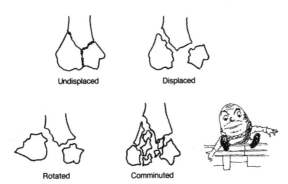

Figure 11.2.   Intercondylar T and Y fractures. (Modified from Riseborough EJ, Radin EL: Intercondylar T fractures of the humerus in the adult. *J Bone Joint Surg* 51A:130–141, 1969.)

Type IV
- severe comminution of articular surface and
- wide separation of condyles, the
- "Humpty Dumpty" fracture of the elbow.

TREATMENT

Type I
- posterior slab for 3 to 4 weeks, with
  —x-rays at Days 3, 7 and 10 to see whether the fragment has displaced;
- then physiotherapy.

Types II and III

Young patient (Fig. 11.3)
- open reduction and internal fixation through a
  —posterior approach (Campbell). Identify and retract gently the ulnar nerve;
  —reduce the condyles first, then fix them with a transverse screw or bolt (this must be centered accurately in the bone or it will cross the articular cartilage or the olecranon or coronoid fossa). Then
  —reduce the condyles and the humerus and stabilize them with two oblique screws or percutaneous pins through the medial and lateral epicondyles or with a malleable plate. The screws or pins must engage opposite cortex of the humeral shaft to prevent rotation;
- very difficult technically. Do not perform this operation if you are not experienced. Instead, treat the patient by nonoperative means, overhead traction with an ulnar pin for 3 weeks, with gentle active mobilization after a few days.

Convert condyles
into one fragment

Fix condylar
fragment to shaft

Figure 11.3.   Internal fixation of the intercondylar Y fracture.

Old patient

- overhead traction with an ulnar pin for 3 weeks;
- gentle active mobilization (never passive) must be started after a few days in traction;
- this method does not reduce the fracture; instead, it attempts to regain mobility and function of the elbow. Complications of decubitus, however, may outweigh those of open reduction.

Type IV

- best treatment is
  —traction and early mobilization because
  —reduction is impossible by any method;
- remember that
  —closed treatment and
  —early movement are better than
  —operative treatment and
  —no movement!

COMPLICATIONS

- neurovascular;
- skin;
- nonunion is not common but
- malunion is;
- reduced mobility almost always occurs;
- myositis ossificans.

Epicondylar Fractures

ETIOPATHOLOGY (Fig. 10.10)

- may be knocked off or pulled off and then displaced by muscle pull;
- medial epicondylar fracture may be associated with

—dislocation of the elbow, with a fragment lodged in the joint after reduction, and with an

—ulnar nerve lesion.

TREATMENT

Medial epicondyle

- if the medial epicondyle is not in the joint (look for this especially after closed reduction of a dislocation), and there is no ulnar nerve lesion, treat with
  —plaster backslab for 10 days, followed by
  —mobilization. Reduction of the fracture is not necessary;
- if the epicondyle is in the joint, it must be removed and excised through the medial approach, and the flexor muscles must be sutured to the humeral metaphysis;
- with ulnar nerve lesion, treat with
  —plaster backslab for 10 days, and if there is no return of muscle function,
  —explore, excise the epicondyle, and free and transpose the nerve anteriorly, as necessary.

Lateral epicondyle

- plaster backslab for 10 days, then
- mobilization; usually heals by fibrous union;
- reduction of fracture is not necessary because a
  —pseudarthrosis of the epicondyle is rarely symptomatic.

Old untreated fracture

- treat a painful pseudarthrosis by
  —excision of the fragment,
- marked collateral instability by
  —ligamentous reconstruction, and
- tardy ulnar nerve palsy by following the principles described in Chapter 10.

Olecranon Fractures

ETIOPATHOLOGY

- results from a fall or direct blow on the elbow;
- violent contraction of the triceps may produce a transverse fracture by avulsion. An
- intact triceps aponeurosis will prevent displacement, but if the
- aponeurosis, collateral ligament and capsule are torn, the triceps pulls the

proximal fragment backward and upward, and the fracture is displaced.
The fracture is
- always intra-articular.

CLASSIFICATION (Colton) (Fig. 11.4)

- undisplaced (with elbow at 90°);
- displaced (more than 2 mm)
  —transverse or oblique,
  —comminuted or
  —fracture dislocation;
- diagnosis is based on a
  —true lateral x-ray. An
  —oblique x-ray may hide the fracture, so insist on a true lateral x-ray.

TREATMENT

Undisplaced

- plaster backslab for 10 days, then
- active mobilization.

Displaced

Oblique or transverse fracture (Fig. 11.5)

- open reduction by
- posterior Boyd approach;
- reduce the fracture and
- fix with two Kirschner wires and a
- figure-of-8 wire (tension band wiring); test stability through full range
  of movement (ROM);

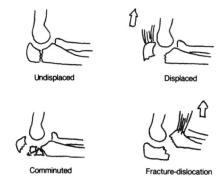

Undisplaced　　　　　　Displaced

Comminuted　　　　Fracture-dislocation

Figure 11.4. Olecranon fractures. (Modified from Colton CL: Fractures of the olecranon in adults: classification and management. *Injury* 5:121–129, 1973.)

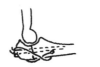

Figure 11.5. Traction-absorbing wiring of olecranon fracture.

- backslab for 3 days, then
- active mobilization.

Small fragment or comminution

- a small fragment, less than one third of the articular surface, can be excised if the elbow joint is not dislocated and there is no other fracture. Excision of a fragment in the presence of a dislocation or other fracture might make the elbow unstable. After excision,
- suture the triceps to the remaining part of the olecranon.

Associated fracture or dislocation

- excision of fragments in an unstable elbow will increase the instability. So
- reduce and fix the fragments as accurately as possible and have the patient start
- early motion.

COMPLICATIONS

- ulnar nerve injury
  —usually recovers spontaneously;
- malunion and nonunion;
- limitation of movement;
- degenerative osteoarthritis.

OLD UNTREATED DISPLACED FRACTURES

Clinical features

- fracture may be nonunited or malunited;
- elbow may be painful, and there may be a
- triceps lag, i.e., an inability to extend fully the elbow against gravity.

Treatment

- if there are one or two large fragments, through a
  —posterior approach
  —remove fibrous tissue from between the fracture surfaces,
  —reconstitute the olecranon with the forearm in extension,
  —fix the fracture with two K wires and a figure-of-8 tension wire, and
  —graft it.

- if the fracture fragment is small or is comminuted and impossible to reconstitute,
  —excise the fragment(s) and
  —reattach the triceps to the stump of the olecranon. If the fracture is
- malunited and this interferes with function,
- excise the end of the olecranon (but not more than 40%, as this will create instability) and
- reattach the triceps.

Radial Head Fractures

ETIOPATHOLOGY

- common fracture, caused by a
- fall on the hand, with the force transmitted up the radius. Occasionally it is
- associated with posterior dislocation of the elbow;
- fracture occurs on impact of the radial head against the capitellum, and the
- articular surface of capitellum may be damaged too.

CLASSIFICATION (Mason) (Fig. 11.6)

- undisplaced;
- marginal fracture with displacement which includes
  —impaction,
  —depression and
  —angulation;
- comminuted fracture of the entire head;
- fracture with elbow dislocation.

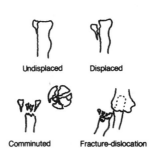

Undisplaced   Displaced

Comminuted   Fracture-dislocation

Figure 11.6. Radial head fractures. (Modified from Mason ML: Some observations on fractures of the radius with a review of one hundred cases. *Br J Surg* 42:123–132, 1954.)

DIAGNOSIS

- localized tenderness over the radial head,
- pain on supination of the forearm, and
- effusion of the elbow joint, seen best in the triangle between the tip of the olecranon, lateral epicondyle and radial head, are cardinal signs.
- Radiologically, an undisplaced fracture may be difficult to see. In this case, with positive clinical signs, assume that there is a radial head fracture;
- examine the x-ray closely, since the capitellum is sometimes fractured too.

TREATMENT

Undisplaced fracture

- plaster backslab for 5 days, or a sling if little pain is present,
- then active ROM exercises.

Marginal displaced fracture

Small fragment

- treat closed, as discussed previously.

Large fragment

- excision of radial head if the
  —fracture is more than one third of the articular surface, or
  —angulation of the fragment is more than 30°, or
  —depression of the fragment is more than 3 mm. If in
- doubt,
  —treat closed and reevaluate at 3 months; then if
  —movement is limited, or the
  —elbow is painful, or
  —crepitus is felt on rotation of the forearm,
- excise the head.

Comminuted fracture

- immediate excision of head and part of neck through a
  —lateral approach;
  —leave the annular ligament attached to stabilize the proximal radius;
- active mobilization from the first day after surgery.

Fracture-dislocation (Fig. 11.7)

- perform immediate closed reduction of the elbow and then
- assess fracture of the radial head and treat as outlined previously. If
- excision of the radial head is indicated,
  —replace it with a prosthesis; otherwise you will
  —destabilize the joint.

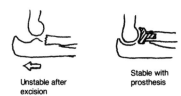

Unstable after
excision

Stable with
prosthesis

Figure 11.7. Fracture-dislocation of the elbow with excision of the comminuted radial head.

COMPLICATIONS

- myositis ossificans, especially with fracture-dislocation;
- stiffness, especially if immobilized too long;
- degenerative osteoarthritis;
- painful subluxation of distal radioulnar joint after excision of the radial head is unusual.

UNTREATED DISPLACED FRACTURES

- incongruity causes osteoarthritis with
- pain, crepitus and
- limitation of forearm rotation and maybe flexion and extension;
- excise the radial head and half the neck and
- mobilize the elbow 5 days after surgery.

Baby Car Fracture

ETIOPATHOLOGY

- the elbow or arm resting on the open window of a car or hanging outside the window of a car is
  —hit by a vehicle passing close or in a
  —side collision or is injured when the
  —car rolls over.

CLASSIFICATION (Shorbe)

- soft tissue injury alone;
- fracture of the tip of the olecranon;
- fracture of the radius and ulna or of the humerus only;
- multiple fractures of the distal humerus and proximal radius and ulna, a "bag of bones," usually
- associated with a Type II or III skin wound and sometimes
  —arterial and nerve injuries too.

TREATMENT
- treat closed fractures as detailed elsewhere. But for
- comminuted, multiple fractures with a Type II or III skin wound, debride the wound and use
  —external fixation across the joint from the humerus to the ulna.

Dislocation

ANATOMOPATHOLOGY
- the ulna can be considered as a distal extension of the humerus, and the radius can be considered as a proximal extension of the wrist and hand.
- dislocation of the elbow joint may be
  —posterior,
  —medial or lateral, or a
  —combination (commonest variety),
  —posteromedial or
  —posterolateral;
  —anterior and divergent dislocations are both rare;
- posterior dislocation may be associated with
  —fracture of the coronoid,
  —fracture of the radial head or
  —fracture of the medial epicondyle.
- extensive soft tissue disruption accompanies all dislocations, especially anterior dislocation. Damaged tissues include the
  —capsule,
  —collateral ligaments and
  —periosteum. In posterior dislocation the
  —brachialis muscle is torn, and in anterior dislocation the
  —triceps may be detached from the ulna.

DIAGNOSIS
- gross swelling may mask all clinical features. So
- confirm the diagnosis by x-ray and look for associated fractures. In
- posterior dislocation the
  —elbow is in slight flexion, the
  —olecranon is prominent posteriorly, the
  —radial head fossa is palpable posteriorly, and the
  —triangle between the two epicondyles and the olecranon is disrupted. In
- anterior dislocation the
  —elbow is in full extension, the
  —olecranon fossa and trochlea are palpable posteriorly, and the
  —biceps and brachialis are tented up anteriorly.

TREATMENT

Posterior dislocation

- closed reduction without anesthesia may be possible if it is a very recent injury, before muscle spasm and swelling have occurred, or
- with general anesthesia or narcolepsy (e.g., ketamine);
- technique:
  - —countertraction on the arm,
  - —reduction of medial or lateral displacement first,
  - —then traction on the forearm with downward pressure on the proximal forearm and
  - —gentle flexion of the elbow;
  - —reduces with a "clunk";
- full range of movement of the elbow after this maneuver confirms the reduction; if
- movement is limited, the elbow is not properly reduced, or there is a fracture fragment in the joint. If
- four or five gentle attempts at closed reduction fail, open reduction is indicated (rarely necessary).

Anterior dislocation

- closed reduction by
  - —traction on the forearm,
  - —countertraction on the arm and
  - —gentle backward pressure on the forearm.

Postreduction care

- if the reduction is stable, treat by
  - —plaster backslab for 10 days, with active graduated ROM exercises daily with the patient out of the splint,
  - —then by a sling for 5 days and active physiotherapy. If the reduction is
- unstable, a dilemma is posed:
  - —prolonged immobilization for stability, with the risk of permanent stiffness, or
  - —early mobilization for function, which risks permanent instability. So
- compromise by use of a
  - —percutaneous Steinmann pin through the olecranon and into the humerus, and a
  - —plaster cast with the elbow at 90° for 2 to 3 weeks, then active (never passive) mobilization after pin removal;
- x-ray to confirm reduction and
- look for fractures that
  - —were not visible before reduction or
  - —that occurred during reduction (iatrogenic).

COMPLICATIONS

- radial head fracture
  —treat as outlined previously;
- coronoid fracture
  —may return to its place after reduction. If it is
  —small, ignore it, but if it is
  —large and displaced more than 1 cm, perform open reduction and fixation
    with wire or a screw, through an anterior approach.
- neurovascular injuries;
- entrapped medial epicondyle should be
  —removed from the joint;
- residual collateral instability may require
  —ligamentous reconstruction;
- myositis ossificans.

OLD UNTREATED DISLOCATION

- closed reduction is usually impossible after 3 weeks. If
- function of the elbow is reasonably good, do nothing. If function is
- poor, treat by
  —open reduction (see Chapter 10), followed at 10 days by
  —active physiotherapy. If function is
- still unsatisfactory or
- articular cartilage is destroyed, a
  —dermis arthroplasty may help.

chapter 12
Injuries of the Forearm, Wrist and Carpals

General Remarks

- the forearm is unique because it affords simultaneous
- —stability and
  —mobility (supination and pronation);
- rotation is made possible by
  —three-dimensional curvature of the radial shaft (Fig. 12.1);
- the axis of rotation passes through the
  —radial head at the elbow and the
  —ulnar head at the wrist, with the distal radius rotating 160° around the ulnar head;
- main factors which may impair rotation are
  —abnormal radioulnar joints,
  —loss of the normal radial curve,
  —radioulnar synostosis or
  —contracture of the interosseous membrane.

Fractures of Radial and Ulnar Shafts in Adults

RADIOLOGICAL FEATURES

- fracture lines may be
  —transverse, oblique, or comminuted;
  —at the same level in both bones or at
  —different levels;
- the ulna is usually displaced with the radius but has less tendency to rotate.

TREATMENT

Nonoperative

Undisplaced fracture

- well-molded long arm cast, with the elbow at 90°, the forearm in neutral rotation, and sling attached at the level of the fracture, for 12 weeks, with active exercises for the shoulder and fingers;

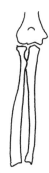

Figure 12.1. Forearm bones are curved for rotation.

- x-rays through plaster weekly for the first 4 weeks, then biweekly for the next 4 weeks. If the fracture
- displaces in the cast, perform
- open reduction.

Displaced fracture

- results of nonoperative treatment are usually unsatisfactory, so
- use this method temporarily only if open reduction and internal fixation are contraindicated by
  —infection or doubtful skin viability,
  —gross edema of the forearm,
  —poor general condition of the patient, or
  —inadequate facilities.

External fixation

- indications are
  —open wound Type III,
  —loss of bone or
  —poor skin;
- external fixation apparatuses such as the Hoffmann and Roger Anderson types are ideal but if one is unavailable, use the
- pins and plaster method with a
  —transverse pin through the proximal ulna,
  —another pin through the distal radius, and a
  —plaster cast which should include both pins;
  —bones are stabilized and held out to length, and wounds can be dressed through windows in the cast.

Operative

Indications

- associated vascular injury;

- displaced fracture, e.g.,
  —angulated,
  —rotated or
  —overlapped.

Technique

- separate incision for each bone to avoid synostosis
  —posterior for the ulna and
  —anterolateral (Henry) for the radius. Use
- plates and screws for both bones with 3 screws on each side of the fracture;
- intramedullary rods, whether Rush rods for either bone or a Küntscher rod for the ulna, are not as good as plates, and the natural curvature of the radius is difficult to reestablish with a rod;
- reduce both bones before fixing either because it is difficult to reduce the second bone once the first is fixed;
- use iliac cancellous bone graft if the fracture is comminuted;
- leave the fascia open to avoid vascular compression.

Postoperative care

- if the fixation is rigid, start joint mobilization within a few days;
- plates should be left at least 18 months;
- if fixation is not rigid, treat with a
- long arm plaster cast for 12 weeks, with the elbow at 90° and the forearm in neutral rotation.

COMPLICATIONS

- open fracture is usually
  —Type I and must be
  —explored and cleaned immediately and left open with the forearm supported by long arm plaster backslab. Treat later by
- delayed open reduction and internal fixation when the
  —open wound has healed, there is
  —no sign of infection, and the
  —edema has subsided.
- major vessel injury should be repaired. Fortunately, the forearm has a
  —good collateral circulation;
- vascular (capillary) compression is an urgent problem and will result in
  —muscle ischemia and
  —Volkmann's syndrome if it is not treated promptly (see Chapter 32).
- radial nerve paralysis may occur particularly after use of the
  —posterior (Thompson) approach for fracture of the proximal third of the radius, due to overenthusiastic use of retractors!
- malunion
  —limits pronation and supination.

- nonunion
    —is especially likely in the
    —distal half of the ulna because this is mainly
    —cortical with
    —few muscular attachments;
    —relative lengths of both bones must be maintained when this is treated.
- radioulnar synotosis prevents forearm rotation and is especially likely to occur with
    —both bones fractured at the same level,
    —open reduction of both bones through the same incision, or
    —injury or tear of the interosseous membrane (IOM);
    —synostosis often recurs if it is excised, so perform an
    —osteotomy of the radius if the forearm and hand are in a nonfunctional position.

Fracture of Radial and Ulnar Shafts in Children

CLINICAL AND RADIOLOGICAL FEATURES

- 60% are greenstick, but there is often a
    —rotational element as well as angulation, especially if the fractures are proximal. The remaining 40% are
- complete. The distal fragment may be in any position, but the position of the proximal fragment is controlled by muscle pull. Theoretically, in
- fracture of the proximal third of the radius the
    —proximal fragment of radial shaft is supinated by the supinator muscle. In
- middle and distal third fractures, the pull of the
    —pronator teres and the pull of the
    —supinator muscles cancel each other, and the proximal radius is in neutral rotation or slight pronation. However, the

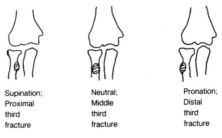

Supination;
Proximal
third
fracture

Neutral;
Middle
third
fracture

Pronation;
Distal
third
fracture

Figure 12.2. Forearm rotation and position of the bicipital tuberosity.

- problem is not always this simple; so
- use your own judgment. On a good anteroposterior (AP) x-ray of the radius, the
- position of the bicipital tuberosity of the radius will show the rotational position of the proximal radius (Fig. 12.2). If the
  —tuberosity is anteromedial, the proximal radius is in supination; if the
  —tuberosity is posteromedial, the radius is in neutral rotation; and if the
  —tuberosity is posterolateral, the radius is in pronation;
  —malrotation is also shown by
  —disparity in the width of the two fracture fragments and
  —angulation at the fracture site. Anterior angulation is usually accompanied by supination, and posterior angulation, by pronation. So
- examine the radiographs carefully to detemine the
  —rotational position of the proximal fragments.

TREATMENT

Closed reduction

Greenstick

- with the patient under general anesthesia,
- break the remaining cortices to avoid angulation in the cast (but do not tear the periosteum) and
- then treat as for complete fracture (see below).

Complete

Reduction technique

- with the patient under general anesthesia, apply
- traction, countertraction and
- manipulation until the fracture feels stable;
- the forearm should be in supination, neutral rotaton or pronation according to the nature of the injury and the rotation of the proximal fragment;
- both bones must be reduced. If one or both are angulated, rotation will be limited.

Cast (Fig. 12.3)

- long arm cast, which must be
- molded flat over the
  —distal triceps posteriorly and the
  —distal biceps anteriorly. It should be
  —straight along the subcutaneous (posterior) border of the ulna,
  —circular over the proximal forearm,
  —oval (anterior to posterior) over the distal forearm, and
  —gently curved concave anteriorly, with the apex of the concavity

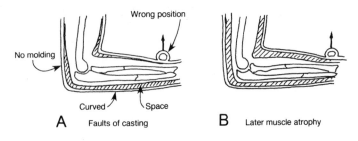

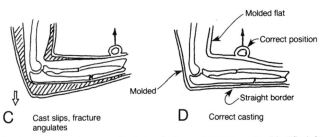

Figure 12.3. Improper and proper techniques for a forearm cast. (Modified from Charnley J: *The Closed Treatment of Common Fractures*, ed 3. Edinburgh, Churchill Livingstone, 1961, p 122.)

at the fracture site (because most forearm fractures have a distal fragment displaced posteriorly; i.e., the apex of angulation is anterior) to give three-point fixation;

— mold the cast between the radius and the ulna to preserve interosseous space;

- cast must come within 2 cm of the axilla and
    — cover the metacarpophalangeal (MP) joints posteriorly but
    — only to the midpalmar crease anteriorly to allow MP joint flexion;
- elbow at 90°. Attach a
- collar and cuff sling to the cast at the level of the fracture to prevent sagging and bowing.

Postreduction care

- split the cast along one edge and
- watch for ischemia;
- complete the cast the next day if neurovascular status is normal, and
- x-ray through the cast weekly for 3 weeks;

- remove the cast at 6 to 8 weeks (depending on age) and reexamine. If the fractures are
- united, do not recast but allow no sports for 4 weeks.

Open reduction

- for failed closed reduction, usually in older
- teenagers with high, oblique fractures. Make
- small incisions to reduce the fractures, then use
- intramedullary Kirschner (IMK) wires to hold the alignment; apply a
- cast and treat as for closed reduction. Remove the K wires at 6 weeks.

Fracture of Ulnar Shaft Alone

- caused by a direct blow (nightstick fracture);
- usually little displacement;
- always look for radial head dislocation or distal radioulnar subluxation, especially if the ulnar fracture is displaced, because this may require open reduction;
- treatment of an adult consists of a
  —cast for an undisplaced fracture and of
  —open reduction and internal fixation, with a bone graft if the fracture is in the distal two thirds of the shaft, for a displaced fracture;
- treatment of a child consists of a
  —cast for an undisplaced fracture and of
  —closed reduction and a cast for a displaced fracture.

Monteggia Lesion

ADULT

Etiopathology

- isolated radial head dislocation in the adult is extremely rare. It is
- nearly always associated with fracture of the ulna, the Monteggia lesion, so look for this;
- caused by a
  —fall on the outstretched hand, with hyperpronation of the forearm, or a
  —direct blow to the forearm.

Classification

- there are many systems of classification;
- the most popular is that of Bado.

Type I (60%)

- anterior radial head dislocation and
- fracture of the ulnar shaft, an extension and pronation injury.

Type II (15%)

- posterior radial head dislocation and
- fracture of the ulnar shaft, a flexion injury.

Type III (20%)

- lateral radial head dislocation with
- fracture of the shaft or proximal metaphysis of the ulna.

Type IV (5%)

- anterior radial head dislocation with
- fractures of the ulna and radius.

Clinical and radiological features (Fig. 12.4)

- pain and tenderness in the elbow and forearm with limited motion and the
- radial head palpable in an abnormal position.
- x-rays must show the
  —entire forearm (AP and lateral),
  —wrist (if not seen on forearm film) and
  —elbow (AP and lateral);
- normally, the longitudinal axis of the radius passes through the center of the capitulum humeri in all positions of the elbow joint. If the
- radial axis is off center, the radial head is subluxed or dislocated. If the
- forearm x-ray shows fracture of the ulna alone, take x-rays well centered on the elbow to look for displacement of the radial head.

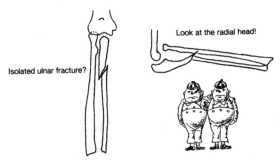

Isolated ulnar fracture?

Look at the radial head!

Figure 12.4.   Bado Type I Monteggia lesion.

Treatment

- lesion in an adult is usually unstable; treatment is surgical through a
- posterior incision along the subcutaneous border of the ulna. Use a
- six-hole plate, a four-hole compression plate, or a Küntscher intramedullary rod for the ulna and
- reduce the radial head by closed manipulation. If this fails,
- continue the incision proximally, as with the Boyd posterior approach, reduce the radial head, and repair the annular ligament, if necessary. For a
- Bado Type IV fracture, treat by
  —open reduction and internal fixation of both fractures through separate incisions, then
  —closed reduction of the radial head, and if unsuccessful,
  —open reduction of the radial head.
- postoperatively, apply a
  —long arm cast with the
  —elbow flexed 110° for Bado Types I, III and IV, with the forearm in 60° of supination (not forced extreme supination). For a
  —Type II lesion (posterior dislocation of the radial head) allow 70° of elbow flexion.
- remove the cast at 6 weeks and start the patient on
- active (never passive) mobilization of the elbow and on forearm rotation if the fracture is healed.

Complications

- palsy of the deep motor branch of the radial nerve, for which recovery is usually spontaneous;
- redislocation of the radial head if the
  —ulna is malaligned, or the ulnar
  —fracture is not properly stabilized, or the
  —elbow was in the wrong position in the cast;
- nonunion of the ulna may occur, especially if the fracture is distal.

CHILD

Etiopathology

- uncommon (2% of all forearm fractures).
- usually caused by
  —hyperpronation injury (anterior dislocation of the radial head) or
  —direct blow to the forearm;
- components of the injury include
- complete or greenstick fracture of the
  —ulnar shaft (transverse or oblique) or of the
  —proximal metaphysis of the ulna and

- dislocation of the radial head from the humerus and from the ulna. The direction of dislocation follows
- Bado's classification (see previous discussion).
- Monteggia-like lesions include
  —ulnar fracture with displaced fracture of the radial neck,
  —radial head dislocation with olecranon fracture (the proximal radioulnar joint may be intact), or
  —bowed ulnar shaft (young children's bones bend a lot before they break).

Diagnosis

- whenever you see an apparently isolated fracture of the ulna, take good AP and lateral x-rays of the elbow because
- radial head dislocation is missed more often than ulnar fracture;
- a line through the long axis of the radius must pass through the center of the capitellum in all radiographic views. If it does not, the radial head is out of position.

Treatment

Closed reduction

- both
  —ulnar fracture and
  —radial head dislocation must be reduced. After
- reduction of the ulnar fracture, the
- radial head is reduced by traction and pressure over the head with the elbow
  —flexed for anterior or lateral dislocation and
  —extended for a posterior dislocation. With
- lateral dislocation, flex the elbow and supinate the forearm; this is often
  —difficult to reduce.
- apply a long arm cast with the elbow in flexion or extension according to the direction of the radial head dislocation.

Percutaneous IMK wire

- an oblique fracture of the ulna is often unstable and may require intramedullary stabilization.
- after closed reduction, insert a Kirschner wire percutaneously through the posterior surface of the olecranon, down the intramedullary canal, and across the fracture;
- bend the wire and cut it off outside the skin;
- apply a long arm cast. Remove this along with the wire at 4 weeks.

Open reduction

- rarely necessary in children;
- indication is failed closed reduction. Use a
- posterior approach,
- reduce the ulnar fracture and hold it with an IMK wire. The
- radial head should reduce with closed manipulation;
- if it does not, extend the incision proximally and do an open reduction of the radial head. If the
- annular ligament prevents reduction, it may have to be cut;
- always repair or reconstruct the annular ligament when it is cut or torn, to avoid recurrent subluxation or dislocation of the radial head.

Prognosis

- excellent if you remember that
  —isolated dislocation of the radial head and
  —isolated fracture of the ulnar shaft are both
  —rare. They usually
- accompany each other, the Tweedledum and Tweedledee of orthopaedics. So
  —when you see one, look for the other (Fig. 12.4).

OLD UNTREATED MONTEGGIA

Pathology

- malunion of the ulna and persistent
- dislocation of the radial head;
- capsule and fibrous tissue are adherent to radial head, capitellum and radial notch of the ulna;
- annular ligament is usually torn, retracted and fibrotic.

Clinical features

- irreducible by closed methods after 10 days in a child or 3 weeks in an adult;
- radial head is prominent, usually anterolaterally;
- ulnar angulation may be evident;
- flexion is usually limited to about 110° with an anterior radial head dislocation, but
- occasionally function is normal.

Treatment

Child

- if the ulna is angulated and prevents reduction of the radial head, perform an osteotomy through the callus (posterior approach). Using a

- posterior approach to the elbow (Boyd), clean the capitellum and radial head and reduce it. Division or excision of the annular ligament may be necessary. To stabilize the osteotomy,
- drill an IMK wire down the ulna or fix the ulna with a plate.
- repair the annular ligament or
- reconstruct it from
  —fascia over the long extensors;
  —leave the fascial strip attached to the subcutaneous border of the ulna opposite the radial neck,
  —wind the strip around the radial neck and
  —suture it to itself with the radial head reduced;
  —ligament should not be too tight (limitation of rotation) or too loose (instability);
- stabilize the reduced radius with a K wire across the lateral humeral condyle into the radius with the elbow at 90°. Then apply a
- long arm cast.
- remove the K wire at 3 weeks. (Do not leave it in longer because it may break at the joint, and the radial part will be difficult to remove!) Remove the cast at 4 weeks if the fracture has healed;
- start the patient on active (never passive) mobilization.

Adult

- if function is good,
  —do nothing. If
- flexion or extension is blocked,
  —excise the radial head. For
- marked ulnar deformity,
  —consider osteotomy, realignment, fixation and cancellous graft for the ulna and
  —excision of the radial head.

Fracture of Radial Shaft Alone

UPPER TWO THIRDS

Undisplaced

- treat by long arm cast with the forearm rotated according to rotation of the proximal radius.

Displaced

- proximal fifth of shaft: treatment consists of a
  —cast with the forearm
  —supinated because the proximal fragment is too short for internal fixation;

- distal to proximal one fifth: in an
- adult, treat by open reduction through Henry's anterior approach and stabilization with a plate. In a
- child, treat by closed reduction and a cast;
- judge the degree of rotation of the proximal fragment, using the criteria mentioned previously. In general, the limb should be immobilized in
    —supination with a fracture of the proximal third and in
    —midrotation with fracture of the middle or distal third, because the pull of the supinators and the pull of the pronators cancel each other;
- mold the cast between the radius and ulna to prevent narrowing of the interosseous space.

GALLEAZI LESION

Clinical and radiological features (Fig. 12.5)

- oblique or transverse fracture at the junction of middle and distal thirds of the radius. The fracture is
- unstable, and the distal radius
    —displaces proximally and anteriorly, due to pull of the
    —pronator quadratus, brachioradialis and thumb abductors, with consequent
- dislocation of the distal radioulnar and carpoulnar joints and disruption of the triangular cartilage. When
- x-rays show a fracture of the
    —distal radial shaft, always look for
    —dislocation of the distal radioulnar joint. The
- Galleazi lesion looks innocuous and easy to treat;
- it is not!

Treatment

Undisplaced

- long arm cast with the elbow at 90° and the forearm in supination;

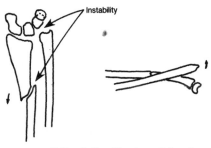

Figure 12.5.   Galleazi fracture-dislocation.

- regular x-rays with the limb in the cast to watch for displacement. If displacement occurs, operate. If this does not occur, remove the
- cast at 8 to 10 weeks.

Displaced

Child

- closed reduction and a cast as for an undisplaced fracture;
- weekly x-rays for 3 weeks, and if the fracture displaces, operate. If it does not displace, remove the
- cast at 6 to 8 weeks.

Adult

- closed reduction gives very
  —poor results because the injury is unstable and will redisplace in the cast with resultant
  —malunion,
  —limitation of forearm rotation and wrist movements, and later
  —osteoarthritis of the distal radioulnar joint.
- open reduction produces the
  —best results. Use
- Henry's anterior approach and
  —dissect the pronator quadratus from the front of the radius;
  —reduce the fracture and fix with a heavy six-hole plate if possible (a compression plate is best);
  —confirm reduction of the radioulnar joint by x-rays before closure;
  —leave the fascia open to avoid a compartment syndrome; treat with a
  —long arm cast for 6 weeks, then with
  —active exercises, particularly to regain forearm rotation.

Malunion

- after the patient has started active physiotherapy to regain as much forearm rotation, wrist and finger movements as possible, perform an
- osteotomy through the fracture. Stabilize it with a
- six-hole plate as discussed previously. If the
- distal radioulnar joint is still subluxed or dislocated,
  —resect the distal 2 cm of the ulna after the radius has united;
  —do not resect the ulna at the same time that you fix the radius or the radius may displace in spite of the plate and screws.

Colles Fracture

ETIOPATHOLOGY

- common in adults, usually the elderly with osteoporotic bone;
- caused by a
  —fall on the dorsiflexed hand with the forearm in pronation. The
- fracture goes through the distal radial metaphysis and sometimes the epiphysis. The distal fragment may be
  —displaced dorsally and radially
  —with or without fracture of the ulnar styloid. The
- fracture line may be
  —simple or comminuted,
  —extra-articular or intra-articular.

CLINICAL AND RADIOLOGICAL FEATURES (Fig. 12.6)

- if the fracture is undisplaced, there may be
  —swelling and pain only. If it is displaced, it will have the classic
- dinner fork deformity with
  —posterior displacement of the distal radius and wrist;
- x-rays show
  —there is posterior and radial displacement of the distal fragment with impaction posteriorly;
  —distal radial articular surface is tilted backward instead of forward;
  —radius is shortened, so that the radial styloid process is at same level as the ulnar styloid;
  —distal radioulnar joint may be dislocated.

TREATMENT

Undisplaced

- below-elbow cast for 6 weeks (less in an elderly patient) with the forearm in neutral rotation. Shape the cast so that

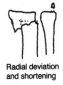

Radial deviation
and shortening

Posterior displacement

Figure 12.6. Colles' fracture tends to be undertreated, creating deformity and disability.

—dorsally it comes to the MP joints and

—anteriorly it comes to the proximal transverse palmar crease to allow flexion of the MP joints, and

—cut the cast around the first metacarpal to allow opposition of the thumb. Start the patient on

- shoulder, elbow and finger exercises from the day of fracture.

Displaced

Noncomminuted

- reduce the fracture with the patient under
- anesthesia which may be
    —general,
    —regional, or
    —local, with the latter injected into the fracture hematoma with use of rigorous, sterile technique.
- technique:
    —increase the angulation of the fracture to disimpact it, then use
    —traction and
    —ulnar deviation to gain length, then
    —push the distal fragment anteriorly;
- an assistant maintains reduction while you apply the below-elbow cast
    —molded concave anteriorly and convex posteriorly, with the
    —apex of the curves opposite the fracture (three-point pressure) and with the
    —wrist flexed 15° and in ulnar deviation. The cast should be
    —circular around the proximal forearm and
    —oval around the distal forearm with the
    —forearm in neutral rotation;
    —cut the cast distally to allow finger and thumb movements. Take
- x-rays through the cast to confirm reduction. On the AP x-ray, the
    —radial styloid process should be 1 cm more distal than the ulnar styloid, and on the lateral x-ray, the
    —distal radial articular surface should face 30° anteriorly.
- instruct the patient to elevate the arm until swelling goes down;
- x-ray through the cast every week for 3 weeks, and if the reduction is completely lost, manipulate the fracture again;
- encourage active movement for joints not immobilized;
- remove the cast at 6 weeks and start the patient on active movements of the wrist.

Comminuted

- position will slip after closed reduction, even in a long arm cast, with resultant

—deformity,

—diminution of function, and the possibility of

—median nerve compression;

- skeletal fixation will avoid this loss of position. Do this for a
  —very comminuted, unstable fracture. An
- external fixation device is ideal, or use
- pins and plaster with
  —one K wire through the second and third metacarpals, retracting the first interosseous muscle with your thumb to avoid spearing the muscle, and the
  —other K wire through the ulna 5 cm distal to the elbow joint, drilling from medial to lateral to avoid the ulnar nerve; use the subcutaneous border of the ulna as a guide.
  —reduce the fracture, then
  —apply a below-elbow cast and incorporate the pins;
  —elevation and physiotherapy are used as discussed previously;
  —remove pins and plaster at 6 weeks.

Intra-articular

- noncomminuted fracture; treat by
  —closed reduction and a cast. If this
  —fails and the fragments are large, perform
  —open reduction through a posterior approach, fix the fragments with several K wires, and apply a cast. Remove the pins and cast at 6 weeks. A
- comminuted fracture is usually
  —unstable, so treat by
  —closed reduction and hold it in place with pins and plaster.

COMPLICATIONS

- more frequent than one may think!
- median nerve compression may occur with a poor reduction due to
  —narrowing of the carpal tunnel and
  —local hemorrhage and edema;
  —treat by operative decompression.
- ruptured extensor pollicis longus tendon at Lister's tubercle should be
  —repaired or the tendon of the
  —extensor indicis propius should be transposed.
- shoulder-hand syndrome with a
  —stiff shoulder and a
  —stiff, swollen, painful hand
  —may be due to an autonomic nervous system disturbance;
  —treat with vigorous, prolonged, active physiotherapy.

- limitation of
  —wrist joint movements and of
  —forearm rotation due to contracture of the interosseous membrane.
- malunion is
  —common with a
  —dinner fork deformity and radial deviation of the hand. This deformity is
  —aesthetically displeasing and is usually the
  —biggest, single cause of a patient's complaints. To correct the deformity by osteotomy through the healed fracture site is not easy. It may be better to treat the
  —painful functional disability by excision of the ulnar head and neck.

Barton's Fracture

ETIOPATHOLOGY (Fig. 12.7)

- adults;
- fracture of dorsal or ventral lip of the distal radius, with the fracture line crossing the articular surface of the radius transversely;
- fragment is usually displaced posteriorly (dorsal fracture) or anteriorly (ventral fragment) with the carpals which therefore
- sublux or dislocate. The
- diagnosis is based on a
  —good lateral x-ray of the wrist.

TREATMENT

Dorsal fragment

- closed reduction may be possible with
  —wrist in neutral. If the
  —wrist is flexed, the fragment will redisplace posteriorly. Put on a
  —well-molded cast and take
  —regular x-rays through the cast. At the
  —first sign of displacement, perform an
- open reduction by the
- posterior approach;

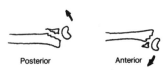

Posterior   Anterior

Figure 12.7. Types of Barton fracture-dislocations.

- open the wrist joint and look at the articular surface to obtain accurate reduction;
- stabilize the fragment with a buttress plate and screws or K wires. Apply a
- below-elbow cast with the wrist in neutral;
- removal the cast and pins at 6 weeks.

Ventral fragment
- treat as for Smith's fracture (see below).

Radial Styloid Fracture

- adults;
- fracture line runs from the middle of the radial articular surface laterally and proximally to the radial metaphysis. Treat by
  —closed reduction in ulnar deviation and a
  —below-elbow cast for 6 weeks. If the fracture is
- unstable, percutaneous K wires along with a cast will hold it;
- remove the wires and cast at 6 weeks.

Smith's Fracture

ETIOPATHOLOGY
- occurs in adults but is uncommon;
- caused by a
  —fall on the dorsiflexed hand with the forearm in supination or by a
  —direct blow on the back of the distal radius;
- fracture line runs through the distal radial metaphysis, with anterior displacement of the distal fragment (reverse Colles deformity). The fracture is
- unstable when it is
  —oblique,
  —intra-articular or
  —comminuted;
- carpals displace with the distal radial fragment;
- do not mistake this for a Colles fracture;
- it is the reverse of a Colles, and the treatment is correspondingly different. Always examine x-rays of any wrist injury very carefully.

TREATMENT
  Stable
- closed reduction and a
- long arm cast with the

—elbow at 90°,

—forearm in supination, and

—wrist in 10° of flexion. Extension of the wrist will displace the fracture.

Unstable

Percutaneous pins

- closed reduction and either
  —percutaneous pins across the fracture site or the
  —pins and plaster technique with one K wire through the second and
    third metacarpals and another across the proximal ulna. These two
    methods are usually
  —unsatisfactory because
  —accurate reduction of the intra-articular fracture is
  —not possible and the carpals will remain subluxed.

Open reduction

- use anterior approach,
- reduce the fracture under direct vision and stabilize it with
  —pins or, better still, an
  —anterior buttress plate (Ellis plate). Apply a
- long arm cast with the
  —elbow flexed to 90° and the
  —forearm in supination. Encourage
- active mobilization of shoulder and fingers;
- remove pins and plaster at 6 weeks and
- start the patient on physiotherapy.

COMPLICATIONS

- similar to those of the Colles fracture; also from
- mistaken diagnosis. If this uncommon fracture is treated as the more
  common Colles fracture, the result will be
  —deformity,
  —limitation of dorsiflexion of the wrist, and a
  —weak grip.

Distal Radius and Ulna Fractures in Children

FRACTURE THROUGH METAPHYSES

Radiological features

- both bones fracture through the distal metaphyses. The
- displacement may be an
  —anterior angulation (and is notorious for redisplacing in the cast) or

—complete posterior displacement of both bones, with overlap and shortening producing a bayonet deformity.

Treatment

Undisplaced

- long arm cast, carefully molded, for 6 weeks.

Angulated

- closed reduction under anesthesia and apply a well-molded
- long arm cast with the forearm in
- supination to neutralize the pull of the brachioradialis. If the forearm is pronated, the fracture may angulate even further in the cast.
- remove the cast in 6 weeks.

Complete displacement (Fig. 12.8)

- attempted reduction by straight traction will fail because the posterior periosteal hinge is intact and will prevent the reduction. This is the
- Red Queen's fracture:
  "With this fracture, you see, it takes all the pulling you can do to keep it in the same place. If you want to move the distal fragment, you must pull at least twice as hard as that!" And even then you will not succeed! The
- secret to reduction of the Red Queen's fracture is manipulation:
  —bend the distal fragment backward until the fracture is angulated 90° and the apex is angulated anteriorly, then
  —push the distal radial fragment distally with your thumb until the dorsal fracture margins engage each other, and

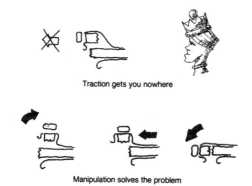

Traction gets you nowhere

Manipulation solves the problem

Figure 12.8. Red Queen's fracture of the distal radius.

—lever the distal fragment anteriorly as far as it will go (posterior periosteum prevents overreduction). Then
—reduce the ulna and apply a
—well-molded long arm cast with the forearm in neutral rotation;
- x-ray through the plaster after reduction and weekly for 3 weeks to check for displacement;
- always compare
   —the most recent x-ray with the
   —first x-ray after reduction to
   —appreciate the total loss of correction. This is a
   —good general rule for all fractures;
- if you compare the recent x-ray with the last one, you will accept small degrees of loss of correction and miss the overall loss. This may be considerable and warrant a second manipulation.
- remove the cast at 6 weeks

Radius only
- usually accompanied by ulnar styloid fracture;
- treatment as discussed previously, but put the forearm in pronation.

EPIPHYSEAL INJURIES

Salter-Harris Type I
- common injury usually involving the radius; occurs in
- young children and is
- often not displaced;
- diagnosis is made on clinical grounds with
   —pain,
   —tenderness over the growth plate, and localized
   —swelling;
- x-rays may appear normal;
- treat on suspicion with a long arm cast for 3 weeks.

Salter-Harris Type II
- common;
- epiphysis is usually displaced backward. The
- triangular ligament frequently avulses the ulnar styloid process.
- treat by
   —gentle closed reduction and a
   —well-molded long arm cast with the
   —wrist in neutral (neither flexed nor extended). If you achieve only
   —partial reduction with 50% apposition or more, accept this because the
   —metaphysis will remodel and

—repeated manipulation may damage the growth plate with consequent
—premature closure and growth disturbance;
• remove the cast at 3 to 4 weeks.

Functional Anatomy and Pathology of Carpals

ANATOMY (Fig. 12.9)

• proximal carpal row consists of the
  —scaphoid,
  —lunate and
  —triquetrum (the pisiform is a sesamoid bone articulating only with the triquetrum);
• distal carpal row consists of the
  —trapezium,
  —trapezoid,
  —capitate and
  —hamate; functionally, the
  —scaphoid should also be included because this links the two rows;
• stability of the carpals depends particularly on
  —volar ligaments, which radiate from the radius to the scaphoid, lunate, capitate and triquetrum;
  —intercarpal ligaments; and
  —collateral ligaments from radial and ulnar styloid processes. On lateral
• radiographs in the neutral position the
  —axes of the radius, lunate, capitate and third metacarpal are colinear, but the
  —scaphoid is angled 45° (30° to 70°) forward and downward in relation to the long axis of the lunate and the carpals, and the
  —articular spaces between the carpal bones are never more than 1 or 2 mm wide anywhere, in any position (more than 3 mm is abnormal).
• changes of these relationships indicate carpal instability.

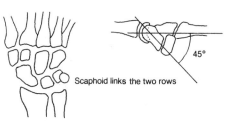

Scaphoid links the two rows

Figure 12.9.   Carpals.

FUNCTION

- scaphoid lies in both rows and acts as a connecting rod between them, stabilizing them during dorsiflexion and palmar flexion;
- dorsiflexion and palmar flexion average 70° each;
- half of each of these movements occurs at the radiocarpal joint and half occurs at the intercarpal joint through concurrent and synchronous movement;
- this range of movement increases the excursion of the long finger flexors and extensors and alters their power;
- no tendons attach to the proximal carpal row, which is an intercalated segment between the radius and the distal carpal row;
- movements of the proximal row are controlled by radiocarpal and intercarpal capsule and ligaments, by the scaphoid and by the geometry of the joints.

MALFUNCTION

- when integrity of the support structures (ligaments, capsules or scaphoid) is interrupted, the stability of the intercarpal joint is destroyed, and the proximal carpal row sags and collapses in zigzag fashion under compressive stress.
- carpal injuries are unusual in children. The following applies mostly to adults.

Scaphoid Fractures

SURGICAL ANATOMY OF SCAPHOID (Fig. 6.2)

- two thirds of the scaphoid bone is covered in articular cartilage;
- vascular supply is through the
  —tuberosity on the distal pole and
  —middorsal surface. In 30% of patients the
- proximal pole depends entirely on intraosseous vessels for its blood supply and may die after a fracture of the proximal third. The scaphoid
- articulates

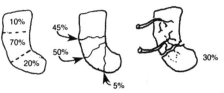

Fracture site   Fracture shape   Ischemia in 30% of
                                       proximal pole fractures

Figure 12.10. Scaphoid fractures.

—proximally with the radius,

—medially with the lunate and capitate, and

—distally with the trapezium and trapezoid.

CLASSIFICATION (Fig. 12.10)

• 60% to 70% of all carpal injuries.

Site of fracture

• proximal third (20%)
   —proximal pole is relatively avascular;
   —healing is very slow, 20 weeks or more;
   —nonunion and
   —avascular necrosis of the proximal pole are common.
• middle third (70%)
   —middle third of the bone is the waist of the scaphoid;
   —proximal pole is avascular in 30% of these fractures.
• distal third (10%)
   —usually heals well with no vascular problems.

Obliquity of fracture line

• transverse fractures (45%) are stable;
• oblique (50%) and
• longitudinal (5%) fractures are unstable, especially the latter.

CLINICAL FEATURES

• pain and swelling over carpals on the radial side with
• well-localized tenderness on pressure over the scaphoid
   —posteriorly,
   —laterally in the "anatomical snuffbox" and
   —anteriorly;
• pain in scaphoid area on forced dorsiflexion of the wrist.

RADIOLOGICAL FEATURES

• scaphoid fractures are often just a hairline crack and are difficult to see;
• if AP and lateral x-rays do not show a fracture, ask for
   —oblique and
   —AP x-rays with the hand in ulnar deviation;
• if you are still in doubt, treat the patient as though he has a scaphoid fracture, then repeat the x-rays out of plaster 2 weeks later.

TREATMENT

Recent fracture

• treat the patient based on clinical signs, whether or not you see a fracture on the radiographs. Apply a

- short arm plaster cast with the
  —wrist in 15° dorsiflexion and radial deviation and the
  —thumb in opposition;
  —include the thumb to the base of the distal phalanx;
- remove the cast at 6 weeks and x-ray. If the
- fracture is united, protect the site for 4 weeks with a bandage and limitation of physical activities. If it is
- not united, apply a new cast for 6 more weeks; if it is still not
- united, consider
  —internal fixation with a lag screw.

Pseudarthrosis

Radiological features

- fracture surfaces have resorbed and may be sclerotic,
- cyst may form within the bone, and
- proximal and distal fragments may move independently, each with its own carpal row.

Treatment

Asymptomatic

- in a young healthy patient,
  —graft the nonunion by the Matti-Russe procedure (see below);
- in an older patient, usually no treatment is required.

Symptomatic

- with no degenerative changes,
- graft the bone by the
  —Matti-Russe technique or with a
  —bone wedge if the scaphoid is angulated posteriorly through the pseudarthrosis due to bony resorption anteriorly. The wedge
  —corrects angulation and
  —improves carpal stability;
- use x-ray control to confirm your position because it may be
  —difficult to find the pseudarthrosis at surgery if the articular cartilage has united (the "peanut" fracture in which the cartilage is the shell and the two fragments are the nuts), and you may
  —mistake the scapholunate joint for the pseudarthrosis.
- with degenerative changes in the radioscaphoid joint,
  —excise the radial styloid and graft the nonunion;
- with degenerative changes of other intercarpal joints, either
  —treat with analgesics, elastic or leather wrist support, or if the patient is very disabled,
  —fusion of the wrist from the radius to the third MC.

Sprains and Subluxations of Wrist and Intercarpal Joints

SPRAIN

- examine carefully AP and lateral radiographs with the wrist in the neutral position and, if in doubt, obliques to eliminate intercarpal subluxations. Compare these x-rays with those of the normal side;
- treat with a cast for 3 to 6 weeks.

SUBLUXATION

- always accompanied by disruption of radiocarpal and intercarpal ligaments;
- rotary subluxation of the scaphoid is commonest.

Diagnosis

- based on the AP x-ray (compare it with that of the normal side) which will show the
  - "Terry Thomas" gap between the lunate and scaphoid to be greater than 3 mm (the key sign), especially on the ulnar deviation film;
  - foreshortened scaphoid (it looks "funny") (Fig. 12.12);
  - with greater degrees of scaphoid rotation, the waist of the scaphoid appears as a bony ring within the bone;
  - the lunate is in the collapsed position with one or other of its horns overlapping the capitate more than normally;
- on lateral x-ray the scaphoid is almost at right angles to the long axis of the carpus.

Treatment

Recent injury

- closed reduction may be possible, with use of an image intensifier, by
  - correcting the zigzag deformity and
  - molding the cast. If this fails, perform an
- open reduction through the anterior and posterior approaches, i.e.,
  - reduction and stabilization of the scaphoid in relation to the lunate, capitate and radius with use of K wires,
  - dorsal and volar capsular and ligamentous repair, and
  - x-ray before closure to confirm accurate reduction (compare it with that of the normal side). Then apply a
  - cast, and send the patient to physiotherapy later.

Old injury

- if it is asymptomatic, no treatment is required. If it is
- symptomatic without widespread osteoarthritic changes,
  - reconstruct the ligaments or

—fuse the scaphoid to the lunate. If it is
* symptomatic with generalized osteoarthritis, consider wrist fusion.

Lunate Dislocations and Perilunar Injuries

ETIOPATHOLOGY (Figs. 12.11 and 12.12)

* dislocations only through the wrist joint (radius and ulna proximally, carpals distally) are rare. The lunate and scaphoid are well protected, and the line of injury usually goes through, around or between these bones. These lunar and perilunar injuries comprise
* 10% of all carpal injuries. On the
* medial side the dislocation is between the ulna and triquetrum, and on the
* radial side it may be
  —around the lunate (perilunar dislocation),
  —around the lunate and the scaphoid (scaphoperilunar dislocation),
  —around the lunate and through the scaphoid, with a fracture of the scaphoid (transcaphoid perilunar fracture-dislocation),
  —around the lunate and through the radial styloid, with fracture of the styloid (transstyloid perilunar fracture-dislocation). The
* carpus may
  —remain dislocated, leaving the lunate (and the proximal part of the scaphoid if this is fractured) in its normal relationship with the radius, or the

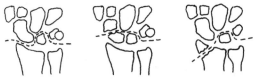

Perilunar   Transscaphoid perilunar   Transstyloid perilunar

Figure 12.11.   Types of perilunar dislocation.

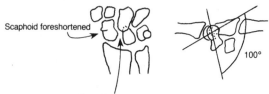

Scaphoid foreshortened

100°

Terry Thomas gap;
rupture of scapholunate ligament

Figure 12.12.   Rotary subluxation of the scaphoid.

—lunate (and proximal scaphoid when fractured) may dislocate, usually anteriorly, with the rest of the carpus remaining in normal relationship with the radius and ulna. The
- palmar radiolunate ligament is nearly always intact, so avascular necrosis of the lunate seldom occurs;
- intercarpal ligaments and capsules are torn, particularly anteriorly, and contribute to chronic instability and recurrent dislocations.

RADIOGRAPHIC FEATURES

- identifying the lunate bone and its relationships with the radius and the other carpals is the key to the diagnosis. The following features are common to the various types of lunar and perilunar dislocations:
- AP x-ray shows
  —soft tissue swelling,
  —shortened wrist and carpus, and an
  —increase in the overlap pattern (look carefully at all wrist x-rays to familiarize yourself with the normal carpal pattern, and if you are in doubt, x-ray the patient's other wrist and compare the two);
  —fracture lines may be present (usually scaphoid or radial styloid);
- lateral x-ray shows that the
  —capitate is absent from the lunate cup; the
  —lunate may be normally aligned with the radius or may be displaced anteriorly or rarely posteriorly;
- fracture lines may be seen better on distraction of the carpus with the patient under anesthesia, before reduction.

TREATMENT

Lunate and perilunar dislocations

Closed reduction

- anesthesia;
- traction on the hand with countertraction on forearm by an assistant. Then for a
- perilunar dislocation
  —hold the lunate in its correct relation to the radius and
  —manipulate the other carpals forward to reduce them around the lunate. For
- anterior lunate dislocation
  —redislocate the other carpals backward, reduce the lunate and hold it in position, then reduce the
  —other carpals. If
- reduction is perfect, apply a
  —below-elbow cast,

—x-ray weekly for 3 weeks, and
—look for redisplacement in the cast. If
- reduction fails, or the
- scaphoid remains subluxed and rotated with a gap between the lunate and scaphoid on the AP x-ray and with the scaphoid lying horizontally, or
- dislocation recurs in the cast,
  —operate.

Open reduction

- anterior and posterior approaches together;
- incise the flexor carpal retinaculum (carpal tunnel release); do not resuture it;
- reduce the dislocation but do not damage further the soft tissue attachments of the carpals, especially the lunate;
- repair the ligaments and capsule, especially the tear in the palmar carpal capsule; use fascia if necessary;
- hold the reduction with K wires through the radius, lunate and scaphoid and into the capitate and hamate.

Transscaphoid and transstyloid perilunar fracture-dislocations

- open reduction and stabilization of the lunate with K wires;
- fixation of fracture with a small scaphoid screw or K wires;
- capsular repair, with fascia if necessary;
- cast for 6 weeks;
- daily physiotherapy for shoulder, elbow and fingers starting immediately postoperatively for all these injuries.

Untreated injuries

- closed reduction is usually impossible after 3 weeks, so
- open reduction is indicated.
- if gross cartilage damage or extensive degenerative changes are present, fuse the wrist if it is symptomatic.

Fractures and Dislocations of Other Carpals

- dorsal chip fracture of any carpal may occur (10% of all carpal injuries). Treat with a cast for 4 weeks.
- fractures and dislocations of other carpals are rare. Follow the same principles of treatment as for perilunar dislocations and fracture dislocations.

Complications of Carpal Injuries

- nerve injuries are uncommon. The
  - —median nerve is the most vulnerable in lunate dislocations, and the
  - —ulnar nerve is the most vulnerable in fractures of the pisiform or hook of the hamate;
  - —reduction relieves the pressure, and recovery is usually complete;
  - —shoulder-hand syndrome is common and can be treated by physiotherapy;
- ischemic contractures are uncommon unless there is an associated crush injury;
- posttraumatic osteoarthritis is often asymptomatic;
- avascular necrosis of the
  - —proximal pole of the scaphoid or capitate, and of the
  - —lunate when soft tissue attachments are completely disrupted, may occur;
  - —revascularization usually occurs after reduction and healing with prolonged immobilization. Necrosis itself is usually not troublesome.

Care after Treatment

- elevate the arm for 48 hours after reduction;
- start the patient on shoulder, elbow and finger exercises as soon as possible;
- x-ray through the cast weekly for 3 weeks to look for loss of position;
- remove K wires at 6 weeks;
- change the cast at 6 weeks, and if the fracture is not healed, continue with serial casts until it is healed. It takes as much time to
- return to full mobility as the fracture was immobilized, and
- return to full power takes 4 times longer, so warn the patient at the beginning.

chapter 13
Soft Tissue Injuries of the Hand

General Considerations

OBJECTIVES OF TREATMENT

- to restore function, notably
  - —pinch and
  - —grip;
- without this, anatomic restoration is useless;
- function depends on
  - —tactile sensation and controlled
  - —joint mobility.

SURGERY

- the anatomical structures are fine and delicate, so the
- instruments and the
- surgery should be fine and delicate too;
- hand surgery is tiring, so
  - —sit down to operate with the
  - —patient's hand on a small table, a
  - —good light shining over your shoulder, and a
  - —good assistant facing you;
- elective surgery should be scheduled early in the day when the operating team is relatively fresh;
- use a pneumatic tourniquet around the arm, not an Esmarch bandage or a band around the base of a finger.

SKIN

Preparation for surgery

- dirt may be ingrained into palmar skin. So before surgery, for prevention of infection,
  - —confirm that the patient has been immunized against tetanus;
  - —cut the patient's nails and
  - —clean them with a file;

- —scrub the hand for 5 minutes with a scrubbing brush and ordinary soap, then
- —prepare the skin in routine manner;
- plan skin incisions in advance, mark them with methylene blue, and "cut along the dotted line."

Skin closure

- early skin closure of a clean traumatic wound, when possible, is important, to
    - —prevent infection,
    - —decrease scarring which would destroy tendon gliding movements, and
    - —ensure survival of tendon, cartilage and bone;
- direct suture of skin, without tension, is the best method and is easy to perform on the dorsum, where skin is mobile, but may be more difficult to perform in the palm, where skin is fixed;
- large, clean defects may be covered with split-thickness skin grafts,
    - —the thinner the graft, the better the take;
    - —graft will not take on bare cortical bone, cartilage or tendon;
    - —graft will die if hematoma forms beneath it or gross infection is present. But
    - —thin graft may contract to one half or one quarter of its original size;
- do not use full-thickness grafts or flaps in acute injuries;
- do not close dirty wounds primarily. Clean and debride the hand carefully, then perform
    - —delayed primary closure at 3 days, if the wound is not infected, or
    - —split-thickness skin grafting later;
- do not allow a granulating area to heal by itself because the resulting scar will contract. Cover the area with split-thickness skin graft as soon as any portion of the granulation is clean. A
- distally-based flap of skin may not survive due to ischemia or insufficient venous drainage (arterioles run distally, veins drain proximally, and in this flap these vessels are cut). If in doubt, excise the flap and replace it with split-thickness skin graft.

Tendon Injuries

CLOSED TENDON INJURIES

Flexor tendon rupture

- not common;
- usually occurs in men 20 to 40 years old at the tendon's insertion into bone;
- often the flexor digitorum profundus (FDP) tendon;
- 20% associated with synovitis;

- proximal tendon retracts into the palm where it curls up and makes a lump;
- if flexor tendon rupture is asymptomatic, no treatment is required; if it is symptomatic,
- excision of the mass in the palm is required. If the
- FDP tendon to the index finger is ruptured, and pinch is impaired, arthrodese the distal interphalangeal (DIP) joint at 25° of flexion.

Extensor tendon rupture (Fig. 13.1)

Insertion

- called
  —mallet finger,
  —cricket ball finger (in Commonwealth of Nations) or
  —baseball finger (in North America);
- common in athletes;
- caused by acute, forced flexion of the DIP joint. Either the
  —tendon is pulled off from its insertion, or the
  —dorsal lip of the base of the distal phalanx (DP) fractures and this flake of bone comes off with the tendon, a Salter-Harris Type III epiphyseal injury in children;
- treatment of recent injury is by splinting of the DIP joint in extension for 8 weeks;
- injury older than 3 months requires
  —advancement of the proximal end of the tendon.

Central slip rupture (Fig. 13.2)

- called buttonhole deformity (boutonnière);
- not common;

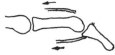

Figure 13.1.   Mallet finger with avulsed extensor tendon.

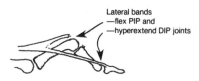

Figure 13.2.   Extensor tendon central slip rupture with buttonhole deformity. *PIP*, proximal interphalangeal; *DIP*, distal interphalangeal.

- causes loss of extension of the proximal interphalangeal (PIP) joint. So the
- PIP joint is permanently flexed with
- hyperextension of the DIP joint;
- treat a fresh injury by
  —splinting of the metacarpophalangeal (MCP) and PIP joints in extension for 6 weeks, followed by a lively extension splint; or
  —reattachment of the central slip through a dorsal approach, with the
  —PIP joint held in full extension for 3 weeks. For an
- old injury,
  —free displaced lateral bands and
  —suture them together and to retracted central slip over dorsum of the middle phalanx (MP).

OPEN FLEXOR TENDON INJURIES

Primary suture

Prerequisites

- a clean, incised wound with little or no edema;
- minimal contamination;
- injury less than 6 hours old with
- no fracture in related area (tendons adhere to callus);
- primary skin closure must be possible without tension.

Indications (Figs. 13.3 and 13.4)

Wrist

- when all tendons and nerves are divided at the wrist,
- in a child under 5, suture all structures;
- in a child over 5 and in an adult, only suture the
  —FDP and the
  —flexor pollicis longus (FPL) tendons and then the

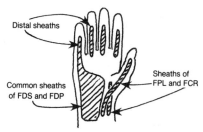

Figure 13.3. Synovial flexor sheaths in the hand. *FCR*, flexor carpi radialis.

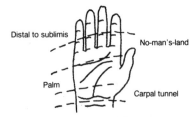

Figure 13.4. Flexor zones of the hand.

—median and ulnar nerves, and divide the flexor retinaculum;
- when all four flexor digitorum sublimis (FDS) and only one or two FDP tendons are cut at the wrist, suture the
    —FDS tendon to the index and middle fingers as well as
    —all the cut FDP tendons;
- palmaris longus (PL) and FDS tendons to the ring and little fingers need not be sutured.

Palm between wrist and distal palmar crease

- when one tendon is divided in the palm,
    —suture it;
- when both tendons of a finger are cut in the palm, suture both in a child but just the FDP in the adult and excise the FDS;
- when multiple tendons are cut in the palm, suture the
    —FDP tendons only and excise the FDS tendons.

"No-man's-land," distal palmar crease to PIP joint

- critical area of pulleys. If the
- FDS tendon alone is cut
    —excise it as far distally as possible without additional incisions;
    —an FDP tendon provides adequate flexion of both interphalangeal (IP) joints, so
    —do not suture the FDS tendon. If the
- FDP tendon alone is cut,
    —start immediate active finger movements to prevent adhesions of the FDS tendon. Do not suture the FDP tendon. If the
    —index finger FDP tendon is cut, the DIP joint can be stabilized later by tenodesis or arthrodesis in 25° flexion. If both
- FDS and FDP tendons are cut,
    —excise the FDS tendon and
    —suture the FDP tendon.

Finger distal to PIP joint

- if the FDP tendon is cut near the PIP joint,
    —suture it;

- if the FDP tendon is cut near the DIP joint,
  —excise the distal part, pull the proximal end of the tendon distally (not more than 2 cm), and suture it to the base of the DP.

Flexor pollicis longus tendon

- if the FPL tendon is cut anywhere,
  —suture it. If the suture line is at the
  —level of the MCP joint,
  —excise the pulley.

Tendon identification

- tendons retract proximally because they are attached to muscles. Incisions may have to be extended for a considerable distance proximally to find the tendon;
- match the proximal and distal tendon ends carefully by comparing their
  —size and shape,
  —angle and level of cut, and
  —relation to other structures;
  —pull on the distal ends to see which tendon moves which joint;
- do not suture the median nerve to a tendon! The nerve
  —is off-white (pale yellowish),
  —does not glisten,
  —has an artery running longitudinally on its anterior surface, and
  —has a sheath (neurilemma), and the
  —axons pout from its severe ends. Use a magnifying glass;
- if you are still in doubt as to whether a structure is a tendon or nerve,
  —trace it proximally to see if it is attached to a muscle and
  —pull the distal end gently to see if it flexes a finger!

Technique of tendon suture

- approximate the ends of a tendon by
  —end-to-end suture with a multiple diagonal stitch (Bunnell crisscross stitch) for a single tendon. A
  —double right-angled mattress suture is easier but less tidy than the crisscross stitch. An
  —end-to-side anastomosis is useful for suturing one tendon to several others, e.g., when one motor must activate several tendons. And a
  —fishmouth end-to-end suture is useful for attaching a small tendon to a large one.
- attach tendon to bone by
  —decorticating a small area of the bone; then
  —drill a small hole into this area and through the bone;
  —put a crisscross stitch in the tendon,

—pass the ends of the stitch through the hole in the bone and the skin, and

—tie it tightly over a button or gauze to pull the end of the tendon into the cortical defect.

Secondary tendon suture

- when primary suture is contraindicated, approximate the tendon ends at the first operation to prevent retraction and order
- daily passive range of movement (ROM) exercises to prevent stiffness of the affected fingers. Repair the tendons secondarily when the
  —skin wound is healed,
  —edema has subsided,
  —no infection is present,
  —fractures are stabilized in good alignment,
  —joints have a useful passive ROM, and
  —sensation in the affected fingers is useful;
- secondary suture is possible in the forearm, wrist and palm
  —up to 4 weeks after injury by
  —flexing the wrist to overcome muscle contracture;
- follow the previously discussed rules relating to zones and which tendons to suture.

Tendon grafting

Indications

- indications for late reconstruction by tendon grafting are: for the
  —FDP tendon when both tendons are cut and the FDP has retracted too far for end-to-end suture, and for the
  —FPL tendon when end-to-end apposition is impossible;
- the prerequisites are similar to those for secondary tendon suture (see previous discussion);
- grafting is not justified for division of the
  —FDS tendon alone, because the FDP tendon can compensate, or the
  —FDP tendon alone, because a flail DIP joint can be stabilized by arthrodesis or tenodesis.

Technique

- use palmaris longus, plantaris or long extensors of toes;
- excise both FDS and FDP tendons from the finger to be grafted;
- shorten the two pulleys by excising half of each, thus exposing a greater area of the graft for revascularization;
- attach the distal end of the graft to bone at the base of the DP, then
- pass the graft through the pulleys and

- suture the graft to the proximal end of the FDP tendon in the palm, wrapping lumbrical muscle around the suture line;
- do not allow the suture line to lie in "no-man's-land" or the carpal tunnel. For the
- FPL tendon, the suture line should lie proximal to the carpal tunnel;
- the graft and the FDP or FPL tendon must be under correct tension, but
  —too much tension is better than too little tension because muscle may stretch later. Allow
  —more tension for the ring and little fingers than for the index and middle fingers.

Tenodesis

- can be used to stabilize the DIP joint of the index finger in flexion when the FDP tendon is cut and cannot be repaired.
- distal attachment of the FDP tendon to the DP is left intact. Leave 1.5 cm of distal tendon.
- anchor the tendon proximally to the anterior surface of the shaft of the MP with the DIP joint in 20° of flexion. The tendon acts as a checkrein and prevents passive or active extension of the DIP joint.

OPEN EXTENSOR TENDON INJURIES

- primary suture anywhere is usually possible;
- if part of the tendon is damaged or destroyed, or the wound is several days or weeks old and the proximal tendon has retracted,
  —transfer the extensor proprius tendon (from the index or little finger) to the distal end of the cut tendon, or
  —suture the distal end of the cut tendon to adjacent, intact tendon, or
  —perform a tendon graft if several extensor tendons are damaged, or
  —if muscle is damaged as well, transfer the flexor carpi ulnaris (FCU) tendon around the ulnar border of the wrist to provide a motor.

TENDON TRANSFER

Prerequisites

- tendon transfer is the final step in reconstructive surgery of the hand; prerequisites include
  —healed skin with
  —no infection;
  —skeletal stability;
  —mobile joints with
  —no fixed deformities; and the presence of
  —sensation. This does not have to be normal, but surgery will fail if the

patient cannot feel with his palm and fingers because he will not use the hand.

Principles of technique

- choose a muscle which
  —does not have an essential function,
  —has normal strength (it will lose one grade of strength after transfer),
  —can be mobilized without damaging its nerve and blood supply, and has an
  —adequate excursion; i.e., the distance through which the muscle moves the tendon must be sufficient to move the joint. The
- transferred tendon should be
  —embedded in fat and be subcutaneous, if possible, to provide a sliding bed and prevent adhesions. It should lie in a
  —straight line from its muscle to its point of suture because bends and pulleys reduce the efficiency of the tendon transfer.

POSTOPERATIVE CARE

- after surgery, immobilize the fingers and wrist in a position which avoids tension on suture lines
  —4 weeks for extensor tendons and
  —3 weeks for flexor tendons. The
- best position for the fingers is the "intrinsic plus," with the
  —MP joint flexed and the
  —IP joints extended to avoid permanent stiffness, and the thumb in
  —wide abduction to avoid adduction contracture of the web space, with the pulp in
  —opposition to the index finger unless contraindicated, because this may not be the optimum position for tendon suture lines. You must strike a nice balance between the two;
- start the patient on gentle active exercises as soon as possible, depending on the surgery performed, supporting the hand between exercises for 5 weeks after surgery.

ADHERENT TENDONS

Etiopathology

- tendons may adhere to
  —a fracture site., e.g., the FDP tendon to the proximal phalanx (PP) or the extensor tendon to the metacarpal (MC) or PP;
  —surrounding scar tissue; or
  —adjacent tendons when two or more have been sutured.

Clinical features

- active movement of the joint for which the tendon is responsible is absent, but passive movement in the direction of the tendon pull is possible;
- passive and active movements of the joint in the opposite direction are prevented by the adherent tendon because this acts like a check-rein;
- e.g., when FDP is stuck to PP,
  —active flexion of DIP joint is absent,
  —passive flexion of DIP joint is possible,
  —active flexion of PIP joint by the FDS tendon is possible,
  —passive flexion of PIP joint is possible, and
  —active flexion of MP joint by the FDS and FDP is possible; but
  —full active and passive extension of PIP and DIP joints is absent;
  —active and passive extension of the PIP joint is increased by passive flexion of the DIP joint, and vice versa, but is not increased by passive flexion of the MP joint;
  —extension of the wrist may initiate flexion of the MP joint.

Differential diagnosis

- includes
  —skin, joint or muscle contracture,
  —severed tendon, and
  —paralyzed muscle or a
  —combination of these;
- accurate diagnosis is essential for correct treatment!

Treatment

- tenolysis with
  —liberation of the tendon by sharp dissection and
  —excision of all scar tissue from the tendon. If the
  —tendon is stuck to bone, interpose fascia or part of the tendon sheath between the tendon and bone. Initiate
- immediate, active mobilization after surgery.

Nerve Injuries
- see Chapter 31.

Shotgun Injuries

- multiple wounds are usually
- very dirty;
- treatment:
  —debride the wounds thoroughly,
  —remove all damaged tissue except nerves and vessels,
  —remove as much shot as possible, especially any in the joints,
  —remove unattached bone fragments and bridge bone defects with K wires;
  —leave the wound open for a few days (not longer than 5), then
  —cover with skin (grafts if necessary);
- reconstruct bone, nerves and tendons as secondary procedures.

Wringer Injuries

ETIOPATHOLOGY

- compression injury, usually due to rollers on a washing machine;
- half the patients are under 5 years old;
- edema and interstitial hemorrhage within the first few hours are the major problems;
- there may be abrasions or even avulsion of skin;
- fracture of epiphyseal plate injuries may be associated.

TREATMENT

- admit to hospital;
- clean the skin;
- do not suture lacerations;
- apply pressure dressings evenly and
- elevate the arm,
  —tying it to an intravenous (IV) pole or to the head of the bed;
  —the limb must remain elevated throughout treatment;
- be alert for vascular insufficiency in the forearm compartment (see Chapter 32);
- change dressings every 24 hours
  —to inspect and clean the wounds and because
  —compression effect is lost after the first few hours;
- debride and close the wounds when swelling disappears.

General Care after Surgery

- for all surgical procedures on the hand, apply a
- compression dressing with the

—wrist in 15° extension,

—MCP joints in flexion (except thumb), and

—IP joints in extension unless contraindicated. Leave the

—fingertips visible to evaluate circulation;

- elevate the hand by tying it to a bar or an IV pole until edema subsides.
- early motion of all joints is important whenever possible, but the
- best physiotherapy and occupational therapy eventually are

—activities of daily living at home and

—the patient's work.

chapter 14

Fractures and Joint Injuries of the Hand

General Remarks

- Fractures in the hand are the most common fractures of the body and account for
  —30% of industrial accidents and
  —10% of all accidents that injure the hand. These fractures are
- sometimes poorly treated because the
  —bones are small and the
  —injuries are common, so they are
  —often relegated to the most junior doctor for treatment.
- hand surgery is not minor surgery. It is difficult and demanding. It should be supervised and taught by an experienced surgeon.
- closed reductions can be done in the
  —emergency room, but
- open wounds should be explored and treated in the
  —operating room under proper conditions;
- anesthesia for the treatment of hand injuries must be adequate;
- local anesthesia is usually sufficient, such as an
  —intravenous block,
  —median and ulnar nerve blocks at the wrist with a dorsal wheal to block the dorsal sensory branches, or a
  —digital nerve block in the palm or the web space;
- do not use a ring block around the base of the finger because this may cause ischemia;
- never use epinephrine (adrenaline).

Initial Evaluation

- the first time the patient is seen is the best time to
  —evaluate the injury,
  —restore the anatomy, and
  —plan for functional recovery.

HISTORY

- important factors are the patient's
  - —age,
  - —hand dominance,
  - —occupation and hobbies, and the
- five Ws (see Chapter 2).

PHYSICAL EXAMINATION

- vascular status of the hand and of individual fingers, i.e.,
  - —color,
  - —temperature and
  - —capillary filling. Compress the pulp, not the nail bed;
- motor and sensory examination for
  - —median and
  - —ulnar nerves, the long
  - —flexor and extensor tendons and the
  - —intrinsic muscles. Know your anatomy!
- evaluate a skin wound with regard to
  - —location and extent,
  - —contamination, and
  - —viability of surrounding skin or flaps.
- swelling and tenderness must be localized by careful examination; e.g., if the interphalangeal (IP) joint is swollen, is the maximum tenderness
  - —dorsal, denoting central slip tear, or
  - —lateral, denoting collateral ligament tear?

RADIOLOGICAL EXAMINATION

- essential in all hand injuries. Ask for
- three views:
  - —anteroposterior (AP),
  - —lateral, especially of an individual finger, and
  - —oblique, especially of metacarpals (MCs) to avoid superimposition.
- obvious injuries are easy to see on a radiograph but
- smaller injuries are not! So
- look for
  - —greenstick fractures,
  - —small intra-articular fractures, and
  - —subluxations.
- compare x-rays of the two hands when necessary, and
- relate radiological to clinical findings to avoid confusion with
  - —soft tissue shadows and
  - —epiphyses.

Metacarpal Fractures (Excluding Thumb)

• common in men, uncommon in children.

METACARPAL BASE

• stable unless it is intra-articular because the latter is often associated with
  —subluxation or
  —dislocation;
• beware of
  —rotation and
  —angulation because these deformities are greatly magnified at the finger-
    tip. The fracture should be
  —reduced and may require
  —pinning with Kirschner wires either obliquely across the fracture or
    transversely through an adjacent metacarpal.

METACARPAL SHAFT (Figs. 14.1 and 14.2)

Transverse fracture

Etiopathology

• usually caused by a direct blow;
• angulates dorsally because the interossei act like a bowstring;
• may rotate;
• once reduced, shortening is not a problem.

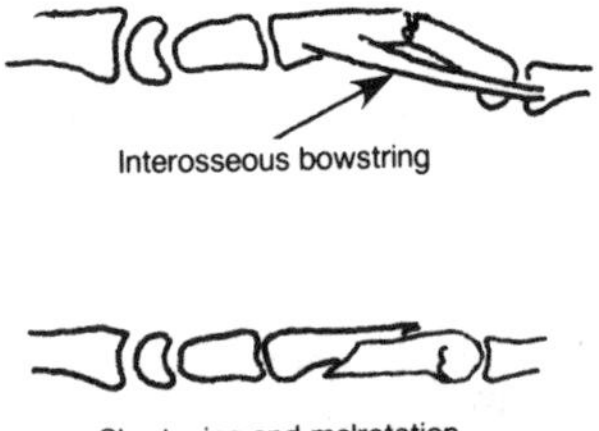

Interosseous bowstring

Shortening and malrotation

Figure 14.1. Metacarpal shaft fractures.

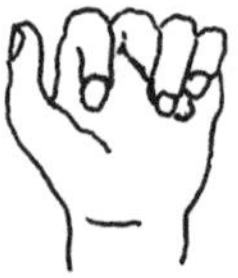

Figure 14.2. Malrotation of the third metacarpal or proximal phalanx.

Treatment

Reduction

- closed reduction is usually possible;
- AP angulation in the midshaft is not acceptable, but minor angulation near the metaphysis can be accepted in the fourth and fifth metacarpals (MCs) because there is compensatory motion at the carpometacarpal (CMC) joints;
- lateral angulation and rotation are not acceptable because they are magnified at the fingertip, and the resultant deformity interferes with grasp. Check for rotational deformity by comparing the
  —angulation of the nail of the injured finger with the nails of the normal fingers, which are all horizontal in the same plane, and by
  —flexing the injured finger to see if the tip touches the same spot on the palm as the other fingers. When each finger is flexed individually, each fingertip normally touches the base of the thenar eminence, and when the fingers are flexed together, the fingers point toward the scaphoid.
- open reduction is rarely necessary unless the fracture is open.

Stabilization   ′

- well-padded (particularly on dorsum) gutter plaster cast
  —incorporating the finger to its tip and adjacent normal finger,
  —immobilizing the wrist, and
  —holding the reduction with three-point pressure.
  —remove the plaster finger extensions at 3 weeks and start the patient on guarded active movements;
  —remove the cast at 5 weeks. If the fracture is
- unstable, use
  —transverse K wires drilled horizontally through the two fracture fragments into an adjacent normal MC;
  —this controls angulation and rotation;
  —remove pins at 4 weeks for a closed fracture and at 6 weeks for an open fracture.
  —start the patient on guarded active finger movements 5 days after reduction.
- do not introduce intramedullary pins percutaneously through the MC head. This causes metacarpophalangeal (MCP) joint stiffness and does not control rotation.
- with open reduction, or an open fracture, use the transverse pin method for fixation because percutaneous crossed K wires across the fracture site may interfere with the extensor tendons.

Oblique fracture

- caused by a twisting force;
- these fractures cause
  —rotation and
  —shortening, especially of the second and fifth MCs because these are only supported on one side;
- angulation is usually not a problem.
- with minimal deformity, treat with a
  —plaster cast, as for transverse fracture. If
- unacceptable rotation or shortening is present, treat by
  —closed reduction and fixation with
  —transverse K wires, as for transverse fractures.

Comminuted fracture

- direct blow;
- usually not displaced but often
- associated with marked soft tissue damage.
- treat with
  —compression dressing and elevation until edema subsides. Then if it is
  —displaced, use a Böhler
  —palmar splint, flexed at the MCP joints and extended at the IP joints, with the
  —finger taped to the splint with rotation and shortening corrected.

METACARPAL NECK

Etiopathology

- often caused by a fist fight, especially a fracture of the fifth MC, the street fighter's fracture;
- angulates posteriorly with the MC head displaced into the palm;
- anterior cortex is comminuted and fracture is
- unstable.
- fourth and fifth CMC joints are mobile, with 15° and 25° of AP mobility, respectively, and may compensate for displacement of the MC head;
- second and third CMC joints are not mobile (move your own and see for yourself), and displacement of the MC head is more disabling.
- fracture is through cancellous bone and usually unites in 3 weeks.

Treatment

Fourth and fifth MCs

- with angulation of less than 50°, accept the deformity and treat by a
  —protective splint;
  —remove the splint at 2 weeks and start the patient on active guarded motion.

- with angulation of more than 50°, if the fracture is
- recent, treat by
  —closed reduction and
  —transverse fixation with two K wires into adjacent MC for 3 weeks.
  If the fracture is
- old, accept the deformity and encourage active mobilization unless
  the head in the palm is very disabling, in which case osteotomy and
  K wire fixation may be necessary.

Second and third MCs

Undisplaced

- radial splint for 3 weeks;
- x-ray through the splint at 4 or 5 days and correct any deformity
  that has occurred.

Displaced

- do not accept angulation in these two MCs.
- treat by
  —closed reduction and
  —fixation with transverse K wires, at least one wire through each
    fragment. If this
- fails, perform
  —open reduction and K wire fixation. Encourage
- early active motion of fingers;
- remove pins at 3 weeks.

METACARPAL HEAD

- rare;
- usually comminuted;
- open reduction and internal fixation are very difficult, so the best
- treatment is
  —protection with a splint for 5 days, then
  —active movement;
- results are poor with
  —loss of movement, and
  —pain may or may not be a problem.

COMPLICATIONS OF METACARPAL FRACTURES

- soft tissue injuries
  —tendons may be damaged by the injury or tethered by adhesions;
  —skin may be damaged, since frequently MC fractures are open, especially
    those due to crush injuries; and
  —massive edema from a crush injury may be present with resultant stiffness
    of the fingers.

- malunion
  —angulation causing clawing of the finger or painful and weakened grasp or
  —malrotation interfering with grasp may require derotational osteotomy.
- stiff MCP joint
  —due to immobilization of the MCP joint in extension with subsequent contracture of the collateral ligaments;
- stiff proximal interphalangel (PIP) joint
  —due to prolonged immobilization of the PIP joint in acute flexion;
- pin tract infection when pins protrude through the skin.

Thumb Metacarpal Fractures

- the thumb is different from a finger, and so are its injuries;
- functionally the thumb is 50% of the hand, equal to the other four digits combined.

THUMB METACARPAL BASE (Fig. 14.3)
- the most common MC fracture.

Bennett's fracture-dislocation

Etiopathology
- often the result of a fist fight, from a longitudinal axial blow on a partially flexed thumb. The
- fracture is intra-articular.
- one third or one half of the palmar lip of the base is fractured off and remains in situ, held there by the very strong anterior oblique ligament which goes from the fragment to the tubercle of the trapezium;
- the other MC fragment dislocates from the CMC joint with
  —posterolateral and proximal displacement due to pull of the abductor pollicis longus (APL) and with

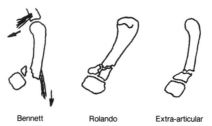

Bennett   Rolando   Extra-articular

Figure 14.3. Fractures of the first metacarpal base.

—abduction of the base and adduction of the head due to pull of the adductor pollicis, which results in

—reduction of the span of the first web space, an important disability.

- the epiphyseal plate of the thumb MC is at the base, whereas in the other four MCs it is at the neck;
- a Salter-Harris Type III or IV epiphyseal plate injury in a child is similar to a Bennett fracture in an adult.

Treatment

- make one attempt at
  - —closed reduction and
  - —immobilization in a well-molded, padded cast or
  - —fixation with two percutaneous K wires passing through the major fragment into the trapezium or into the second MC;
  - —do not attempt to transfix the small fragment and
  - —do not hyperextend the MCP joint, a common error. This will cause pain and stiffness;
  - —x-ray control is essential.
- if closed reduction fails, perform
  - —open reduction through a curved posterolateral incision and
  - —fix the fracture with two K wires passing from the larger fragment to the smaller. If it is still unstable,
  - —pass a third K wire through the major fragment across the CMC joint into the trapezium. To fix the fracture with a wire loop passed through both fragments is difficult and time-consuming.
- whether reduction is closed or open, treat with a below-elbow cast incorporating the thumb for 6 weeks.
- treatment for a Type III epiphyseal plate injury is similar. Do not hyperextend the MCP joint; this should be in slight flexion.

Rolando's fracture

- is an intra-articular T or Y fracture of the MC base, but it may be more comminuted than this.
- treat a T or Y fracture by
  - —open reduction and fixation with K wires, as for Bennett's fracture. If the fracture is
- comminuted,
  - —immobilize it in plaster splint for 10 days, then treat with active mobilization;
  - —do not attempt open reduction.

Extra-articular fracture

- is the most common fracture of the base of the MC. It
- may be transverse or oblique. In a

- child the injury is a Salter-Harris Type II epiphyseal plate injury.
- treat by
  —closed reduction and by a cast for 4 weeks;
  —angulation of 20° can be accepted, but
  —do not hyperextend the MCP joint in plaster.

THUMB METACARPAL SHAFT AND HEAD

- these fractures are similar in pathology and treatment to those of other MCs, but the MCP joint should generally be immobilized in extension.

Fractures of Proximal and Middle Phalanges

ETIOPATHOLOGY

- transverse and comminuted fractures are caused by a direct blow;
- oblique and spiral fractures are caused by torsion.
- angulated midshaft fractures involve the flexor tendon sheath and may cause tendon adhesions.

Proximal phalanx (PP) (Fig. 14.4)

- direction of the angulation in unstable fractures is anterior because the
  —interossei pull the proximal fragment forward and the
  —distal fragment is pulled into hyperextension by the central extensor slip acting on the middle phalanx.

Middle phalanx (Fig. 14.5)

- uncommon fractures;
- fracture through the base angulates posteriorly because the
  —proximal fragment is extended by the central extensor slip and the
  —distal fragment is flexed by the flexor digitorum sublimis (FDS);
- fracture through the distal shaft or neck angulates anteriorly because the
  —proximal fragment is flexed by the FDS and the
  —distal fragment is extended by insertion of extensor digitorum communis (EDC) into the distal phalanx;
- fracture through the midshaft may
  —angulate in either direction or
  —remain undisplaced.

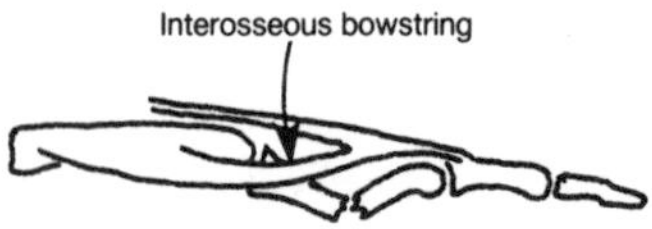

Interosseous bowstring

Figure 14.4.   Transverse fracture of the proximal phalanx.

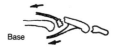

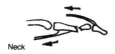

Figure 14.5.   Extra-articular fractures of the middle phalanx.

TREATMENT
Undisplaced and impacted extra-articular fractures
- tape the finger to its largest neighbor, leaving the IP joints free (buddy taping). In children in particular, do not immobilize one finger alone; always immobilize two fingers together to prevent angulation, rotation and displacement.
- encourage active movements of both fingers and normal daily use while the fracture heals;
- you must be positive that on examination of good AP and lateral x-rays there is no displacement, angulation or rotation before this method of treatment is chosen;
- careful clinical and radiological follow-up is important for detection of displacement during treatment.

Displaced extra-articular fractures
Stable after closed reduction
- treat by closed reduction with traction and manipulation, followed by
- immobilization in a malleable, padded aluminum splint or in a
- plaster splint if the patient is not likely to cooperate. For fracture of the
- PP, immobilize the
  —MCP and PIP joints in some flexion. For fracture of the
- middle phalanx distal to insertion of the FDS,
  —flex the PIP joint and the distal fragment. For fracture of the
- middle phalanx proximal to the FDS insertion,
  —extend the PIP joint;
- correct rotational alignment by comparing the plane of the nails of the two fingers immobilized. Malrotation is a far greater disability than shortening or even AP angulation.
- you will not see callus on x-rays, so

- remove the splint at 3 weeks, tape the finger to its neighbor, and start the patient on active movements;
- remove tape 2 weeks later.

Unstable after closed reduction

- an oblique or spiral fracture of the PP may be unstable;
- treat by
  —closed reduction and
  —percutaneous K wires perpendicular to the fracture line (difficult to do). Check for malrotation. Apply a splint because K wires are not usually sufficient.
- remove the splint and pins at 3 weeks and tape the finger to its neighbor for 2 more weeks to allow active movements. If
- closed reduction fails,
  —approach the fracture through a dorsal incision splitting the extensor longitudinally. After reduction,
  —stabilize the fracture with K wires and start the patient on
  —early movement.
- treat comminuted fractures closed with a cast or splint and then early mobilization.

Greenstick fractures and Type I or II growth plate injuries

- usually at base of PP with lateral angulation;
- treat by closed manipulation, either
  —placing a pencil vertically in the web space on the side of the apex of the angulation and using the pencil as a fulcrum to lever the phalanx over it and correct the angulation or, better still,
  —flexing the MCP joint to 95° to tighten the collateral ligaments and thus stabilize the epiphysis and then manipulating the distal fragment. With a
  —greenstick fracture, break the intact cortex. After reduction, apply
  —buddy taping for 2 weeks.
- angulation in any direction at the base of the PP may remodel with growth, but
- lateral angulation at the base of the middle phalanx will not, nor
- will rotation anywhere.

Intra-articular fractures

Undisplaced

- usually at the base of the phalanx;
- if fracture is displaced less than 2 mm, treat by
  —buddy taping with early active movements.

Displaced

Condyles

- fractures of the neck or condyles of a phalanx do not remodel in any direction because there is no growth plate;
- one or both (T or Y fracture) condyles of the head of the PP or middle phalanx may be fractured and are usually displaced;
- treat by
  —accurate open reduction through a lateral approach for one condyle or by dorsal midline incision, splitting the central slip but not detaching it, for both condyles;
  —internal fixation with two fine K wires;
  —do not detach soft tissues from the condylar fragments to avoid avascular necrosis;
  —central slip must be sutured. This is difficult surgery, especially for the middle phalanx. Postoperatively, encourage
  —early, active motion under supervision;
  —remove pins at 3 weeks for an adult and at 6 weeks for an adolescent and buddy tape for 2 more weeks.

Base

- usually the PP;
- fragment may be avulsed by collateral ligament;
- in children this is a Salter-Harris Type III growth plate injury. A
- small fragment requires
  —buddy taping and early active motion. A
- large displaced fragment should be treated by
  —open reduction through a middorsal approach, splitting the extensor hood, and by
  —fixation of the fragment with two K wires. Then
  —suture the extensor hood and
  —start the patient on early motion;
  —remove pins at 3 weeks and buddy tape for 2 more weeks.

Comminuted

- grossly comminuted fractures cannot be reduced accurately;
- treat by closed reduction and encourage early motion.

Fracture-dislocation of PIP joint

Etiopathology (Fig. 14.6)

- either a fragment of bone is avulsed from the
  —dorsum of the base of the middle phalanx by central extensor slip and the

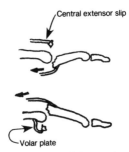

Figure 14.6. Fracture-dislocation of the proximal interphalangeal joint.

—middle phalanx dislocates anteriorly. This is a
—Type III growth plate injury in a child. The
—triangular ligament is usually ruptured. This ligament is a dorsal
  band which joins the two lateral slips of the extensor tendon and
  prevents them from dislocating anteriorly.
- or a fragment may fracture from the
  —anterior lip of the base of the middle phalanx with
  —posterior subluxation or dislocation of the middle phalanx. Both
    these injuries are
- unstable.

Treatment

- for posterior lip fracture,
- open reduction through a dorsal, S-shaped incision;
- fix the fragment with fine K wires or sutures;
- suture the triangular ligament with correct tension. If tension is
  —too tight, it will prevent full flexion of the PIP joint; if tension is
  —too loose, the lateral slips will remain anterior to the axis of flexion of
    the PIP joint and will flex it when the long extensor contracts. For
- anterior lip fracture,
  —reduce the joint and
  —transfix it with K wire. In both injuries,
- postoperative immobilization with a short plaster splint of the
  —PIP joint only, leaving the
  —MCP and distal interphalangeal (DIP) joints free for guarded active
    movement;
- remove the K wire at 4 weeks and buddy tape the finger for 2 more
  weeks to allow active movement of PIP joint.

Follow-up care

- always watch for redisplacement, angulation or rotation during the first
  3 weeks and correct it as soon as it occurs;

- encourage early active motion whenever possible, because a stiff finger in extension is a functional amputation;
- supervise treatment and encourage the patient;
- do not immobilize a finger for longer than 3 weeks because
  —clinical healing occurs before
  —radiological healing, and prolonged immobilization causes
  —stiffness;
- protect the finger by buddy taping for 2 or 3 more weeks and encourage active motion and use of fingers during this time.

Distal Phalangeal Fractures

ETIOPATHOLOGY

- more than 50% of all hand fractures;
- swelling and hematoma in the tight, closed fibrous compartments of the pulp cause great pain.
- longitudinal fracture is
  —usually undisplaced;
- transverse fracture is
  —near the base and
  —often angulated posteriorly;
- comminuted fracture is
  —due to crushing, usually involves the
  —distal tuft, and is
  —associated with gross soft tissue damage, edema and pain. This is the
  —most frequent type of distal phalangeal fracture.

TREATMENT

Subungual hematoma

- decompress this for pain relief by
  —burning a hole in the nail with a heated paper clip or pin.

Undisplaced and comminuted tuft fractures

- require protection only, to relieve pain;
- do not put on a tight splint, as this increases the pain;
- a hairpin splint, taped to the sides of the middle phalanx and curving around the distal phalanx like a bumper curves around a car, will give adequate protection for 3 to 5 weeks;
- the fingertip may remain painful or tender for several months, so warn the patient.

Displaced fracture

- closed reduction and
- immobilization by

—splint or

—longitudinal K wire. A

- Salter-Harris Type I epiphyseal fracture may disrupt the nail bed. This is an

  —open fracture;

  —debride and

  —reduce the fracture, and

  —preserve the nail and

  —replace it under the nail fold;

  —immobilize in extension for 2 weeks.

Fracture-dislocation of distal interphalangeal joint

Etiopathology (Fig. 5.2)

- similar to mallet deformity (see Chapter 13), but there is an unstable

  —intra-articular fracture of the dorsal lip of the base of the distal phalanx (DP), involving a third or more of the articular surface and

  —anterior subluxation or dislocation of the DP. In a

- teenager, the injury is a Salter-Harris Type III ephiphyseal fracture. These fracture-dislocations are unstable.

Treatment

- closed reduction and transarticular pinning, or
- open reduction through a dorsal incision and
- fixation with K wire or sutures.
- if the fragment cannot be fixed with a K wire through it,

  —immobilize the DIP joint in extension with a longitudinal wire through the DP and across the joint into the middle phalanx;

- immobilize with a plaster splint the

  —DIP joint in extension and the

  —PIP joint in 60° flexion to reduce pull of the extensor tendon on the bone fragment;

- remove the splint from the

  —PIP joint at 3 weeks to allow active motion, but

  —do not remove the K wire until the fracture is healed on x-ray. This may take up to 8 weeks. If the K wire is removed too soon, subluxation may recur.

Carpometacarpal Dislocation (Excluding Thumb)

ETIOPATHOLOGY AND DIAGNOSIS

- uncommon;
- MCs usually dislocate dorsally;

- dislocations may be multiple and are
- often associated with MC fractures;
- gross swelling masks the clinical deformity, and the diagnosis may be missed;
- diagnosis is based on good AP, lateral and oblique x-rays;
- whenever there is a
  —displaced MC fracture, look carefully for an associated
  —CMC dislocation.

TREATMENT
Recent injury

- closed reduction by
  —traction on the fingers, then
  —manipulation, pushing on the dorsal surface of the bases of the dislocated MCs;
- fixation by percutaneous K wires
  —through the dislocated MCs and either
  —into adjacent normal MC or
  —into the carpals;
- the injury is unstable, so hold the MCs reduced while drilling the K wires across.
- forearm cast for 6 weeks, then remove the K wires.

Old untreated injury

- if the injury is painful with functional disability but there are
- no degenerative changes in the CMC joints, perform
  —open reduction through a dorsal approach,
  —fix with K wires, and
  —repair capsule and ligaments. If there are
- degenerative changes, perform
  —open reduction and
  —CMC arthrodesis.

Thumb Carpometacarpal Dislocations
ETIOPATHOLOGY

- pure dislocation without fracture is uncommon,
  —Bennett's fracture-dislocation is more common;
- mechanism of injury is similar to that of Bennett's, i.e.,
  —longitudinal force on a slightly flexed thumb.

TREATMENT
- closed reduction and
- percutaneous pin fixation for 4 weeks with a plaster cast, then
- graduated active movement.

RESULTS
- residual
  —instability,
  —pain and
  —functional deficit are common;
- treatment for this is
  —arthrodesis (trapezium to first MC) with the thumb in opposition.

Metacarpophalangeal Subluxation and Dislocation (Excluding Thumb)

ANATOMY OF MCP JOINT
- volar plate is the
  —thick fibrocartilaginous anterior part of the joint capsule;
  —distally, it is attached firmly to the anterior surface of the base of the PP,
  —proximally, it is attached loosely to the anterior surface of the neck of the MC, and
  —laterally, it is continuous with the deep, transverse MC ligament. The
  —volar plate folds on itself in MCP flexion and allows some hyperextension.
- collateral ligaments are attached
  —proximally to the neck of the MC posterior to the axis of rotation,
  —distally to the base of the PP, and
  —anteriorly to the lateral borders of the volar ligament by the accessory collateral ligament;
  —the collateral ligament is stretched in flexion and loose in extension because the
  —MC head is broader anteriorly than posteriorly and the
  —center of rotation of the MC head is eccentric, being closer to the distal articular surface than to the anterior surface. So immobilize MCP joints of the fingers in flexion to avoid stiffness.
- movements at the MCP joint are
  —flexion and extension,
  —some hyperextension,
  —abduction and adduction when the MCP joint is in extension, and
  —limited circumduction.

PATHOLOGY, CLASSIFICATION AND CLINICAL FEATURES

- tear of radial collateral ligament of index finger may lead to instability during pinch-grip if it is not treated properly.
- dislocation of MP joint occurs only in the index (more common) and little fingers. It is a
- hyperextension injury and
- the PP dislocates dorsally;
- dislocation may be
- simple with the
  —PP displaced and angulated dorsally at nearly 90°,
  —puckering of palmar skin, and the
  —head of the MC palpable in the palm. Or the dislocation may be
- complex (Fig. 14.7)
  —usually the second MCP joint. Clinical features are
  —slight hyperextension (20° to 30°) of the MCP joint, with the
  —skin puckered in the proximal palmar crease overlying the dislocated MCP joint;
  —MC head is buttonholed through the anterior capsule. Reduction is prevented by the
  —volar plate, which is torn from the MC and interposed in the joint, and by the
  —superficial transverse ligament of the palmar fascia proximally and the
  —flexor tendons and lumbrical muscle medially and laterally, which close around the neck of the MC;
  —MC head is palpable in the palm;
- sesamoid bone appearing in the joint on x-ray is pathognomonic of a complex dislocation. The sesamoids lie in the volar plate. Do not confuse a sesamoid bone with an avulsion fracture.

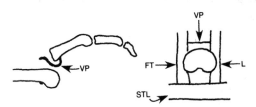

Figure 14.7. Complex dislocation of the second metacarpophalangeal joint. *VP*, volar plate and natatory ligament; *L*, lumbricals; *STL*, superficial transverse ligament; *FT*, flexor tendons and pretendinous band of midpalmar fascia.

TREATMENT

Collateral ligament tear

- immobilize with a splint or K wire in the overcorrected position for 3 weeks. Then start the patient on active motion.

Dislocation

Closed reduction

- always attempt gentle closed reduction first. With the patient under
- good anesthesia,
- dorsiflex the PP to 90°, then
- push distally on the base of the PP to lever it over the head of the MC;
- do not apply traction on the finger, as this may convert a simple dislocation into a complex dislocation by allowing the volar plate to become trapped in the joint space. If reduction is
- successful, apply
  —buddy taping for 3 weeks, with
  —early active motion. If reduction
- fails, operate.

Open reduction

- make anterior transverse incision 2 mm distal to palmar crease,
  —the MCP joint is not situated at the palmar-digital crease where the finger joins the palm but is
  —more proximal. Examine your own hand.
- beware of the digital neurovascular bundle which is stretched tightly over the MC head and is easily cut by the skin knife!
- remove the volar plate from the joint and reduce the joint. Then treat with
- buddy taping for 2 weeks and early active motion.

Thumb Metacarpophalangeal Subluxation and Dislocation

COLLATERAL LIGAMENT INJURY

Etiopathology

- the ulnar collateral ligament may be
  —stretched (gamekeeper's thumb),
  —partially torn or
  —completely torn (ski pole injury) and may be curled on itself beneath the adductor tendon or may lie superficial to it.
- less often, the radial collateral ligament is injured.

Diagnosis

- pain, tenderness and swelling over the injured ligament;
- x-ray may show avulsion fracture of the base of the PP.
- differentiate a stable lesion from an unstable lesion by injecting local anesthetic into the painful area and stressing the ligament in
  —abduction or valgus for the ulnar ligament and
  —adduction or varus for the radial ligament. If the lesion is
- unstable, take
  —stress x-rays and compare them with x-rays of the noninjured side to assess the
  —degree of instability and to
  —differentiate between partial tear and complete tear.

Treatment

Partial tear

- forearm scaphoid type plaster cast to the tip of the thumb with the MCP joint in slight flexion;
- remove 4 weeks later.

Complete tear

- indications for open reduction of recent injury are a
  —displaced avulsion fracture of the base of the PP or a
  —positive stress film showing wide unilateral opening of the joint space.

Ulnar collateral ligament

- open reduction through a
  —medial approach. If the
  —ligament is folded beneath the adductor tendon, release the tendon and suture it afterward; if an
  —avulsion fracture is present, replace and pin the fragment with two K wires; if the
  —ligament is torn through its center, suture it; if it is
  —torn from the attachment to bone, suture it to bone or use a pullout wire stretched over a button;
- scaphoid cast for 4 weeks.

Radial collateral ligament

- open reduction through a
  —lateral approach with a
  —technique of repair similar to that used for repair of the ulnar collateral ligament;
- cast for 4 to 6 weeks.

Old untreated injury

- clinical features include
  —pain, tenderness and swelling with weakness and instability, with the thumb "giving way" during pinch.
- for a symptomatic joint, either
  —reconstruct the ligament with a fascial graft or
  —fuse the joint.

DORSAL DISLOCATION

Etiopathology

- more frequent than in all other MCP joints together;
- caused by forced hyperextension;
- volar plate is torn from its attachment to the neck of the MC;
- collateral ligaments are often intact, but if one is torn, lateral instability after reduction will result;
- if the volar plate is interposed in the joint, consider this a complex dislocation which is irreducible by closed methods.

Diagnosis

- simple dislocation
  —phalanx angled at nearly 90° to the MC;
- complex dislocation
  —phalanx nearly parallel with the MC or angled at 20° to 30°, and there is a
  —skin dimple over the anterior surface of the thenar eminence;
  —sesamoid bone may be seen in the joint on x-ray. Sesamoids are incorporated into lateral margins of the volar plate and into tendons of thenar muscles.

Treatment

Simple dislocation

- closed reduction with the patient under anesthesia
  —hyperextend the MCP joint to 90°, then
  —push distally on the base of the PP and slide it over the head of the MC;
- do not pull on the thumb because
- traction may allow the volar plate to enter the joint and convert the simple, reducible dislocation into a complex, irreducible one;
- test collateral ligament stability immediately after reduction. If there is a rupture of collateral ligament with instability, treat this as outlined previously.
- cast for 3 weeks.

Complex dislocation
- make one attempt at closed reduction, and
- if you are succesful, continue as for simple dislocation;
- if you are not, perform
  —open reduction as for MCP dislocation in a finger. The
  —tendons of the flexor pollicis brevis (FPB) or the flexor pollicis longus (FPL) may also be interposed. Encourage
- early, protected active movement after surgery.

Proximal Interphalangeal Subluxation and Dislocation

ANATOMY
- PIP joint is important because the
  —normal PIP joint motion can compensate for stiffness of other small joints, whereas
  —the converse is not true; i.e., normal MCP and DIP joints cannot compensate for a stiff PIP joint.
- PIP joint quickly becomes stiff
  —if it is injured or
  —if it is normal but immobilized for too long, especially in the adult;
- PIP joint is a
  —hinge joint with flexion and extension but with no abduction, adduction or rotation;
  —collateral ligaments are tight in flexion and extension because they are attached proximally at the axis of rotation of the joint;
  —volar plate and accessory collateral ligaments are similar to that of the MCP joint;
  —extensor hood covers the joint dorsally and dorsolaterally.
- DIP joint subluxation or dislocation without a fracture is rare and is not considered here.

COLLATERAL LIGAMENT INJURIES OF PIP JOINT

Etiopathology
- caused by an adduction or abduction force with the finger extended;
- common in ball sports and wrestling;
- may be
  —stable, a sprain or partial tear, or
  —unstable, a complete tear;
- ligament is usually torn from its proximal attachment and may be folded into the joint;

- avulsion fracture of the base of the middle phalanx may occur too, especially in adolescents, as a Type III epiphyseal injury.

Diagnosis

- swelling and local tenderness with pain on lateral stress. If you
- suspect instability due to a complete rupture, take comparison stress x-rays.

Treatment

Stable

- buddy taping for 2 to 3 weeks, but warn the patient that pain and swelling may persist for 6 months or more.

Unstable

Recent

- closed reduction, splinting for 4 weeks, then buddy taping and active motion.
- indication for surgical repair is marked instability with either
  —interposition of ligament in the joint or a
  —displaced avulsion fracture at the insertion of the ligament. Through a
- collateral midline incision
- extract ligament from the joint and
- reattach it to bone or reduce and fix the epiphyseal fragment.
- cast for 3 weeks in 30° flexion, then
- guarded active movement.

Untreated, older than 6 weeks

- if the injury is symptomatic, with significant pain and disability,
  —reef the ligament if it is elongated, or
  —resuture it if that is possible, or
  —reconstruct it with a fascial graft.

VOLAR PLATE INJURIES OF PIP JOINT

Etiopathology and Diagnosis

- caused by a hyperextension force. The plate may be
- torn from its attachment to the base of the middle phalanx or the neck of the PP.
- local swelling and tenderness are present with
- pain on passive hyperextension;
- PIP joint may hyperextend and DIP joint may flex, i.e., the swan neck

deformity, when the patient actively extends the finger; or a flexion deformity may develop;
- pinch is weakened if the index finger is involved;
- x-rays are not helpful.

Treatment

Recent, within 6 weeks

- splinting of the PIP joint in 30° flexion for 3 weeks,
- then buddy taping with active movements for 2 weeks.

Old

- if the injury is symptomatic, with pain and disability, either
  —advance and reattach the volar plate, if possible, or perform
  —tenodesis with one limb of the FDS to prevent the last 15° of PIP joint extension.

DISLOCATIONS OF PIP JOINT

Etiopathology

- usually posterior due to a
  —hyperextension force;
  —volar plate and sometimes the collateral ligament are torn.
- anterior dislocation is rare. The central slip of extensor tendon tears and the extensor mechanism or the interposed volar plate may prevent reduction. With improper immobilization after reduction, a buttonhole deformity may develop (PIP flexed, DIP extended).

Treatment

Posterior dislocation

- closed reduction by traction, and if the joint is stable,
- buddy taping with active movements for 3 weeks; but if it is
- unstable after reduction, treat with a
  —splint for 3 weeks, with the PIP joint flexed 30°, then
  —buddy taping and active movements for 2 weeks.

Anterior dislocation

- try closed reduction first, and if this fails due to buttonholing or interposition of the volar plate, perform
- open reduction through a dorsal incision;
- immobilize the PIP joint in full extension for 5 weeks after reduction to allow central slip of the extensor tendon to heal, and thus prevent a buttonhole deformity;
- always verify reduction of both types of dislocation with x-rays.

Multiply-injured Hand

- apply basic guidelines as outlined previously.
- stabilize all unstable fractures and joint injuries with K wires, with the MCP joints (except the thumb) in flexion and the IP joints in extension;
- multiple MC fractures can be treated with external fixation by
  —transverse K wires glued to
  —longitudinal wires by acrylic cement.
- do not close the skin if the wound is
  —dirty, or
  —more than 6 hours old, or due to an
  —animal or human bite (teeth are always very dirty), or caused by a
  —firearm, or associated with a
  —severe crush injury;
- change the dressing in the operating room 2 or 3 days later, and if the wound is then clean,
  —close it without tension on the skin edges or cover it with a
  —split-thickness skin graft;
- if the wound is still dirty,
  —debride the wound further and
  —change the dressing 2 or 3 days later in the operating room. Repeat the process until the wound is clean and can be closed.
- after surgery, apply a
  —bulky, soft compression dressing,
  —elevate the arm, and start the patient on
  —early, active movements of the fingers to reduce edema and prevent permanent stiffness.

chapter 15

Fractures of the Pelvis and Pelvic Ring

Introduction

- 3% of all fractures are pelvic fractures;
- more common in adults than in children;
- road accidents, mainly motor vehicle accidents involving pedestrians, cause 75% of pelvic fractures;
- the pelvis is like a motor cyclist's helmet; when it is damaged, you worry more about the contents than about the helmet itself. This is because the
- danger to the patient is
  —not usually from the pelvic fracture but from
  —associated injuries to pelvic and abdominal viscera and small vessels;
- consequently, pelvic fractures have complications and a mortality rate second only to skull fractures;
- hemorrhage from a pelvic fracture alone may be severe enough to cause
  —hypovolemic shock, but because of the
- severity of the trauma, a patient with a pelvic fracture often has other major injuries too.

Mechanical Anatomy and Functions of the Pelvis

MECHANICAL ANATOMY

- the pelvis forms a ring. The
- upper half of the pelvis forms the femorosacral arch and
  —supports the spine and trunk. The arch is
  —supported by the two legs. A
- tie beam, the pubic rami, prevents the arch from spreading outward and being flattened. The
- arch is under compression while the
- tie beam is under tension.

- weak areas of the pelvic ring are the
  —symphysis pubis,
  —pubic rami and
  —ilium just lateral to the sacroiliac (SI) joint.

FUNCTIONS

- the pelvis protects viscera that lie inside it or pass through it. The ilia particularly are a source of hematopoietic bone marrow and a
- repository of
  —calcium,
  —phosphorus,
  —sodium and other minerals. The pelvis serves as an
- anchor for muscles of trunk and lower limb and
- supports the trunk.
- Howell (1944) summarized the functions of the pelvis:
  "Within its borders are housed a portion of the urinary and intestinal systems and the female genitalia; through its foramina pass the great nerve trunks and blood vessels, while beneath its arches pass all mankind with few exceptions, the most notable Julius Caesar."

General Clinical and Radiological Features

GENERAL

- for every motor vehicle accident victim, think of the pelvis. Unlike long bone fractures, pelvic injuries are rarely obvious. So
- assume that every victim of a serious accident has a pelvic fracture until you are sure that he does not.
- resuscitate the patient first, as necessaary; i.e., check the
  —airway,
  —breathing and
  —circulation, especially with an unstable pelvic injury in which hemorrhage may be massive. Then take a
- brief history and perform a
- complete clinical examination of the
  —head and neck,
  —chest,
  —abdomen and pelvis,
  —limbs (do not forget the peripheral neurovascular status) and
  —thoracic and lumbar spine, since
- major accident victims have a high incidence of multiple injuries;
- do not stop the examination when you find a fracture or a definite injury. Always complete every examination because
- there may be other injuries.

CLINICAL FEATURES

- swelling, ecchymoses, pain, tenderness and crepitus;
- palpate gently the subcutaneous parts of the pelvis, the
  —iliac crests and spines,
  —pubic and ischial rami and ischial tuberosity,
  —sacrum, coccyx and sacroiliac joints (under the dimple in women and children). If the patient is
- semiconscious, pelvic compression may elicit a pain response.
- examine both hips for pain and range of movement and measure the leg lengths. If both legs are intact, perform the
- FABER test by placing the
  —heel of one of the patient's feet on the patella of the other leg and
  —pushing the flexed leg outward. The hip is then in
  —*F*lexion,
  —*AB*duction and
  —*E*xternal *R*otation (*FABER*). This stresses the pelvic ring and causes
  —pain if the ring is broken. Perform a
- rectal examination and insert a
- urethral catheter if the patient has not passed clear urine since the accident.

RADIOLOGICAL EXAMINATION (Figs. 15.1 and 15.2)

- always ask for an anteroposterior (AP) radiograph of the pelvis if you
  —suspect a pelvic fracture or if the patient has been in a

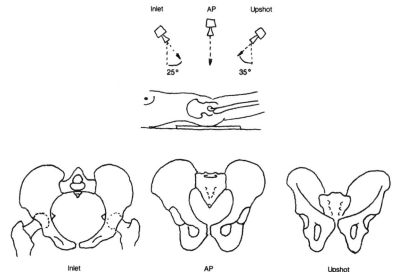

Figure 15.1. Three standard radiological views of the pelvic ring.

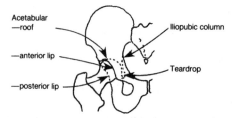

Figure 15.2. Five radiological pelvic landmarks.

—serious accident and is
—unconscious or has a
—fracture of the patella or femur or an
—abdominal injury. If
- major pelvic ring fracture can be seen on the AP view, take an
  —inlet view to show lateral or medial displacement and rotation and an
  —upshot view to show proximal or distal displacement or rotation. When
- examining x-rays of the pelvis,
  —compare one side with the other and
  —scrutinize all bony components and their relationships with each other, the
  —roof,
  —anterior and
  —posterior margins of the acetabulum, and medially the
  —iliopubic column and the
  —"teardrop." Compare the
  —sacroiliac joints and the
  —symphysis pubis, and
  —look at margins of the sacral nerve root foramina;
- in children, fractures at the
  —symphysis pubis or the
  —sacroiliac region may be
  —epiphyseal injuries at the chondroosseous junction.

Etiology and Treatment

STABLE FRACTURES OF PELVIS (Fig. 15.3)

- isolated fracture or
- single break in the pelvic ring.

Avulsion of apophyses

- usually occurs in young athletes;
- anterosuperior or inferior iliac spines may be avulsed by the sartorius or

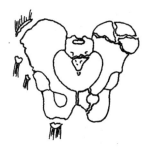

Avulsion injuries   Fractures

Figure 15.3. Stable pelvic injuries. Avulsion injuries, usually in adolescents.

the straight head of the rectus femoris;
- ischial tuberosity can be pulled off by hamstrings, the biceps femoris, the semimembranosus and the semitendonosus.
- treatment is symptomatic with
  —analgesics and
  —rest.
- all heal well within 8 weeks.

Fracture of single ramus

- isolated fracture of the pubic or ischial ramus is the
- most common fracture of the pelvis and often occurs in
- elderly people. Differentiate carefully between this and a hip fracture because the treatment is different!
- treat symptomatically, with weight-bearing as tolerated.

Fractures of ipsilateral rami

- isolated fractures of both rami on the same side do not displace;
- FABER test is positive;
- treat symptomatically.

Isolated fracture of iliac wing

- called Duverney's fracture,
- caused by a direct blow,
- often comminuted but
- usually not displaced because the surrounding muscles splint the bone;
- treat symptomatically.

Isolated sacral fracture

- usually horizontal at the distal end of SI joints;
- fracture is difficult to see, so examine carefully the superior margins of anterior sacral foramina through which the sacral nerve roots exit. This fracture is

- occasionally associated with sacral nerve root damage, i.e., S1 and S2, so examine the motor function and sensation of the lower limbs, particularly
  —glutei muscles, which extend and abduct the hip,
  —hamstrings, which flex the knee,
  —calf muscles, which plantar flex the ankle,
  —Achilles tendon reflex, and
  —sensation over the outer border of the foot;
- treat symptomatically. Nerve injuries usually recover spontaneously unless the fracture is very displaced.

Coccyx

- occurs more frequently in women than in men;
- treat symptomatically;
- a rubber ring is helpful during sitting, preventing pressure over the coccyx;
- if pain persists more than 2 months, infiltrate the area with local anesthetic and steroid;
- removal of the coccyx is seldom indicated and is not helpful.

Others

- subluxation of the symphysis pubis or SI joints is
- rare;
- FABER test is positive;
- treat symptomatically.

UNSTABLE FRACTURES OF PELVIC RING

General observations

- comprise about one third of all pelvic ring fractures in adults but are much less common in children;
- are usually caused by severe trauma, either direct or indirect, through the lever arm of the femur and hip joint;
- occult hemorrhage is usual and
- associated injuries are common.
- displacement of the fracture is due to
  —original trauma and to
  —muscle pull on the floating segment, but it is
  —less common in children due to a thicker periosteum and incomplete fracture through cartilage.
- most of these unstable pelvic fractures in adults can be treated closed by
  —femoral traction or
  —hip spica. But if the fracture is
  —very unstable or

—abdominal or peripheral surgery is necessary, stabilization by
—external fixation may be indicated;
• open reduction and internal fixation of pelvic ring fractures are seldom indicated because
• accurate reduction is
—difficult,
—hazardous, and
—usually unnecessary. But a
• woman of child-bearing age with
—malunion of a pelvic ring fracture may require
—cesarean section for childbirth, and
—you must warn her of this.
• children require only bed rest. Closed reduction is rarely indicated and open reduction is exceptional.

Anteroposterior compression injury (Figs. 15.4 and 15.5)

Etiopathology

• caused by a violent blow to the front of the pubis;
• common associated injuries are to the

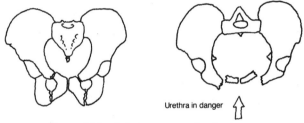

Urethra in danger

Figure 15.4. Anterior compression fractures.

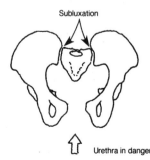

Subluxation

Urethra in danger

Figure 15.5. Diastasis of the pubis by anterior compression.

—urethra, especially in men, and the

—rectum.

- two types of injury are common:

Straddle fracture

- bilateral fracture of both pubic rami;
- the central portion is displaced backward, carrying the membranous urethra with it;
- the amount of displacement is seen on the inlet view.

Separation of symphysis pubis

- diastasis is always associated either with
  —subluxation or dislocation of one or both sacroiliac joints or with
  —fractures around one or both SI joints. The
- two halves of the pelvis open like a book, and one or both legs are in external rotation. The
- amount of displacement is seen best on the AP view.

Treatment

Bilateral pubic fractures

- bed rest,
- analgesics and
- weight-bearing when the fractures have healed.

Diastasis less than 3 cm

- treat with bed rest and analgesics, followed by
- physiotherapy and graduated weight-bearing after 12 weeks.

Diastasis more than 3 cm

- use a pelvic sling, but
  —take x-rays with the patient in the sling to avoid overcorrection and overlap, and
  —watch for pressure sores beneath the sling;
  —remove the sling at 6 weeks and treat with
  —physiotherapy, with progressive weight-bearing begun at 12 weeks.
- alternative method is
  —closed reduction of diastasis with the patient under general anesthesia and on his side
  —and bilateral plaster spica with the hip in
  —15° abduction and
  —full internal rotation.
- if the pelvis is very unstable, or the fracture is open, or surgery or wound care in the abdomen, pelvis or perineum is necessary, or there are fractures of the lower limbs, use external fixation with

    —three vertical pins in each iliac crest and
    —two crossbars tightened after reduction.
- failure of these methods may be an indication for
    —open reduction of the symphysis and
    —internal fixation with a plate through
    —Pfannenstiel's incision.
- if pain over the symphysis persists for 6 to 12 months and is disabling, fusion of the symphysis with iliac bone block may be necessary.

Lateral compression injury (Fig. 15.6)

Etiopathology

- caused by a violent lateral force;
- anteriorly, both rami break on one side and
- posteriorly, on the same side, and either the
    —SI joint dislocates or the
    —ilium or sacrum fractures;
- then the large fracture fragment which contains the acetabulum and the hip joint swings inward on the posterior hinge, like a door opening into a room. The amount of displacement is seen only on the inlet view.
- a commonly associated injury is
    —extraperitoneal rupture of the bladder, especially if it is full, as, for example, on Friday night! The rupture is caused by
    —sharp ends of fractured rami moving inward to pierce the distended and immobile bladder wall;
- sacral nerve roots may also be injured.

Treatment

- skeletal traction through the supracondylar region of the ipsilateral femur with the hip and knee flexed 20°;
- when the hemipelvis is reduced, either

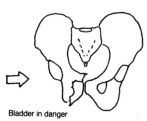
Bladder in danger

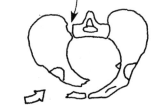
Subluxation

Figure 15.6. Lateral compression fracture.

—continue with traction for 6 weeks, then apply a spica for 6 weeks, or apply a

—spica with the hip in abduction and external rotation to maintain reduction for 12 weeks;

- then start the patient on physiotherapy and graduated weight-bearing;
- external fixation is excellent when indicated, as discussed previously;
- when the SI joint is dislocated, delay weight-bearing for 16 weeks after fracture. Pain at the SI joint may persist even then, and unilateral SI fusion may be necessary at 6 months to 1 year, depending on the severity of the symptoms.

Vertical shear injury (Fig. 15.7)

Etiopathology

- Malgaigne fracture;
- anterior component of the injury is
  —fracture of the rami or
  —dislocation of the symphysis pubis;
- posterior component of the injury is
  —dislocation of the SI joint or fracture of the ilium or sacrum on the same side as the fractured rami, which is similar to lateral compression injury, but the
- hemipelvis is
  —displaced en bloc proximally or distally in the sagittal plane or
  —swings upward or downward on an anterior or a posterior hinge, creating an apparent leg length discrepancy;
- hemipelvis may also displace posteriorly as well.
- the amount of proximal or distal displacement is seen only on the upshot view; backward displacement is seen on the inlet view.

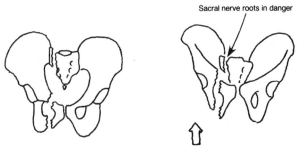

Sacral nerve roots in danger

Figure 15.7. Vertical shear injury.

Treatment

Upward displacement

- skeletal traction with the hip in slight flexion,
- pin just proximal to the femoral condyles, then
- spica after 6 weeks.

Downward or backward displacement

- femoral supracondylar skeletal traction with the
  —hip flexed 90° and the
  —knee flexed 90°, the so-called 90/90 traction;
- 6 weeks later, spica with the hip and knee semiflexed;
- then physiotherapy and graduated weight-bearing.

External fixation

- similar indications for other pelvic ring fractures (see previous discussion).

Combined vertical shear and AP compression injury (Fig. 15.8)

Etiopathology

- the "bucket handle" injury;
- posteriorly there is SI dislocation or fracture of the ilium or sacrum on the same side as the trauma, whereas
- anteriorly both rami break on the opposite, contralateral side;
- hemipelvis swings upward and medially, like a bucket handle, with one hinge at the SI joint and the other hinge at the fracture of the contralateral rami;
- fractured rami displace and may overlap, puncturing the wall of a full bladder or tearing the bladder wall during reduction. There is an
- apparent leg length discrepancy.

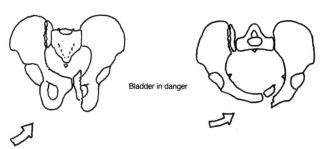

Bladder in danger

Figure 15.8.   Combined vertical shear and anterior compression injury.

Treatment

- skeletal traction through the femur on the affected side for 6 weeks, with the hip and knee slightly flexed; then
- spica with the ipsilateral hip in
  —abduction and
  —external rotation. Or
- reduction with the patient under anesthesia and spica as discussed previously.
- external fixation for the same indications as discussed previously.
- physiotherapy at 12 weeks with graduated weight-bearing.

"Humpty Dumpty" pelvic fracture

- combination of fractures with total disruption of the pelvic ring;
- caused by very severe trauma;
- likelihood of other injuries and complications is very high;
- treat the fracture with
  —bed rest,
  —traction where necessary, and
  —no weight-bearing for 16 weeks.

Complications and Associated Injuries

EARLY

Hemorrhage

- all pelvic fractures bleed, and this is the major cause of death;
- blood may fill the extraperitoneal space in the pelvis and the retroperitoneal space in the abdomen.
- initial treatment of a severe pelvic fracture must be
  —fluid volume replacement with
  —whole blood or with
  —plasma volume expanders until blood is ready;
- do not wait until the patient is in shock before ordering and giving blood;
- monitor the vital signs, especially
  —hourly urine output, and
- reexamine the patient frequently.
- laparotomy to arrest hemorrhage is not advised because it may
  —increase morbidity and mortality by
  —releasing the tamponade effect and increasing the risk of
  —infection;
- ligation of one or both internal iliac arteries is rarely indicated because the rich pelvic anastomoses bypass the arteries.

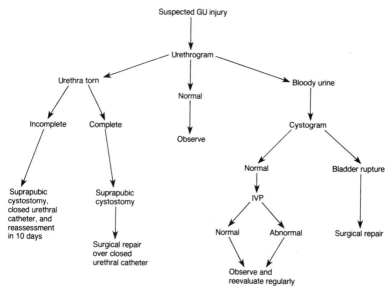

Figure 15.9. Flow chart for diagnosis and treatment of suspected genitourinary injury. *GU*, genitourinary; *IVP*, intravenous pyelogram.

Intrapelvic visceral injuries (Fig. 15.9)

- urinary bladder and urethral injuries are common with disruptive pelvic injury;
- untreated bladder rupture always kills, usually by infection;
- suspect a urinary tract injury when the patient
- fails to urinate or there is
- blood in the
  —urine (kidney or bladder injury) or in the
  —urethral meatus (urethral injury);
- difficulty or inability to catheterize the patient suggests a urethral injury. A
- displaced prostate on rectal examination indicates
  —urethral transection above the perineal diaphragm, whereas a
- perineal hematoma confined by attachments of Buck's or Colles' fascia signifies
  —urethral disruption below the diaphragm.
- management is outlined in Figure 15.9
- primary elements of treatment of bladder or urethral injuries are
  —suprapubic drainage,

—repair of intraperitoneal bladder rupture and inframembranous urethral transection;

—alignment over a Foley catheter for disruption of the supramembranous urethra, and

—adequate local drainage of the retropubic space of Retzius;

- posterior urethral injury is often followed by impotence.
- the rectum is seldom injured other than by perineal laceration. Treat initially with a
  —defunctioning colostomy.

Neurological injuries

- uncommon unless the patient has a sacral fracture or a SI disruption;
- fifth lumbar and first and second sacral roots are the most vulnerable;
- no initial treatment, but record initial findings and
- reexamine the patient regularly for a change in status.

LATE

Loss of reduction

- if traction is removed or the patient bears weight too soon, reduction may be lost. This may lead to
- malunion which is
  —common but rarely causes symptoms;
- vaginal childbirth may be dangerous for both the mother and the child.
- nonunion is rare and does not need surgery unless the injury is symptomatic, in which case a graft is used.

Thrombophlebitis

- infrequent, but because it may cause a fatal embolus, you must
  —recognize it early and

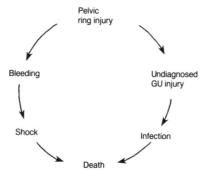

Figure 15.10. Major complications of pelvic ring injuries. *GU*, genitourinary.

—treat it promptly. It may be
- prevented by
  —elastic stockings or a bandage and by
  —daily, active muscle exercises of both legs.
- do not use anticoagulants.

Sacroiliac arthritis
- associated with SI joint subluxation or dislocation;
- fuse if symptoms are uncontrolled by nonoperative measures.

Summary (Fig. 15.10)
- the pelvic fracture itself will not kill the patient, but
- hemorrhage and
- associated injuries might;
- avoid these complications by
  —immediate blood volume replacement and
  —early recognition and treatment of bladder or urethral injury.

chapter 16
Acetabular Fractures and Traumatic Dislocations of the Hip

Introduction

- acetabular fractures
  —functionally involve the hip more than the pelvis and are
  —often associated with hip dislocations;
- they are caused by major trauma, so
  —associated injuries and
  —injuries to other systems, e.g., the head, chest and abdomen, are common;
- an acetabular fracture may be missed if there are other fractures of the same leg, e.g., of the femur or tibia, so
- with any patient with severe trauma from a motor vehicle or industrial accident,
  —think of the
  —pelvis and hips and
  —x-ray them.
- acetabular fractures are less common in children, and
- posterior dislocation of the hip in a child is rarely accompanied by a posterior lip fracture.

Acetabular Fractures

SURGICAL ANATOMY (Fig. 16.1)

- the acetabulum is built of two columns, anterior and posterior, joined by an arch which forms the roof. The
- anterior column is built from the anteroinferior part of the ilium and the superior pubic ramus. The
- posterior column consists of parts of the ilium and ischium and is thicker and stronger than the anterior column. The
- roof is hard iliac bone.

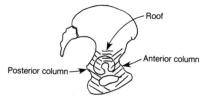

Figure 16.1. Acetabular columns.

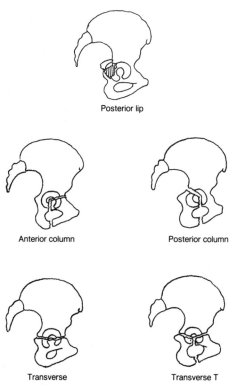

Figure 16.2. Acetabular fractures.

ETIOLOGY (Fig. 16.2)

Anterior blow on knee

- force is transmitted along the femur from a blow on the flexed knee with the hip flexed; e.g., a

—passenger in a car hits his knee on the dashboard or a
—motorcyclist hits another vehicle with his knee. With a
- hip in adduction, there is usually a
  —posterior hip dislocation but no acetabular fracture. With a
- hip in neutral rotation, there may be a
  —fracture of the posterior acetabular lip, which is often associated with a posterior hip dislocation. With a
- hip in moderate abduction, there is a
  —fracture of the posterior column, usually without dislocation. With a
- hip in wide abduction, there is a
  —transverse fracture of the acetabulum and central dislocation of the hip.

Lateral blow on greater trochanter

- force is transmitted along the femoral head and neck to the acetabulum. With a
- hip in internal rotation, a
  —fracture of the posterior column results. With a
- hip in neutral rotation, there is a
  —central fracture-dislocation. With a
- hip in external rotation, the
  —anterior column may fracture.

PATHOLOGY

Hemorrhage

- pelvic bones and surrounding soft tissues are very vascular and bleed a lot, so
- hemorrhage is moderate or severe, causing
- hypovolemic shock, and may even
- kill the patient if it is untreated.

Cartilaginous damage

- articular cartilage of the acetabulum and femoral head is
  —usually damaged with undisplaced fractures and is
  —always damaged with displaced fractures, due to the compressive force of the injury;
- small flakes of cartilage may be knocked off and may lodge in the synovial cavity, causing later symptoms of
  —intra-articular foreign bodies and
  —chronic synovitis;
- cartilage damage is a prelude to
  —degenerative osteoarthritis.

- cartilage nutrition is improved and the risk of degenerative changes and stiffness is reduced if the joint is not immobilized for too long. For hip dislocations and acetabular fractures,
  —traction or surgery, followed by
  —early mobilization and
  —physiotherapy, is the key to reasonable functional recovery.

Blood supply of femoral head

- is delicate and easily damaged, with resultant
- partial or complete avascular necrosis. The probability of this complication
  —increases with the delay between injury and treatment.

CLASSIFICATION (Fig. 16.2)

- is based on the position of the fracture line;
- posterior lip fracture is usually associated with posterior dislocation of the hip; with fracture of the
- posterior column, the fracture line usually crosses the
  —ilioischial column, then runs down through
  —both pubic rami across the obturator foramen; with fracture of the
- anterior column, the fracture line crosses the
  —iliopubic column and
  —both pubic rami;
- the transverse fracture line proceeds
  —straight across both columns;
- the transverse T fracture line crosses
  —both columns with the stem of the T down through
  —both pubic rami.

RADIOLOGICAL DIAGNOSIS (Fig. 16.3)

Anteroposterior (AP) x-ray of pelvis

- you should be able to see or at least suspect a fracture of the acetabulum on an AP x-ray of the pelvis;
- to determine the exact position and configuration of the fracture, order two lateral oblique views.

Lateral oblique x-rays

- the internal oblique x-ray shows the
  —anterior column and the
  —posterior lip of the acetabulum;
- the external oblique x-ray shows the
  —posterior column and the
  —anterior lip of the acetabulum.

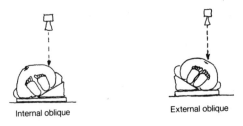

Internal oblique   External oblique

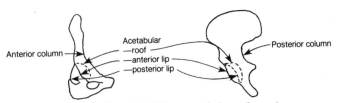

Figure 16.3. Standard oblique acetabular radiographs.

Tomography and CAT scan

- helpful both preoperatively and postoperatively in visualizing bone or cartilage fragments lodged in the acetabulum.

Interpretation

- answers to the following questions are important because they affect the treatment and prognosis:
  —where is the fracture?
  —what is fractured?
  —does the fracture cross the acetabular roof which is the weight-bearing area of the acetabulum?
  —are the fragments displaced?
  —is the fracture comminuted? (There may be fragments in the joint.)
  —is the femoral head subluxed or dislocated?

TREATMENT OF UNDISPLACED FRACTURES

- bed rest, analgesics, and
- longitudinal traction with gentle active and passive exercises for 6 weeks, then mobilization with
- non-weight-bearing (NWB) on the injured side for 6 weeks. If the patient

- walks on the hip too soon, he is more likely to have
  - —pain and
  - —degenerative osteoarthritic changes later.

TREATMENT OF DISPLACED FRACTURES

Posterior lip fracture (Fig. 16.4)

With hip dislocation

- associated hip dislocation must be reduced as soon as possible to diminish the likelihood of avascular necrosis of the femoral head;
- test the reduction for stability, then put the leg in
- traction to maintain reduction, and plan treatment of the acetabular fracture.

Stable reduction

- if the hip is stable and there are no fracture fragments in the acetabulum, treat with
  - —3 weeks of traction with exercises, or
  - —spica, followed by
  - —9 weeks of NWB.

Unstable reduction

- if the hip is unstable, with the femoral head dislocating posteriorly in flexion and adduction, or the hip is
- not completely reduced, perform
  - —open reduction through the posterior approach,
  - —dislocate the hip gently, and
  - —irrigate the acetabulum to remove flakes of bone and cartilage; then
  - —reduce the hip,
  - —reduce the posterior lip, and
  - —fix it with a molded plate and screws;
  - —make sure that the screws are not in the acetabulum!

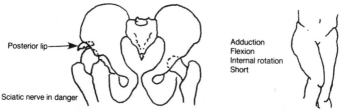

Posterior lip

Sciatic nerve in danger

Adduction
Flexion
Internal rotation
Short

Figure 16.4.   Posterior fracture-dislocation of the hip.

—then treat with traction and exercises for 6 weeks or with a spica, followed by NWB for 6 more weeks.

Without hip dislocation

- is unusual. Treat by
- traction for 4 weeks, then
- NWB for 8 weeks. But if there is an associated
- sciatic nerve lesion,
  —explore the nerve without delay and
  —reduce or excise the bone fragment.

Central fracture-dislocation (Fig. 16.5)

Intact acetabular roof

Without hip dislocation

- the femoral head is in normal relationship with the acetabular dome. Treat by
- longitudinal traction with exercises for 4 weeks, then NWB for 6 weeks.

With hip dislocation

- the femoral head is subluxed relative to the intact portion of the acetabular roof;
- attempt
  —closed reduction and
  —maintain the reduction by longitudinal and lateral traction of up to 20% of the patient's body weight. If this is successful,
- reduce traction to 10% of the patient's body weight after a few days and
- continue traction for 6 weeks and NWB for 6 more weeks. Start the patient on

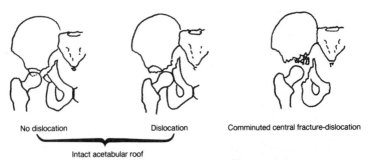

No dislocation   Dislocation   Comminuted central fracture-dislocation

Intact acetabular roof

Figure 16.5. Central fracture and fracture-dislocations.

- active and passive exercises early or
- apply a hip spica for 6 weeks, followed by NWB for 6 weeks;
- take x-rays at regular intervals to monitor the position of the femoral head. If
- attempted closed reduction is
- unsuccessful, consider
- open reduction and internal fixation of the fracture through an
  —anterior or
  —posterior approach for the respective column or
  —both approaches or a triradiate approach for both columns. This is difficult surgery, so be thoughtful and careful!

Comminuted acetabular roof fracture

- the "Humpty Dumpty" pelvis;
- ignore the fracture-dislocation and try to
- restore function early;
- treat with
  —longitudinal traction with
  —exercises for 4 weeks, then NWB for another 8 weeks;
- do not attempt to reduce the hip or to reduce or fix the fracture.

Traumatic Hip Dislocation in Adults

ETIOPATHOLOGY

- usually is caused by severe trauma, with hip in adduction or wide abduction;
- there is major disruption of the soft tissues, the
- capsule is torn, and
- retinacular vessels which supply the femoral head may be
  —ruptured or
  —contused and thrombosed or
  —compressed. The dislocation may be accompanied by
- cartilaginous or bony fractures of
  —acetabulum or
  —femoral head;
- the sciatic nerve is vulnerable, as it lies directly behind the head;
- posterior dislocation is caused by a blow on the knee, with the knee and hip flexed at the time of injury. If the hip is
  —adducted, there is usually no fracture, but if the hip is in
  —neutral rotation or slight abduction when injured, the
  —posterior acetabular lip fractures (see previous discussion).
- for central fracture-dislocation, see the previous discussion.

- anterior dislocation is rare and is caused by leverage on the thigh with the hip in
  —abduction,
  —flexion and
  —external rotation.

POSTERIOR DISLOCATION

Clinical and radiological features

- the leg is in
  —adduction,
  —15° to 30° of flexion, and
  —internal rotation and is
- shortened (Fig. 16.4);
- sciatic nerve injury, especially of the lateral part which contains fibers of the common peroneal nerve, occurs in 10% of posterior dislocations, so test for motor power and sensation in the leg and foot;
- the acetabulum is empty and the
- femoral head is
  —lateral and
  —superior to the acetabulum on an AP x-ray and
  —behind it on a lateral x-ray of the pelvis;
- a posterior lip fracture is best seen on the
  —internal oblique view;
- dislocation is classified by Stewart and Milford according to whether there is
  —no associated fracture (Grade I), a
  —fracture of the posterior acetabular lip (Grades II and III), or a
  —fracture of the femoral head (Grade IV).

Treatment

Without fracture

Closed reduction

- immediate closed reduction with the patient under anesthesia;
- place the patient on his back on a low stretcher or on the floor, and with a
- strong assistant holding the pelvis,
- put traction on the leg in the line of the deformity and gradually
- flex the hip and knee to 90°, then
- pull gently upward on the leg with the hip in neutral;
- if the head does not reduce, gently rotate the hip internally and externally until it does;
- reduction is signified by a "clunk."

- then test for stability with the hip in abduction, neutral rotation and adduction and in extension and flexion.

Stable closed reduction

- if the reduction is stable, put the hip in traction (4 or 5 kg) in
  —15° flexion,
  —25° abduction, and
  —neutral rotation. Start the patient on
- isometric, active muscle exercises.
- maintain skin traction for 3 weeks, then treat with
  —active mobilization of the hip, NWB for 3 more weeks, and afterward,
  —graduated weight-bearing with use of crutches.

Instability

- if the reduction is unstable and the hip easily dislocates again, there may be a fracture that you have missed, so
  —reexamine the x-rays carefully and
  —take new views if necessary, including
  —tomograms and a
  —CAT scan. Follow the plan outlined previously for a fracture-dislocation.

Failed closed reduction

- if closed reduction fails, usually due to a fracture fragment, button-holing of the capsule, or other soft tissue interposition, perform
  —open reduction, fixing the fracture as necessary, followed by
  —traction as discussed previously.

Associated with fracture

Posterior acetabular lip fracture

- with a small fragment, treat as if there were "no fracture";
- with a large fragment but with stable reduction (Grade II), maintain traction or a spica for 6 weeks, then treat with NWB for 6 weeks;
- with a large fragment and instability (Grade III) in spite of 4 weeks of traction, perform
  —open reduction of the fracture and
  —internal fixation (see previous discussion).

Femoral head fracture

- fortunately this is rare;
- the fragment may reduce spontaneously as you reduce the dislocation. If so, treat with a
  —spica for 8 weeks and

—NWB for 8 more weeks;
- if the fragment is still displaced after reduction,
- open the hip joint through a posterior approach and either
  —excise the fragment, if it is very small, or reduce and fix it with countersunk screws, if it is large and on the weight-bearing surface;
- prognosis for this injury is poor.
- for a comminuted fracture, treat with traction and early mobilization.

CENTRAL FRACTURE-DISLOCATION
- see the previous discussion.

ANTERIOR DISLOCATION
Clinical and radiological features
- less than 10% of all hip dislocations are anterior;
- the femoral head may lodge near the
  —obturator foramen or in front of the
  —superior pubic ramus or the
  —ilium;
- the leg lies in
  —abduction and external rotation and is either
  —flexed with obturator dislocation or
  —extended with iliac or pubic dislocation. The
- femoral artery, vein and nerve may be compressed, so neurovascular examination of the leg is important.
- on x-ray the
  —acetabulum is empty. The
- femoral head is
  —always medial to the acetabulum and will be
  —superior in the iliac position or
  —inferior in the obturator position.
- fractures of the anterior acetabular lip or femoral head are rare.

Treatment
- early closed reduction. With the patient on a low table or on the floor, under anesthesia, and an assistant stabilizing the pelvis, apply
- gentle traction in the direction of the thigh, then
- gradual flexion of the hip and knee with the hip in neutral rotation. If the dislocation does not reduce, gently rotate the thigh, but
- do not force the reduction. If gentle manipulation fails, perform
  —open reduction through the lower half of an iliofemoral (Smith-Peterson) approach;

- treat an acetabular or femoral head fracture the same as a posterior fracture-dislocation;
- after reduction, put the leg in traction or a spica for 3 weeks with the hip in
  —15° flexion,
  —15° internal rotation, and
  —neutral abduction, followed by
- mobilization with NWB for 3 more weeks.

UNTREATED POSTERIOR DISLOCATION

2 to 8 weeks old

Traction

- transfemoral traction for 1 week with 10 to 15 kg, then x-ray of the hip.
- do not manipulate the hip because you might break the femoral neck.
- if the hip does not reduce with traction, perform open reduction.

Surgery

- open reduction through an
  —anterior approach;
  —beware of the sciatic nerve! Do not strip soft tissue attachments from the femoral neck;
  —gently reduce the hip in flexion and adduction, using a lever on the head and traction on the femur;
  —if soft tissues are still too tight, release muscle attachments to the lesser and greater trochanters and try again.

Postoperative care

- postoperative traction with the hip in abduction and internal rotation for 6 weeks, and early motion in traction to avoid stiffness;
- NWB for 12 weeks. The
- head is almost certainly dead and may ultimately require an
  —extra-articular fusion or a
  —replacement arthroplasty.

More than 8 weeks old

- traction for 1 week, then
- soft tissue release. If the hip does not reduce easily, close the wound,
- continue skeletal traction, and verify the position of the femoral head with x-rays. If the hip does not reduce with traction but the head is opposite the acetabulum, perform
- open reduction at the second operation. The patient may need
  —fusion or
  —arthroplasty at a later date.

More than 1 year old

- if the hip is painless and mobile, but there is a marked flexion and adduction deformity, perform
  —intertrochanteric osteotomy to correct this. If the hip is
- stiff and painful,
  —resect the head and neck.
- do not attempt open reduction.

Traumatic Hip Dislocation in Children

- only three joints commonly dislocate in children, the
  —hip, which dislocates more frequently than the femoral neck fractures, the
  —metacarpophalangeal joint, and the
  —patellofemoral joint. The
- hip dislocates easily in a child under 5 years old but requires more severe trauma as a child grows older.
- clinical features are similar to those in an adult.
- treatment is
  —gentle, closed reduction as soon as possible with the patient under general anesthesia with good muscle relaxation. If reduction is rough, the femoral capital epiphysis may be knocked off;
  —test hip movements for crepitus and take
  —x-rays to confirm concentric reduction and to be sure that there is no epiphyseal plate injury with displacement of the femoral head epiphysis. Follow this with
  —skin traction for 5 days, then a
  —hip spica for 4 to 6 weeks. The
- femoral head and acetabulum are mainly cartilaginous in a young child and seldom fracture. Radiolucent fragments may lodge in the joint and
  —prevent complete reduction. They can be seen on a CAT scan or an arthrogram. If they are left in the joint, they will
  —cause pain and
  —limit movement after the cast is removed;
- avascular necrosis is less common in children than in adults and occurs in about 10% of older children. It is rare in children under 5 years old. Major predisposing factors of necrosis are
  —severe injury and
  —delayed reduction. In general, the
- results and prognosis are better for children than for adults.

Complications of Acetabular Fractures and Traumatic Hip Dislocation

EARLY

Sciatic nerve injury

- occurs with posterior dislocations and especially with fracture-dislocations because the nerve passes directly behind the posterior acetabular lip and the femoral head;
- its incidence is about 10%;
- reduction of the dislocation to relieve pressure on the nerve is urgent to avoid permanent nerve damage;
- explore and decompress the nerve when there is a large fracture fragment;
- partial or complete recovery may occur in half of the patients. Meanwhile,
- prevent
  —equinus by holding the ankle at a right angle and prevent
  —pressure sores.

Infection

- the infection rate after open reduction is high.

Thrombophlebitis

- is a common complication in pelvic and leg veins, no matter how the injury is treated.

LATE

Avascular necrosis of femoral head

- the incidence of necrosis with a dislocation is between 10% and 15% if reduction is early and up to 100% if reduction is delayed;
- the incidence is increased by
  —severity of the trauma,
  —associated fractures of the acetabulum or femoral head,
  —difficulty in closed reduction,
  —open reduction, and
  —long delay between the injury and the reduction. The
- radiological evidence may not appear for 2 years after injury.

Degenerative arthrosis

- incidence is
  —10% with a simple dislocation and
  —25% with a fracture-dislocation;
- incidence is increased by

—severity of the trauma, partly due to cartilage fractures and death of chondrocytes,

—fracture into the dome of the acetabulum, the weight-bearing part,

—fracture of the femoral head,

—comminuted acetabular fracture,

—poor reduction, and

—instability of the hip joint. Arthrosis

- usually appears early but may not appear before 5 or more years after injury.

Premature closure of triradiate cartilage

- may occur in a young patient with acetabular fracture and will result in a
- disparity of growth and size between the
  —femoral head and the
  —acetabulum;
- pelvic osteotomy to improve coverage of the head may be necessary.

chapter 17

Femoral Neck and Intertrochanteric Fractures

Femoral Neck Fractures in Adults

SURGICAL ANATOMY

Femoral head

- the femoral head is not a perfect sphere. It is
- congruous with the acetabulum only in the weight-bearing position;
- malunion of a proximal femoral fracture alters this congruity.

Trabecular pattern (Fig. 17.1)

- trabeculae are aligned along lines of stress:
  —medial trabeculae are almost vertical, strengthen the calcar femorale, and are under compression;
  —arcuate trabeculae are almost horizontal, are arched with the convexity cephalad, and are under tension;
- malunion causes realignment of trabeculae;
- medial cortex of the femoral neck, the calcar femorale, is thick and strong;
- lateral cortex is thin and weak.
- force across the hip joint is
  —2½ times the body weight if a person is standing on one leg,
  —½ the body weight if a person is lying flat in bed, due to muscle tone, and
  —1½ times the body weight if a person is lying in bed and lifting the other leg.

Blood supply (Fig. 6.2)

- blood supply of the femoral head is mainly through posterior retinacular arteries which lie beneath the capsule and synovium directly on the surface of the neck and are easily injured by fractures, with consequent avascular necrosis of the head;
- these vessels arise from rich anastomoses around the intertrochanteric and basal neck areas;

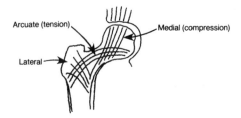

Figure 17.1. Femoral trabecular pattern.

- the artery of the head, in the ligamentum teres, is of little significance in the adult. It enters the head through the fovea.

Soft tissue attachments

- there are no periosteal or muscle attachments on the neck, so there is no subperiosteal callus in neck fractures. The neck grows in width through a layer of physeal growth cartilage on the posterosuperior part of the neck. The
- capsule is attached to the
  —middle of the neck posteriorly and to the
  —intertrochanteric line in front, so
- most of the neck is intracapsular. The
- abductors and external rotators of the hip are attached to the
  —greater trochanter and to the
  —intertrochanteric crest posteriorly.

ETIOPATHOLOGY

- a major predisposing factor of hip fractures is osteoporosis. The fracture
- may start as a stress fracture in this pathological bone and is completed by a minor twisting injury or fall.
- fractures of the neck are classified by region:
  —subcapital, separating the head from the neck,
  —cervical, through the neck, and
  —basicervical, through the base of the neck;
- they are further classified into
  —incomplete or impacted,
  —complete undisplaced,
  —displaced and
  —comminuted fractures. Comminution is usually of the posterior cortex and makes reduction very unstable. The
- fracture line is usually spiral, caused by
  —rotational forces, and even an
- undisplaced or impacted fracture is

—potentially unstable and can

—displace on bed rest alone.

CLINICAL AND RADIOLOGICAL FEATURES (Figs. 17.2 and 17.3)

Impacted and undisplaced subcapital fractures

- the patient may have mild pain or discomfort in the groin, or pain may be referred to the knee through the sensory branch of the obturator nerve;

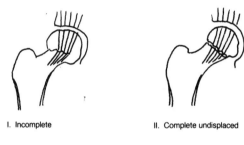

I. Incomplete   II. Complete undisplaced

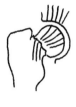   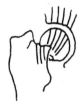

III. Partial displacement   IV. Complete displacement

Figure 17.2. Classification of subcapital fractures. Anteroposterior view. (Modified from Garden RS: Low angle fixation in fractures of the femoral neck. *J Bone Joint Surg* 43B:647–663, 1961.)

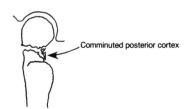

Comminuted posterior cortex

Figure 17.3. Unstable subcapital fracture. Lateral view.

- walking without help may be possible, but it will be with a limp;
- passive and active movement produces a little discomfort, and there may be
- pain on pressure anteriorly or posteriorly over the femoral neck.
- x-rays and tomograms may not show a stress fracture, and a radioactive isotope scan may not be positive, so be prepared to make the diagnosis on clinical grounds;
- a stress fracture starting in the superior border of the femoral neck may be visible on x-rays after 14 days.
- an impacted subcapital fracture is visible on anteroposterior (AP) x-ray with the hip in neutral rotation; the head is usually tilted into valgus and angled posteriorly;
- but beware: most x-ray technicians leave the hip in external rotation for the AP, thus the
  —neck appears short, the
  —whole of the lesser trochanter is visible, and the
  —fracture may be invisible! So
- supervise the x-ray yourself by holding the leg in neutral rotation on the x-ray table. In an impacted fracture the
- trabeculae of the head are
  —misaligned with those of the
  —acetabulum, and the
- trabeculae along the
  —medial side of the neck appear to be
  —bent. This is the Garden Type I fracture. In a
- complete, undisplaced subcaptial fracture, the Garden Type II, the
  —femoral trabeculae are
  —well aligned with the head, but there is
  —discontinuity of the trabeculae across the fracture.

Displaced and comminuted subcapital fractures

- there is a history of a fall, but whether that or the fracture occurs first is open for discussion;
- the patient usually has severe pain and cannot walk. The
- leg may be a little short and externally rotated. An
- AP x-ray with the hip in neutral rotation shows an obvious displacement. In a
- complete fracture with partial displacement, the Garden Type III, the
  —head is in varus and the
- trabeculae of the head are
  —misaligned with those of the
  —acetabulum and the

—femoral neck. All the trabeculae crossing the fracture are broken. With

- complete displacement, there is no longer any contact between the head and the neck, the Garden Type IV, and the
- trabeculae of the head are in
  —normal alignment with the
  —acetabulum.
- lateral x-ray is important to assess degree of
  —angulation and
  —comminution of the posterior cortex.

Transcervical fractures

- are really variants of the subcapital fracture, and the same general principles regarding classification and treatment apply.
- Pauwel's classification, based on the obliquity of the fracture, is not helpful except to say that
  —after reduction
  —the more horizontal the fracture, the greater is its inherent stability.

Basicervical fracture

- is a variant of the intertrochanteric group and should be treated as such.

TREATMENT

Impacted and undisplaced fractures

- internal fixation, with x-ray control during surgery, by
  —short, lateral incision and
  —threaded pins across the fracture to prevent completion of a stress fracture or displacement of an impacted one;
- allow partial weight-bearing (PWB), with gradual increase to full weight-bearing (FWB) within 5 to 10 days after surgery

Displaced fractures

Patient under 70 years old

- the patient's own femoral head is better than a metal prosthesis. This fracture
- requires operative treatment as soon as possible to
  —promote union,
  —reduce the risk of avascular necrosis, and
  —prevent the complications of prolonged bed rest;
- if surgery cannot be performed immediately, put the leg in
  —skin traction and slight
  —internal rotation to reduce the risk of necrosis.

Closed reduction and internal fixation

- reduce the fracture by
  —pulling laterally on the thigh, in the direction of the femoral neck, with the
  —hip flexed to 90°. Then bring the leg into
  —extension and internal rotation to lock the fragments in the reduced position;
  —fix the foot on the fracture table to hold the position, and take AP and lateral x-rays or use the image intensifier to confirm the position;
- reduction should be anatomic or in slight valgus. Repeat the maneuver if reduction is not perfect;
- the fracture can then be pinned through a lateral incision with
  —4 or 5 threaded pins or a
  —compression screw and plate.
- impact the fracture. If the fracture is distracted, it will not unite.

Open reduction and internal fixation

- if closed reduction fails, perform open reduction through the
- Watson-Jones anterolateral approach to avoid damaging the posterior retinacular vessels to the head. Then
- immobilize the fracture as discussed previously;
- apply skin traction for 5 days and have the patient perform isometric exercises, then permit
- non-weight-bearing (NWB) until the fracture has healed, usually about 12 weeks.

Patient over 70 years old

- replace the head with a Moore or Thompson prosthesis through a
- posterolateral approach;
- provide 10° of anteversion and
- seat the prosthesis in a little valgus.
- if the stem is loose in the medullary canal, pack it around with bone from the femoral head; a Thompson prosthesis can be cemented;
- suture the posterior capsule and short rotator muscles to prevent postoperative dislocation.
- postoperatively, apply an
  —abduction cushion for 5 days to prevent posterior dislocation, which would occur in flexion, internal rotation and adduction; and start the patient on
  —physiotherapy with hip mobilization and then
- progressive weight-bearing. The patient can bear full weight at 2 weeks.

- this procedure has a higher morbidity and mortality rate than does use of reduction and internal fixation.

Comminuted fractures

- if the fracture is displaced and the posterior cortex is very comminuted, the reduction will be unstable even with internal fixation. The
- best treatment is either
- prosthetic femoral head replacement or, in a
- young patient,
    —open reduction through a posterolateral approach,
    —internal fixation as discussed previously, and a
    —posterior pediculated graft from the greater trochanter, let into a slot cut posteriorly along the line of the neck across the fracture. Screw the graft into its bed;
- this surgery is difficult.

COMPLICATIONS

Infection

- a disaster because it usually
    —destroys the hip joint and may
    —kill an older patient;
- infection rate is
    —higher with a posterolateral approach and prosthetic replacement than with an
    —anterolateral approach and internal fixation;
- before surgery, treat infection elsewhere, e.g., the chest or urine, and
- give prophylactic broad spectrum antibiotics
    —before,
    —during and
    —after surgery when indicated;
- prophylactic antibiotics after surgery alone are
    —less effective because the antibiotic
    —does not get into the hematoma,
    —the time lag allows pathogenic bacteria to reproduce, and the antibiotics
    —encourage infection by secondary organisms. Antibiotics may also be
    —dangerous because the surgeon is lulled into a false sense of security;
- perform the surgery carefully but do not waste time;
- pay attention to hemostasis, prevent a hematoma from forming, and drain the wound postoperatively;
- treatment of infection includes
    —debridement, lavage, wide drainage and

—appropriate systemic antibiotics. It may be necessary to
—remove the prosthesis, converting the hip to a Girdlestone resection.

Malunion

- the untreated or poorly treated fracture nearly always unites in varus, external rotation and shortening. In
- young patient, perform an
  —intertrochanteric osteotomy with blade plate fixation if the deformity is severe and disabling. In an
- older patient,
  —treat symptomatically or perform
  —total replacement arthroplasty.

Nonunion

- is often associated with a
  —delay between injury and treatment, a
  —displaced fracture,
  —poor reduction and fixation and
  —avascular necrosis.
- treatment for nonunion of a subcapital fracture in an
  —older patient is
  —symptomatic if the pain is mild or the disability is minimal, and consists of
  —replacement arthroplasty if symptoms are severe. In a
- young patient, perform an
  —intertrochanteric valgus osteotomy with blade plate fixation to reduce shear stress on the fracture line, and move the shaft medially beneath the fracture to give added support.

Avascular necrosis

- whether the head lives or dies is usually decided within the first 12 hours after fracture, but early, accurate reduction, avoidance of an acute valgus position, and firm fixation may reduce the incidence of necrosis.

Radiological features

- x-ray changes may not be visible for 2 years or more;
- the head appears dense relative to adjacent osteoporotic bone because the loss of blood supply prevents removal of calcium from the head. The
- superior weight-bearing segment collapses, crushing trabeculae together and increasing the density still further;
- as dead bone is revascularized, it becomes denser because new bone is deposited on dead trabeculae.

Treatment

- ideally the patient should not bear weight on the leg until the head has revascularized, but this is unrealistic, so prescribe
- aspirin and the use of a cane for mild symptoms;
- prosthetic replacement of the femoral head alone as a secondary procedure usually has
  —poor results with a
  —painful, stiff hip and a
  —higher infection rate;
- total replacement arthroplasty is the best alternative in an older person with severe symptoms.

Femoral Neck Fractures in Children

TRAUMATIC PROXIMAL FEMORAL EPIPHYSEAL SEPARATION (Fig. 17.4)

Etiopathology

- requires only moderate trauma for occurrence in an infant, but in older children the epiphyseal separation is
  —caused by greater force, so the
  —child often has other injuries too. In the
- adolescent it
  —represents one end of the spectrum of "slipped upper femoral epiphysis" which may be associated with other disease. The separation is a
- Salter-Harris Type I epiphyseal plate injury, with the fracture line crossing the plate from one side to the other and separating completely the head from the neck. The capital femoral epiphysis
- may be
  —undisplaced, with the only sign being a widened growth plate,

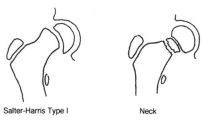

Salter-Harris Type I   Neck

Figure 17.4. Hip fractures in children.

—partially displaced or
—completely displaced. The epiphysis
- slides backward and downward in relation to the femoral neck, so that the limb comes to lie in
    —external rotation,
    —extension and
    —adduction, and the child has a
- painful limp. The
- key sign is
    —limitation of internal rotation.
- radiographically the diagnosis is confirmed mainly by the
    —lateral view.

Treatment

Patient under 9 years old

- if the head is undisplaced, treat with
    —skin traction for 4 weeks, with the hip flexed 30°.
- if it is partially displaced, attempt progressive,
    —gentle, closed reduction by traction, and then apply a
    —spica for 6 weeks with the leg in 15° of abduction, 15° of internal rotation and 30° of flexion.
- complete displacement requires
    —open reduction through a Watson-Jones anterolateral approach and
    —fixation with threaded pins if gentle, closed reduction fails. Results are uniformly poor! Remove the pins later. Do not use a trifin nail, as this knocks the head off again.

Patient over 9 years old

- reduce the epiphysis slowly, by 4 or 5 days of skin traction with the leg in internal rotation and the hip flexed 30°, then perform
- internal fixation with threaded pins;
- do not perform closed manipulation because this may cause avascular necrosis in the older child. For an
- untreated injury older than 3 weeks, do not try closed reduction or operate on the neck, since the incidence of avascular necrosis after femoral neck osteotomy is nearly 100%. Correct the deformity of the leg by an
- intertrochanteric osteotomy and stabilization of the head.

Complications

- avascular necrosis, which occurs in 100% of patients after open reduction,
- malunion and

- premature closure of the growth plate, which may cause problems in the younger child.

FRACTURES OF FEMORAL NECK (Fig. 17.4)

Treatment

Undisplaced

- fracture of the femoral neck is the most common hip fracture in children. If the fracture is undisplaced, apply a
- spica for 8 to 12 weeks;
- results are usually good.

Displaced

- treat by closed reduction or, if this fails, by open reduction;
- fix the fracture with 3 or 4 threaded pins without crossing the growth plate. If the fracture is proximal and the pins must cross into the epiphysis, use smooth pins and remove them when the fracture is healed. Pins are better than a trifin nail because the nail may distract the fragments.

Complications

Loss of reduction

- always results in coxa vara.

Avascular necrosis of femoral epiphysis

- the incidence varies from 5% to 50% and is related to the
  —age of the child, with a higher percentage occurring in the older age groups, to the degree of
  —force of the injury, and to
  —closed manipulation and casting;
- early signs appear in less than a year in a child and include
  —failure of the ossific nucleus of the head to grow (compare with the normal side), and consequent apparent
  —widening of the radiolucent joint space because the unossified cartilaginous anlage of the head does continue to grow;
- later during revascularization, the
  —head becomes radiologically denser than the normal hip. Then the ossific nucleus
  —fragments and becomes
  —deformed, flattened and widened (coxa magna) and may
  —sublux. A
- radioactive isotope bone scan is positive within 3 to 4 months.
- avascular necrosis also causes
  —premature closure of the growth plate which leads to a

—short neck and shortening of the leg and

—relative overgrowth of the greater trochanter with consequent

—coxa vara and

—abductor weakness.

Nonunion or delayed union

- is common if a displaced fracture is not accurately reduced and properly stabilized. Treat by
- subtrochanteric abduction osteotomy and a bone graft.

Premature physeal closure

- may be due to the
  - —initial force of the injury,
  - —avascular necrosis or
  - —threaded pins crossing the growth plate. Treat by
- epiphysiodesis of the greater trochanter to avoid coxa vara.

Intertrochanteric Fractures

ETIOPATHOLOGY (Fig. 17.5)

- common in aged people with osteoporotic bone;
- usually caused by a fall with secondary displacement of the fragments due to muscle pull. The
- medial cortex of the femoral neck and proximal shaft is the
  - —key to stability. If this cortex is
- not comminuted, the fracture is
  - —stable after reduction. But if this cortex is
- comminuted or a large fragment including the lesser trochanter is broken off, the fracture is
  - —unstable. Fracture of the
- greater trochanter does not influence stability.

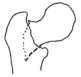

Stable fractures   Unstable four-part fracture

Figure 17.5. Intertrochanteric fractures.

CLINICAL FEATURES

- with an undisplaced fracture, there is
  —pain on movement and palpation and the
  —patient has difficulty walking, but there is
  —little or no deformity.
- with a displaced fracture, there is marked
  —shortening due to pull of the hip extensors, adductors and hamstrings, and the leg is in
  —external rotation due to pull of the psoas. The
  —deformity is more marked with a displaced intertrochanteric fracture than with a femoral neck fracture.

TREATMENT

Traction

- fracture will heal after 8 weeks in traction, followed by 4 weeks PWB, but the
  —fracture often heals in varus, and the
    rest in old people.
- surgery and early mobilization halve the mortality rate and are preferable if the patient can withstand an operation.

Reduction and internal fixation

General remarks

- reduction and internal fixation
  —prevent prolonged bed rest and enable
  —physiotherapy, PWB and rehabilitation to start sooner, and the
  —mortality rate is reduced to less than 20%.
- always use the fracture table because it is easy to maintain reduction;
- if the patient is on his side, with the fractured hip uppermost, the surgery is technically easier to perform.

Stable fracture

Undisplaced

- fix the fracture as it is, through a
  —lateral approach, with a
  —nail and plate or, better still, a compression screw and plate.

Displaced

- reduce the fracture by
  —traction,
  —5° of abduction, and
  —neutral rotation of the leg, if the greater trochanter is attached to the distal fragment, or

—external rotation, if the greater trochanter remains with the proximal fragment. Verify that the

- medial cortex is well reduced. Then
- nail the fracture as discussed previously;
- start PWB as soon as comfort allows.

Unstable fracture

- anatomical reduction is usually impossible and is not necessary;
- convert this to a stable fracture by the Dimon procedure, i.e.,
  —osteotomy of the greater trochanter,
  —medial displacement of the shaft beneath the neck,
  —insertion of a calcar spike into the medullary canal of the shaft, and
  —valgus positioning of the head and neck. This compensates for the shortening of the shaft and adds stability;
- the nail is driven directly into the neck and head without going through the lateral cortex, so the nail must be short;
- insert the nail into the center of the neck but the inferior part of the head so that the head and neck will be in valgus when the plate is attached to the shaft;
- this operation is not easy, but if it is done well, the results are good.

Postoperative care

- respiratory physiotherapy. The
- patient should be sitting up in a chair the next day, and if the
- fracture and fixation are stable, she can start PWB with a walker or parallel bars at 5 to 10 days and can progress to
- FWB as discomfort subsides.
- if the fixation is unstable, NWB is necessary until the fracture is united.

Complications

- poor reduction or
- inadequate fixation may lead to
  —displacement of fragments and
  —malunion or may even lead to
- nonunion if the fracture is distracted by the nail plate. Broken screws or a bent or broken nail plate are signs of pseudarthrosis;
- inadequate penetration of the head by the nail which cuts out of the head anteriorly due to the natural tendency of the leg to fall into external rotation when the patient lies on her back;
- protrusion of the nail through the head, across the hip joint and into the acetabulum as the fracture fragments collapse and impact, due to insufficient impaction at surgery.

CHILDREN

- intertrochanteric fracture is an uncommon injury in children and is
- often comminuted, making open reduction difficult. So
- treat with
  —skin or skeletal traction for 4 weeks, then apply a
  —spica for 4 weeks.

chapter 18
Subtrochanteric and Femoral Shaft Fractures

Surgical Anatomy of Femoral Shaft

- the femur is the largest and strongest bone in the body, and
  —the greatest force is required to break it. The
- shaft is cylindrical and resists angulation forces well but not torsional stress. It is
- surrounded by the largest muscles in the body with
  —excellent blood supply, and in femoral shaft fractures
  —nonunion is uncommon. The
- muscle groups that cause deformity after fracture are the
  —abductors and
  —iliopsoas, which abduct, flex and externally rotate the proximal fragment,
  —adductors, which adduct the distal fragment, and
  —gastrocnemius, which flexes the condyles in a supracondylar fracture. The
- major blood vessels which may be injured where they lie close to bone are
  —three to five perforating arteries from the profunda femoris artery, where they pass across the linea aspera from medial to lateral and the
  —femoral artery, where it passes through the adductor hiatus just proximal to the adductor tubercle. This artery is vulnerable in supracondylar fractures.
- for practical purposes the femoral shaft in the adult starts 5 cm below the lesser trochanter and ends 5 cm above the femoral condyles.

Subtrochanteric Fractures
ETIOPATHOLOGY (Fig. 18.1)
- the subtrochanteric region extends from the superior margin of the lesser trochanter to 5 cm below the lesser trochanter. These fractures occur in a
- younger age group than do intertrochanteric and femoral neck fractures and are

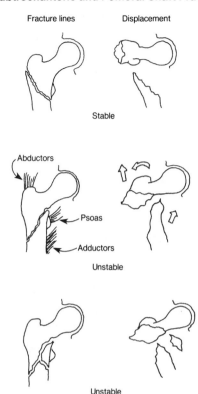

Figure 18.1.   Subtrochanteric fractures.

- caused by severe trauma, so they may be associated with other injuries. The
- medial cortex and the
- direction of the fracture line are the
  —keys to
  —stability. If the fracture is
- oblique downward and inward and there is only
- one fracture line in the medial cortex, the fracture is
  —stable after reduction and fixation. Buf if the medial cortex is
- comminuted or the
- fracture line is oblique downward and outward, the fracture is
  —unstable. The
- fracture may be
  —transverse,

—oblique or spiral or may be

—comminuted with a butterfly fragment and may

—extend into the intertrochanteric region or even be an

—extension of a femoral shaft fracture. The

- fracture line usually extends from

  —cancellous bone of the proximal metaphysis distally to

  —cortical bone of the shaft.

- if the lesser trochanter remains attached to the head and neck fragment, this fragment is pulled into

  —flexion and

  —external rotation by the psoas and into

  —abduction by the gluteus medius. But if the

- lesser trochanter is separate, the proximal fragment is pulled into

  —abduction and

- external rotation only. The

- femoral shaft is displaced proximally and adducted by the adductors.

TREATMENT

Traction (Fig. 4.4)

- almost all subtrochanteric fractures unite with

  —transfemoral traction for 8 weeks, followed by a

  —double hip spica for 8 weeks. But this method is

- only useful for stable fractures. The

- shaft must be in

  —flexion and

  —abduction to align it with the proximal fragment. This requires a Thomas splint and a Pearson knee piece with overhead frame;

- if the proximal fragment is flexed more than 50%, use

- 90/90 traction; i.e.,

  —knee and hip flexed 90°, hip abducted 30°,

  —vertical traction through the distal femur, and the

  —leg supported in a sling. This works especially well in young children for stable and unstable fractures.

Open reduction and internal fixation

Indications

Stable fractures

- to facilitate nursing and the treatment of other injuries and to enable the patient to be

- mobilized early, thus

- preventing the complications of prolonged recumbency and

- accelerating the patient's social reintegration.

Unstable fractures

- to provide the only practical means of
  - —achieving and
  - —maintaining adequate reduction.

Technique

- through a lateral approach with the patient on his side
  - —reduce the fracture and
  - —stabilize it with a Zickel intramedullary nail and signal arm device;
  - —graft the medial side of the fracture with autologous cancelous bone from the iliac crest.
- nail plates are not recommended in adults because they frequently fail in the unstable fracture. But in
  - —adolescents in whom the fracture cannot be treated by traction, a nail plate or nail and screw should be used instead of an intramedullary nail because the
  - —epiphyses are still open. In adults, an
- intramedullary nail without the signal arm does not gain sufficient purchase in the proximal fragment to dispense with auxillary traction or a spica.

Postoperative care

- partial weight-bearing (PWB) until the fracture is united;
- physiotherapy with
  - —isotonic muscle exercises and
  - —active knee mobilization.

Complications

Pseudarthrosis

- nonunion is fairly common with a nail plate, because the varus forces across the fracture are stronger than this fixation device.

Malunion

- frequent when the fracture is treated in traction;
- correct it by osteotomy and sound internal fixation.

OLD UNTREATED FRACTURES

- corrective surgery is often difficult and has complications, especially when there is already marked shortening at the fracture site. Reserve it for young people;
- precede surgery by physiotherapy for knee stiffness.
- use the fracture table and
- put a spica on after surgery. Correct the following deformities by appropriate intertrochanteric osteotomy, rigid internal fixation and bone graft:

- —varus deformity of more than
  - —30° in the trochanteric region, i.e., a neck to shaft angle of 105°, or
  - —25° in the subtrochanteric region;
- anteroposterior (AP) angulation, with the apex always anterior, of more than
  - —40°;
- malrotation of more than
  - —45° of external rotation or
  - —15° of internal rotation.
- shortening of more than 6 cm should be corrected by an
  - —oblique osteotomy at the fracture site and
  - —skeletal traction for 10 days, with the hip and knee flexed to avoid ischemia from arterial spasm. Then use
  - —internal fixation, a bone graft and a hip spica. If the
  - —traction is continued and internal fixation is not used, the
  - —deformity always recurs.
  - —2 or 3 cm of shortening in a child usually corrects itself after 2 years by overgrowth of the fractured femur due to hyperemic stimulation of the proximal and distal femoral growth plates.

Femoral Shaft Fractures in Adults

CLINICAL AND RADIOLOGICAL FEATURES

- femoral shaft fractures usually occur in young patients. A
- single, closed fracture is caused by moderate trauma, but a
- comminuted or segmental open fracture is caused by severe and violent trauma, and there may be
  - —other injuries. The
- clinical diagnosis of the femoral fracture is usually obvious but do not forget to examine the
  - —vasculoneurological status of the leg and foot and to order
  - —x-rays of the hip and knee because dislocation of the hip or fracture of the femoral neck is often associated with a femoral shaft fracture;
  - —examine the knee and tibia for ligament injury or fracture. A
- vascular complication is an emergncy and must be treated without delay (see Chapter 32). If arterial repair is necessary, skeletal traction is quite sufficient for immobilization of the fracture;
- ischemia is less obvious if the patient is unconscious, so look for it. The
- fat embolism syndrome occurs more often with fracture of the femur than with fracture of any other bone, both before and during treatment. You must
  - —think of it to
- diagnose it.

TREATMENT

Emergency department

- examine carefully all systems because femoral shaft fractures are often associated with injuries to the
  —brain or spinal cord, the
  —chest, abdomen or pelvis;
- resuscitate the patient if necessary. Remember that a
  —closed femoral fracture may bleed
  —1½ liters into the thigh;
- splint the fractured leg, preferably with a
  —Thomas splint and fixed skin traction, and
- when the patient's general condition permits, send him for x-rays.

Long distance transportation

- if it is necessary to transport the patient to another center, put the leg in a
- Thomas splint bent 20° at the knee with
- skin traction fixed firmly to the distal end of the splint and tightened with a windlass made from two tongue depressors. Pack the thigh around with cotton wool or soft bandages and
- wind two or three rolls of plaster bandage around the thigh and the splint. This is the
- "Tobruk splint" and enables the patient to be transported easily without fear of increasing soft tissue damage or pain or of movement at the fracture site.

Balanced traction and cast (Figs. 4.4 and 18.2)

Traction

- almost all femoral shaft fractures will unite in traction and can be treated very well by this method,
- except fractures of the proximal third for which the
  —tendency to varus deformity by muscle pull must be
  —countered by lateral slings.
- traction techniques are generally more difficult to manage and more time-consuming than are open reduction and internal fixation, but in a
- situation in which
  —neither the proper facilities
  —nor the trained personnel are available for safe and careful surgery, the
  —advantages of nonoperative methods are overwhelming.
- the best method is
  —closed reduction with the patient under general anesthesia and

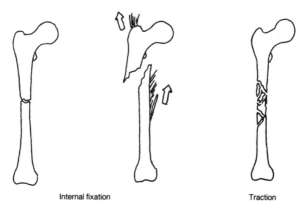

Internal fixation   Traction

Figure 18.2. Indications for treatment in femoral shaft fractures.

—immobilization by skeletal traction with a transtibial pin, with the reduction maintained by a
—Thomas splint and Pearson knee piece and with the traction balanced with string, pulleys and weights to facilitate nursing care and, later, to allow mobilization of the knee.

- do not use skin traction for prolonged period in an adult because this will cause skin problems, especially if more than 4 kg of traction are required.
- the knee should be flexed about 25° to
  —control rotation and
  —lessen the possibility of knee stiffness.
- many satisfactory methods of balanced traction have been described. All follow the same principles of
  —traction and countertraction, correcting
  —alignment and angulation with pads and slings,
  —allowing the patient to move in bed, and
  —permitting knee movement. The methods differ only in detail.
- check the traction daily, paying particular attention to the
  —neurovascular status of the limb,
  —length and alignment of the injured thigh compared with the normal thigh,
  —position and alignment of the entire traction apparatus, and
  —skin over the pressure areas and around the traction pin;
- order x-rays of the patient in traction at regular intervals;
- start the patient on active physiotherapy early with
  —isometric exercises and isotonic foot exercises several times a day;
  —mobilize the knee actively when the fracture is "sticky."

Spica or cast brace

Spica

- apply a hip spica at 6 weeks unless the fracture is still mobile;
- remove the spica 6 weeks later and evaluate the fracture
  —clinically and
  —radiologically.

Cast brace

- can be used for fractures of the midshaft or distal shaft;
- should not be used for fractures of the proximal third because these will drift into varus.
- allows
  —flexion of the knee and
  —weight-bearing and
- can be applied as soon as the fracture is "sticky."
- has certain advantages:
  —rapid fracture healing,
  —less muscle and bone atrophy,
  —greater mobility of the knee,
  —quicker and better rehabilitation and
  —earlier return to home and to work.
- details of application are important and include a well-fitting plaster thigh corset joined to a below-knee cast by two loose hinges at the knee;
- remove the cast brace 6 weeks later if the fracture is clinically and radiologically united.

Weight-bearing

- when the fracture is
  —clinically and
  —radiologically united, start progressive, protected weight-bearing out of plaster;
- the patient should use crutches for about 4 weeks after removal of the spica or cast brace, increasing the amount of weight on the leg day by day.

Advantages of traction

- excellent method for comminuted fracture;
- no infection of fracture site;
- does not interfere with the blood supply to bone and fracture site; there is a
- high union rate, and
- ultimate knee and muscle function is nearly as good as that after internal fixation.

Disadvantages of traction

- prolonged bed rest, but this is usually well tolerated by young patients;
- needs more daily attention by nurses and doctors than does internal fixation. The
- length of time in hospital is longer, averaging
  —10 weeks compared with
  —6 weeks for open reduction and internal fixation, and the
- length of time off work is longer, averaging
  —13 months compared with
  —9 months for operative treatment.

Complications of traction

- pin tract infection;
- peroneal nerve palsy due to external rotation of the leg in the splint with pressure on the nerve at the neck of the fibula, usually with recovery;
- pressure sores;
- nonunion is rare and is usually caused by
  —soft tissue interposition or
  —distraction of the fracture by traction;
- malunion may occur, usually with a lateral varus bow. Accept
  —5° of varus or valgus in the midshaft and less in the distal shaft,
  —10° AP angulation,
  —5° internal rotation, 10° external rotation and
  —2 cm shortening. It is much better to avoid malunion by careful, daily attention to alignment of the limb in traction.
- stiffness of the knee is more incapacitating than stiffness of any other joint in the lower limb. It may be caused by adhesions
  —in the suprapatellar pouch, especially with a distal femoral fracture,
  —between the quadriceps and the femur, particularly in an open or infected fracture,
  —in the knee joint or the patellofemoral joint, especially with an associated intra-articular injury;
- prevent knee stiffness by
  —early isometric quadriceps exercises and
  —passive lateral mobilization of the patella daily,
  —active knee movements as soon as the fracture is "sticky," usually at 4 to 6 weeks, and the use of a
  —cast brace. The fracture is "sticky" when it may angulate slightly on manipulation but can no longer shorten;
- treat knee stiffness by
  —intensive active physiotherapy for several months and

—judicious and gentle manipulation with the patient under anesthesia when indicated. Then

—surgical release or quadriceps lengthening will rarely be necessary.

Internal fixation

- is not urgent, provided that the limb is in traction to maintain femoral length. Wait until the patient is in good general condition before operating.

Indications (Fig. 18.2)

Intramedullary nail

- a transverse or short oblique fracture of proximal or middle third of the femoral shaft without comminution is ideal for closed or open intramedullary nailing. A
- segmental shaft fracture is also an indication for an intramedullary nail. The
- Küntscher cloverleaf nail is still the most satisfactory type.

Intramedullary nail and circumferential banding or plate

- a long, spiral or oblique fracture or a fracture with
- gross comminution is best treated by traction unless this is impractical because the patient is
    —restless, uncooperative or convulsing, e.g., a head injury, or there are
    —multiple injuries, or the patient has a
    —dislocation of the hip, fracture of the femoral neck, a patellar fracture on the same side, or there is an
    —associated vascular injury requiring surgery, or
    —closed reduction fails. In these instances, perform
- open reduction and internal fixation with an intramedullary nail and Parham bands or a long compression plate to
    —control definitively the femoral fracture,
    —allow other injuries to be treated, and
    —facilitate nursing.

Postoperative care

- active knee mobilization and isometric muscle exercises as soon as possible;
- PWB at 2 weeks if the fracture has been stabilized with an intramedullary nail, then full weight-bearing (FWB) when the fracture has healed;
- non-weight-bearing (NWB) until the fracture has healed, if a plate has been used, then
- graduated weight bearing. A

- cast brace gives added support if the
  —solidity of the fixation is dubious or the fracture is
  —comminuted.
- do not remove the nail or plate before 1 year.

Complications of operative treatment

Infection

- the incidence ranges from 1.2% to 20%, depending on the series, but it is 100% for the patient who has it. The
- first aim is to
  —attain bony union, since
  —infection will persist as long as the fracture is ununited and mobile;
- when treating a patient with nonunion due to infection around the intramedullary nail, either
  —leave the nail, if it is stabilizing the fracture, or
  —remove the nail, if it is too small, and replace it with a larger one, or
  —use external fixation;
- a plate which is stabilizing the fracture should also be left in situ.
- drainage of the fracture site, at one or both ends of the nail if this is the site of the infection, debridement, sequestrectomy, closed irrigation and antibiotics are important to control the infection.
- fresh, autologous cancellous bone graft can survive in an infected environment and should be used judiciously to promote union. Always remember that
- malunion due to poor traction technique is preferable to an
- infected nonunion due to poor operative technique!

Errors of technique

- the intramedullary nail may be
  —too short or too narrow to immobilize the fracture, so a spica is necessary;
  —too long, with intrusion into the knee or patellofemoral joint; or
  —too wide and may become stuck in the medullary canal. To remove it you will need a large vice grip (the nail extractor will break) and a heavy hammer. The experience will be unforgettable!
- driving the nail through the femoral neck may fracture the neck. The nail should come out through the greater trochanter;
- distraction of the fracture;
- further comminution of a fracture with undisplaced, hairline fractures undetected before surgery.

Delayed union and nonunion

- open reduction is the greatest cause of delayed union or nonunion in femoral shaft fractures because of increased devascularization of the bone and surrounding soft tissues engendered by the surgery;
- refracture is usually a sign of inadequate union, premature weight-bearing, or weakening of the shaft at screw holes;
- failure of the implant is a certain sign of nonunion;
- treat with
  - —cancellous, iliac bone graft and either an
  - —intramedullary rod or a
  - —long and large compression plate.

Nail migration

- associated particularly with
  - —infection or
  - —osteoporosis. The nail may
- slide distally into the patellofemoral or knee joint or proximally, in which case it becomes painful and develops a bursa over its proximal end.

Knee stiffness

- the etiology is similar to that after treatment in traction (see previous discussion), but
- prevention is generally simpler because the patient can
- start active knee movements within a few days of surgery.

External fixation

Open fracture

- external fixation can be used to
  - —neutralize the fracture and
  - —facilitate treatment of the skin wound.
- once the skin is closed, the fracture can be treated by
  - —continued external fixation or
  - —another, more appropriate method.

Infected nonunion

- external fixation stabilizes the fracture and promotes union if it is used with either
  - —Judet's technique of osteoperiosteal decortication or
  - —cancellous grafting. The fixation device is not likely to spread the infection because the
- pins are placed at a distance from the site of infection.

Femoral Shaft Fractures in Children

GENERAL REMARKS

- a child does not lose sufficient blood into the thigh from a closed femoral fracture to cause shock. So if the
- child is in shock and apparently has only a fractured femur, there is internal hemorrhage too, so look for it.
- temporarily immobilize the femur and treat the shock and serious injuries first.

TREATMENT OF FRACTURE

Traction (Figs. 4.2, 4.3 and 4.4)

- all femoral shaft fractures in children heal well with traction in a Thomas splint;
- general principles of treatment for adults apply to children, with the following exceptions:
- for children under 2 years old weighing less than 10 kg
  —Bryant's balanced gallows traction with the sacrum just off the bed is satisfactory, but it can be dangerous, so
  —check the neurovascular status of both limbs regularly. After 3 weeks, place the child in a
  —1½ spica for 6 to 8 weeks. A
  —safer alternative is a double spica without preliminary traction. Treat children
- between 2 years old and puberty with 4 to 5 weeks of
  —fixed skin traction in a Thomas splint with the knee bent 25° and the distal end raised off the bed, followed by a
  —hip spica for 4 to 6 weeks.
  —alternatively, a 1½ or double hip spica with the knee and hip in extension can be applied immediately with use of anesthetic, thus shortening the hospital stay. This requires careful attention to detail and close follow-up.
- adolescents and heavy children are best treated by
  —skeletal 90/90 balanced traction. Insert the femoral traction pin well away from the physis and the growth plate. When the fracture is sticky, apply a
  —1½ hip spica until the fracture is clinically and radiologically healed, usually 6 to 12 weeks later depending on the patient's age.
- bayonet apposition with slight overlap is acceptable in midchildhood because
- shortening of less than 2 cm is often corrected spontaneously by over-

growth over the following 2 years, depending on how much growth the child has left.

- physiotherapy is rarely needed for children. They mobilize themselves.

Open reduction and internal fixation

- an associated arterial injury requiring repair or a
- restless or convulsing child with a head injury are the major indications for internal fixation with a plate because traction would be too difficult to manage. An intramedullary nail is contraindicated in growing children. An
- open fracture per se is not an indication for internal fixation. It can be managed well by wound toilet and traction.

COMPLICATIONS

- children have very few complications. The
- commonest is a leg length discrepancy which may be caused by
  —overriding or overdistraction of the fracture,
  —subsequent overgrowth, or a
  —traction pin through or too close to the growth plate.
- a difference of
  —1 cm in a small child causes a limp, but when the
  —child becomes an adult, the limp disappears and the discrepancy is undetectable.
  —use a shoe lift for a discrepancy of 2 to 4 cm.
  —a discrepancy of more than 4 cm may require epiphysiodesis of the contralateral femur at the appropriate age. But if the child is already too old for this, consider treatment with a shoe lift, since surgical lengthening and shortening operations have many complications.

UNTREATED FRACTURE WITH MALUNION

- angulation of more than
  —15° anteriorly, 5° posteriorly, or
  —10° in the coronal plane and
- rotational deformity of more than
  —10° of external rotation or 5° of internal rotation are
- not acceptable and may require correction. If the fracture is
- less than 3 weeks old,
  —break callus with the patient under anaesthesia, and treat it as a fresh fracture. If it is
- more than 3 weeks old
  —make several drill holes percutaneously across callus, then
  —break the femur and treat it as a fresh fracture.

chapter 19

Distal Femoral Fractures and Patellar Injuries

Distal Femoral Fractures in Adults

SUPRACONDYLAR EXTRA-ARTICULAR FRACTURES

- the general principles of shaft fractures apply.

Pathology (Fig. 19.1)

- the popliteal vessels may be injured, so look for this. The
- fracture may be
  —displaced or
  —impacted. The
- gastrocnemius and quadriceps muscles may pull the distal fragment into flexion and shorten the thigh;
- knee stiffness is more common with supracondylar extra-articular fractures than with shaft fractures because the
  —proximal fragment tears the suprapatellar pouch and quadriceps, disrupting the gliding mechanism, and the
  —quadriceps tendon sticks to the callus.

Treatment

Open reduction (Fig. 4.4)

- open reduction through a
  —lateral incision and
- internal fixation with a
  —blade plate have the advantages of
  —dispensing with traction and plaster and permitting
  —early knee movement and
  —faster rehabilitation.
- use this method for a simple fracture or a slightly comminuted fracture.

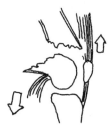

Figure 19.1. Supracondylar femoral fracture.

Traction

- is the best treatment for a very comminuted fracture; use a proximal tibial pin;
- after the patient has been in traction for 3 days, take anteroposterior (AP) and lateral x-rays (do not remove the traction). If the fracture is not reduced, even with the knee flexed, place a
  —second pin through the distal femur at the level of the adductor tubercle and
  —pull vertically. This two-pin traction should reduce the fracture. Verify the reduction with x-rays.
- knee mobilization can be continued with the two-pin technique.
- after the patient is in traction for 4 to 6 weeks, apply a spica or a cast brace for 4 more weeks.

External fixation

- use external fixation for type III soft tissue wounds.

INTRA-ARTICULAR FRACTURES

"T" and "Y" fractures (Figs. 19.2 and 19.3)

- if the fracture is
  —undisplaced (Neer Type I) or
  —very comminuted (Neer Type III), the best
- treatment is
  —proximal tibial pin traction and
  —early, gentle knee movement. If the fracture is
- not very comminuted (Neer Types IIA and IIB), treat by
  —open reduction and
  —internal fixation with a blade plate, fixing the condyles first with a cancellous screw or bolt to form a single fragment, then reducing and stabilizing this with the femoral shaft. Then start
- early knee motion.

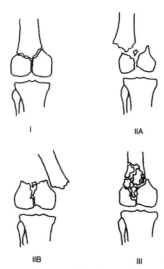

Figure 19.2. Classification of intercondylar femoral fractures. (Modified from Neer CS II, Grantham SA, Shelton ML: Supracondylar fractures of the adult femur. *J Bone Joint Surg* 49A:591–613, 1967.)

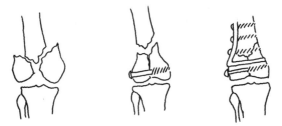

Figure 19.3. Fixation of supracondylar T or Y fracture.

Condylar fractures

- fracture of a single condyle is uncommon. If the fracture is
- undisplaced, treat with
  —tibial traction, then a
  —spica. Do not treat with a long leg cast because the knee may drift into varus or valgus. If the fracture is
- displaced, treat by
  —open anatomic reduction and internal fixation with bolts or cancellous screws, fixing the fractured condyle to the normal one, and by
  —traction with
  —early knee movement.

Chondral and osteochondral fractures

Etiopathology (Fig. 19.4)

- these fractures are partial or complete fractures of the articular cartilage which may contain a piece of underlying bone as well. The
- cartilage lives because it is nourished by synovial fluid, but the attached bone may die because it is nourished by blood vessels from adjacent bone. In a
- partial fracture, the fragment is still attached along one edge and may heal. But in a
- complete fracture, the fragment is free, becomes a joint mouse ("souris articulaire"), and may cause symptoms. The fracture may be caused by direct trauma or indirect shear stress;
- common areas of fracture are the
  —lateral lip of the lateral femoral condyle or the medial edge of the patella in lateral dislocation of the patella,
  —medial margin of the lateral femoral condyle, or
  —weight-bearing surface of either femoral condyle.

Clinical and radiological features

- a patient with a recent fracture has a
  —history of trauma and pain and
  —maybe an effusion of blood containing fat. The latter may be seen if the blood is aspirated and allowed to stand for 1 hour in a bottle or tube; the fat will form a layer on top of the blood, which is a good sign of a fracture. There may be
  —tenderness over the fracture if this is palpable.
- old injury causes
  —persistent pain and crepitation,
  —recurrent effusion and
  —intermittent locking mimicking a meniscal tear.
- good x-rays may
  —show the fragment, if the fracture contains bone, and
  —the defect of the femoral condyle or patella;
  —oblique and tunnel views may also help. An

Figure 19.4. Osteochondral fractures in the knee.

- arthrogram will show whether the fragment is
  —partially or totally detached.

Treatment

Adult

- arthrotomy. If the fragment is
- large and has a little bone attached,
  —freshen the surfaces,
  —replace the fragment and fix it with Smillies' pins;
- postoperatively, encourage active knee mobilization but non-weight-bearing (NWB) until the fracture has healed. If the fragment is
- small,
  —remove it and trim the edges of the defect with a knife until they are smooth and vertical and no loose or separated cartilage remains;
  —drill several holes in the floor of the defect to encourage the growth of fibrocartilage;
  —after surgery, encourage knee movement, quadriceps exercises and weight-bearing. For a
- young patient with a
  —large defect on a weight-bearing surface, use an
  —osteochondral graft from the extreme posterior part of the femoral condyle. This trades a
  —small loss of knee flexion for a more
  —congruous weight-bearing surface.

Child

- if the fragment is still attached, apply a cylinder or long leg cast with NWB for 2 months. If the fragment is
- free in the joint,
  —reduce and fix it if it is large or
  —remove it if it is small.

Distal Femoral Fractures in Children

DISTAL METAPHYSEAL FRACTURES

- relatively common in young children and are
- usually torus or greenstick fractures;
- beware of the angular deformity in the coronal plane;
- displaced fractures may injure vessels, as in the adult;
- treatment for an

—undisplaced fracture is a cast for 6 to 8 weeks and for a

—displaced fracture is closed reduction and a cast;

• x-ray regularly to check for varus or valgus deformity and correct it immediately.

DISTAL FEMORAL GROWTH PLATE INJURIES

Salter-Harris Types I and II (Fig. 19.5)

• common, especially Type II, often a
  —hyperextension injury, and may
  —reduce spontaneously with
  —no indication of fracture on the x-ray except for a metaphyseal flake in Type II injuries. Take a
  —stress x-ray with the patient under anesthesia to confirm a suspected diagnosis.
• treatment is
  —closed reduction by manipulation or traction, followed by
  —a cast for 4 to 8 weeks with the knee flexed or extended according to the original direction of displacement;
• if closed reduction is unstable, fix the epiphysis with percutaneous K wires. If
• closed reduction fails, perform open reduction and internal fixation with K wires.
• take x-rays through the cast at regular intervals so that loss of reduction can be recognized and treated early.

Types III and IV

• less common;
• may be difficult to diagnose. If in doubt, order
  —oblique films and take a
  —stress x-ray.

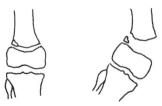

Spontaneous reduction   Stress film

Figure 19.5.   Salter-Harris Type II growth plate injury of the distal femur.

- treat by accurate open reduction and internal fixation with transverse pins or screws. Open the knee joint to ensure congruence of the articular surfaces.
- treat with a plaster cast for 4 to 8 weeks postoperatively.

Complications

- angulation with malunion, especially in the coronal plane, can be avoided by careful reduction and follow-up.
- growth disturbance including angulation and shortening is a high risk in
  —distal femoral plate injuries. So
  —warn the parents and
  —follow the patient until the end of growth with
  —appropriate treatment as necessary;
- stiffness of the knee and quadriceps atrophy are rarely permanent problems in children.

Patellar Injuries

SURGICAL ANATOMY

- the patella is the largest sesamoid bone in the body.
- quadriceps muscle inserts into the superior pole of the patella by three laminae:
  —rectus femoris forms the anterior lamina,
  —vastus medialis and lateralis combine to form the middle lamina, and
  —vastus intermedius forms the posterior lamina. Quadriceps muscle has
- lateral expansions or retinacular fibers which extend from the vastus medialis and lateralis into the
  —tibial condyles and
  —medial and lateral patellar borders. A
- thin layer of quadriceps tendon passes over the front of the patella. The
- patellar tendon extends from the inferior pole to the tibial tuberosity.
- beware of the bipartite patella, a result of twin ossification centers which unite with fibrous tissue. This line is proximal, looks like a fracture, and is bilateral.

FRACTURES

Clinical features

- common in adults, rare in children;
- caused by a
  —direct blow or a
  —fall, with sudden quadriceps spasm tearing the bone apart and sometimes rupturing the retinacular fibers too. The

- clinical diagnosis is usually obvious with
    —skin damage, if the fracture is due to direct trauma;
    —pain and tenderness; and
    —localized swelling and intra-articular effusion. There may be a
    —deformity. Note that the patient
    —can extend the knee if the retinacular fibers are intact.

Treatment (Fig. 19.6)

Transverse undisplaced fractures

- treat with a long leg cast for 4 weeks and
- start the patient on isometric quadriceps and straight leg raising exercises in the cast;
- if the cast is a cylinder, it should be stuck to the skin of the leg with a nonirritant adhesive and should extend from the groin to 5 cm proximal to the malleoli to avoid pressure sores over the malleoli and Achilles tendon.
- knee mobilization and unresistive quadriceps exercises for 2 weeks after cast removal, then graduated resistive exercises.

Transverse displaced fractures and extensor mechanism rupture

Fracture through body of patella

- if displacement is 4 mm or less and the patient can extend the knee, treat with a cylinder or long leg cast as discussed previously.

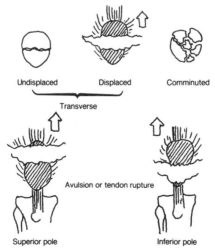

Figure 19.6. Patellar fractures and tendon ruptures.

- if displacment is more than 4 mm or active knee extension is impossible, open reduction is indicated. Through a transverse incision,
  —irrigate the knee,
  —inspect the femoral articular cartilage,
  —repair the retinacular tear, and
  —use K wires and a tension band to maintain reduction of the patella.
- postoperatively, treat with a
  —posterior splint for 4 weeks with daily active knee mobilization out of the splint and
  —isometric exercises;
  —no resistive exercises are allowed for 8 weeks.

Fracture of distal pole

- with 4 mm of displacement, treat the fracture with a cast;
- with more than 4 mm of displacement, treat it surgically and fix the fragment with wire sutures passed through the patellar tendon around the small fragment, then through holes drilled in the main fragment. Do not make these holes through articular cartilage.
- postoperative care is the same as that discussed previously.

Rupture of patellar tendon

- uncommon;
- usually ruptures at its insertion either at the patella or at the tibial tuberosity.
- usually occurs in
  —young athletes, sometimes with a history of cortisone injections into the tendon, or
  —open wound when the tendon is cut;
- clinical features are similar to a fracture of the lower pole plus a
  —gap between the patella and tibial tuberosity. The
  —patella is higher than that of the normal side, the key sign. The tendon
  —may avulse a small fragment of bone from the patella or tibial tuberosity.
- acute rupture needs
  —capsular repair and
  —suture of tendon to bone, and
  —if the tendon has avulsed a bony fragment, suture this to the patella or the tibia with the ligament;
  —relieve tension on the suture line by pulling the patella down and

temporarily wiring it to the tibial tuberosity. This wire must be removed at 6 weeks when the tendon has healed. Treat with
—postoperative cast and isometric quadriceps exercises for 6 weeks, followed by physiotherapy with mobilization and graduated resistive exercises after removal of the wire.

- in an old untreated rupture, the patella is usually retracted too far proximally for surgical repair, so treat with physiotherapy to strengthen the quadriceps.

Proximal pole avulsion and quadriceps tendon rupture

- may be caused by violent quadriceps contraction with the knee flexed;
- usually occurs in an abnormal, degenerating tendon, often in older people;
- a partial tear involves the anterior lamina alone, but a
- complete tear involves all three laminae, sometimes at different levels, and the synovial membrane of the suprapatellar pouch.
- diagnosis is often missed;
- clinical features include
    —pain and tenderness at the top of the patella,
    —a gap between the quadriceps muscle and patella,
    —hemarthrosis if the tear is incomplete (blood escapes into surrounding soft tissues in a complete tear), and
    —inability to straighten the knee actively (quadriceps lag).
- for a recent injury, treatment consists of
    —a cast for 6 weeks for a partial tear and minimal extensor lag;
    —surgical repair for a complete tear, with repair starting with the synovium and reinforcing the quadriceps tendon with a fascial slip or turning a quadriceps tendon flap distally;
    —if a fragment of bone has been avulsed, suture this to the patella with the attached tendon because bone unites with bone better than tendon unites with bone;
    —relieve tension, if necessary, by wiring the quadriceps muscle to the patella. Remove the wire before the knee is mobilized.
- for an old untreated tear, surgical repair is usually not possible because
    —the quadriceps muscle retracts too far proximally; so treatment consists of
    —physiotherapy.

Comminuted fractures

- often stellate;
- if the fracture is undisplaced,

- treat with a cast, physiotherapy and early weight-bearing.
- if it is displaced, treat by
- patellectomy, cutting on bone to leave a thin anterior layer of quadriceps tendon for suturing, with a
- postoperative cast for 4 weeks, then physiotherapy;
- patellectomy weakens the quadriceps mechanism by about 30%.

Complications

- if a displaced fracture is untreated, the result is
- malunion or nonunion with weakened quadriceps power,
- chondromalacia and
- patellofemoral arthrosis, which is often followed by
- degenerative arthrosis of the knee;
- extensor lag with difficulty in walking occurs if a tendon or muscle rupture is untreated.

TRAUMATIC DISLOCATION OF PATELLA

Etiopathology

- uncommon;
- usually occurs in the athlete by a
  —direct blow or,
  —indirectly, by a violent contraction of the quadriceps when the knee is flexed, the foot is fixed on the ground, and the tibia is in external rotation, e.g., when a football player changes direction quickly;
- the patella nearly always dislocates laterally and the
- vastus medialis attachment, retinacular fibers and synovium are torn off the patella margin medially.

Clinical and radiological features (Fig. 19.4)

- diagnosis is usually obvious if the patella is still dislocated. The
  —knee is locked in flexion, the
  —patella lies on the lateral side of the knee, and the
  —femoral condyles and patellar groove are palpable if there is not too much swelling.
- after spontaneous reduction the
  —diagnosis is more difficult and may
  —easily be mistaken for a medial meniscus tear; the
  —patient says the "knee gave out" or "popped," there is
  —tenderness over the medial margin of the patella, and the
  —patient is very apprehensive if you push the patella laterally.
- take AP and lateral x-rays and a skyline view;
- x-rays may show an osteochondral chip fracture of the
  —medial margin of the patella or of the
  —lip of the lateral femoral condyle.

Treatment
- usually easily reduced by flexing the hip to relax the rectus femoris, extending the knee and gently pushing the patella medially.
- x-ray after reduction and look for a fracture fragment. Then treat with a
- cylinder cast with the knee extended for 6 weeks and daily quadriceps exercises.
- surgery is necessary only if a chip fracture is in the joint.

Complications

Recurrent dislocation
- may be associated with
  —generalized joint laxity or a
  —weak vastus medialis, or a valgus knee with increased angle between the axes of the quadriceps and the patellar tendon (the Q angle), a
  —small hypoplastic patella or a high-riding patella (patella alta), or a
  —hypoplastic lateral femoral condyle.
- reconstruct the patellar mechanism in the adult by the
  —Hauser procedure, moving the patella tendon insertion medially but not distally,
  —cutting the lateral retinacular fibers of quadriceps, and
  —repairing or overlapping the medial retinacular fibers. Then treat with a
  —cast and daily quadriceps exercises for 6 weeks.
- in the child, transposition of the patella tendon insertion may damage the growth plate and cause genu recurvatum. It is better to
- treat the child with
  —semitendinosus tenodesis,
  —lateral retinacular release and
  —medial plication.

Loose body
- if a loose body is in the knee, it gives symptoms of
  —recurrent effusion, the
  —sensation of "something moving about in the knee," and
  —locking.
- treatment is arthrotomy, exploration and removal.

Chondromalacia
- clinical features are
  —pain or discomfort around the patella,
  —catching or even locking of the knee,
  —patellofemoral crepitus and
  —pain which increases on walking up or down stairs.

- treatment is
  —symptomatic with
  —quadriceps exercises, especially to strengthen the vastus medialis;
- surgery is rarely necessary and generally produces poor results.

Osteoarthrosis of knee

- develops secondarily to patellofemoral incongruence.

chapter 20

Ligamentous Injuries of the Knee

Surgical Anatomy

- the knee is a complex joint. In order to treat ligamentous and meniscal injuries you must understand the functional anatomy of the knee.

EXTRA-ARTICULAR STRUCTURES (Fig. 20.1)

- the capsule of the knee is reinforced by ligamentous and tendinous structures.

Anterior aspect

- the quadriceps expansions from the retinacula of the vastus lateralis and medialis insert into sides of the patella and patellar tendon with expansions to tibial condyles anteriorly, medially and laterally.

Medial aspect

- the medial (tibial) collateral ligament originates from the medial epicondyle and condyle of the femur and splits into two laminae;
  - —deep fibers (also called the medial capsular ligament) insert into the medial meniscus and edge of the medial tibial condyle, and
  - —superficial fibers run downward and forward to the tibial shaft well distal to the condyle beneath the tendon of the pes anserinus. The ligament
  - —glides backward and forward over femoral and tibial condyles in flexion and extension and
  - —stabilizes the knee against valgus stress (superficial part) and rotation (deep part). Posterior to this ligament is the
- posterior oblique ligament, a thickening in the posteromedial capsule blending with the deep part of the medial collateral ligament in front and with the oblique popliteal ligament behind. This resists rotary stress on the knee. The
- pes anserinus inserts into the medial side of the proximal tibial shaft and protects the knee against rotary and valgus stress.

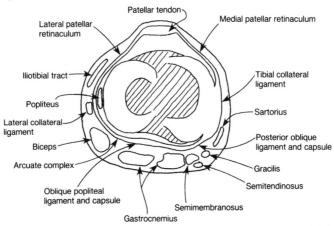

Figure 20.1. External support structures of the knee. (Modified from Nicholas JA: The five-one reconstruction for anterior instability of the knee. *J Bone Joint Surg* 55A:899–922, 1973.)

Posterior aspect

- semimembranosus inserts into the
  - —posteromedial corner of the medial tibial condyle (direct head);
  - —lateral femoral condyle as the oblique popliteal ligament, reinforcing the posterior capsule centrally;
  - —posterior horn of the medial meniscus and adjacent capsule;
  - —medial rim of the medial tibial plateau and, by a
  - —distal expansion, into the tibial metaphysis and popliteus fascia. The semimembranosus
  - —rotates the tibia internally and
  - —tightens the capsule posteriorly and posteromedially, thus stabilizing the knee against rotary stress; it also
  - —pulls the posterior rim of the medial meniscus backward during flexion.
- posterior oblique ligament reinforces the posteromedial capsule, as described previously.
- arcuate complex at the posterolateral corner of the knee consists of the
  - —posterior capsule, lateral part of the
  - —oblique popliteal ligament,
  - —short fibular collateral ligament and expansions from the
  - —popliteus muscle origin (arcuate ligament) and
  - —biceps femoris tendon. This complex
  - —reinforces the posterolateral capsule and
  - —stabilizes the knee against rotary and varus stress.

- meniscofemoral ligaments pass upward and medially from the
  —posterior horn of the lateral meniscus to the
  —medial femoral condyle, with one on each side of the posterior cruciate ligament. These two ligaments
- add stability to the knee through meniscal attachments to the capsule and arcuate complex.

Lateral aspect

- lateral (fibular) collateral ligament runs from
  —lateral epicondyle of the femur to the
  —head of fibula;
  —no capsular attachments;
  —separated from lateral meniscus by popliteus tendon;
  —provides stability against varus stress, especially with the knee extended.
- short fibular collateral ligament lies
  —posteromedial to and parallel with the fibular collateral ligament;
  —reinforces the posterolateral corner of capsule.
- iliotibial tract inserts into the
  —lateral femoral epicondyle, then passes between the lateral border of the patella and biceps tendon to insert into the
  —lateral tibial tubercle (Gerdy's tubercle);
  —stabilizes the knee against varus stress.
- popliteus tendon originates by the
  —main head from the lateral femoral condyle, separating the lateral meniscus from the capsule and lateral collateral ligament; by a
  —fibular head which passes up and posteromedially to join the main tendon and form the arcuate ligament; and by a
  —medial head from the posterior capsule and posterior horn of the lateral meniscus;
- inserts by muscle belly into the posterior tibia above the soleal line;
  —reinforces the posterolateral corner and provides rotary and anteroposterior (AP) stability.
- biceps tendon inserts into the
  —fibular head superficial to the lateral collateral ligament and
  —enhances lateral stability against varus and rotary stress.

INTRA-ARTICULAR STRUCTURES

Menisci

- menisci are made of
- fibrocartilage and contain no blood vessels or nerves. They are
- attached at the periphery to the tibia by the joint capsule (coronary ligaments) except where the popliteus tendon intervenes laterally;

- medial meniscus is also attached to deep fibers of the medial collateral ligament medially and to the semimembranosus tendon posteriorly;
- the posterior horn of the lateral meniscus is attached to the popliteus fibers and the meniscofemoral ligaments;
- anterior and posterior horns of each meniscus are attached firmly to the intercondylar area of the tibia;
- menisci move back and forth (lateral menisci are more mobile than medial menisci) during movements of the knee;
- functionally the menisci
  - —increase anatomical stability of the knee by deepening the tibial condyles (like the glenoid labrum of the scapula),
  - —guide the femoral condyles in gliding and rotary movements on the tibia,
  - —improve the efficiency of joint lubrication,
  - —enlarge weight-bearing surfaces to distribute the weight more evenly,
  - —act as shock absorbers, and seem to
  - —protect the underlying articular cartilage from degenerative changes.

Cruciates

- surrounded by synovial sleeve;
- anterior cruciate ligament runs from the
  - —anterior intercondylar fossa of the tibia
  - —to the posterior part of the medial surface of the lateral femoral condyle in the intercondylar notch;
  - —the small anteromedial portion is tight in all positions of the knee, particularly flexion, while the
  - —large posterolateral part is taut only in extension and prevents hyper-extension.
- posterior cruciate runs from the
  - —extreme posterior end of the intercondylar area of the tibia to the
  - —posterior part of the lateral surface of the medial femoral condyle, crossing posteromedially to the anterior cruciate; the
  - —bulk (anterior portion) is tight in flexion and loose in extension, whereas the
  - —smaller posterior part is loose in flexion and tight in extension. This cruciate is
  - —larger and twice as strong as the anterior cruciate,
  - —lies at the axis of rotation of the knee, and
  - —guides the "screw-home" movement to lock the knee in full extension.
- cruciates
  - —prevent anterior-posterior displacement of the tibia on the femur (maximum normal displacement is about 5 mm);
  - —wind around each other and tighten in internal rotation of the tibia on the femur, thus limiting internal rotation, and

—unwind in external rotation, thus permitting greater external rotation and more AP displacement in this position.

Traumatic Synovitis of Knee

ETIOPATHOLOGY

Synovial effusion

- response of synovium to irritation or injury is to produce more synovial fluid. The
- normal knee contains 2 cc of fluid;
- excess fluid in the knee distends the
  —synovium,
  —capsule and
  —ligaments;
- more than 50 cc, a moderate effusion, may cause
  —pain and limit
  —flexion and extension.

Hemarthrosis

- occurs when the synovium is torn and bleeds;
- fat is usually mixed with the blood when there is an intra-articular fracture (see p. 317).

CLINICAL FEATURES

- joint effusion or hemarthrosis is not a diagnosis but is a sign that indicates an underlying injury which you must diagnose.

Small effusion

- 10 to 30 cc;
- signs are subtle. The effusion
- can be detected by
  —gently pressing the hollow behind and to one side of patella and watching the other side fill up.

Moderate effusion

- 30 to 60 cc;
- signs are
  —fluid thrill transmitted across the knee by flicking one side and palpating the other, and
  —patellar tap, i.e., obliteration of the suprapatellar pouch by pressing it with one hand and tapping the anterior surface of the patella with a finger of the other hand to feel it bouncing off the femoral condyle.

Large effusion

- is obvious because the
  —joint is swollen,
  —fluctuates, and the
  —suprapatellar pouch bulges around the top and sides of the patella like an inverted horseshoe.

Underlying injury

- look for underlying injury by
  —a good history,
  —careful clinical examination,
  —AP and lateral x-rays and other appropriate views.
  —aspiration of the joint if necessary, examination of the fluid, and reexamination of the joint with the patient under anesthesia if necessary.

TREATMENT

- if you have not found a specific injury other than the effusion, treat the patient with a
  —well padded compression bandage (never wrap an elastic bandage around a swollen joint or limb) or a
  —posterior plaster splint;
  —crutches, non-weight-bearing (NWB) on the injured leg, and
  —physiotherapy with isometric quadriceps exercises (the patient can do these at home);
- as swelling subsides, reexamine the knee. This becomes easier when the initial pain and swelling have disappeared. If there is an underlying ligamentous or meniscal injury, you should be able to find it now.
- if there are no signs of other injury, the patient probably had a synovial tear which is healing; in this case,
- start knee mobilization and allow partial weight-bearing (PWB), with progression to full weight-bearing (FWB) when the patient has recovered good quadriceps control. Do not allow weight-bearing if the quadriceps muscle is weak.

Ligamentous Injuries without Instability (First and Second Degree Sprains)

CLINICAL EXAMINATION

- all ligament injuries are called sprains;
- examine the knee carefully;
- the best and often the least painful opportunity for examination of the knee is immediately after the injury;

• if you suspect instability, aspirate the effusion and reexamine the knee, if necessary with the patient under local or general anesthesia (the knee may be too painful to examine without anesthesia).

First degree sprain

• mild point tenderness (use the blunt end of a pen or pencil to elicit this sign) over the ligament where it is injured,
• little or no swelling,
• no instability and
• very little disability;
• very few fibers are torn.

Second degree sprain

• more localized tenderness, maybe
• small effusion and
• some disability, but the patient can walk, albeit with a limp;
• no instability, although more fibers are torn.

RADIOLOGICAL EXAMINATION

• AP and lateral x-rays to rule out fractures;
• stress x-rays (of both knees for comparison) if you are not sure of stability.

TREATMENT

• first degree sprain is treated symptomatically;
• second degree sprain requires
  —ice, elevation, bandage and rest until the pain and swelling have diminished. Then
  —reexamine the knee to rule out a meniscus tear and ligamentous instability. You may need to use a
  —splint or cast with the knee bent for 4 weeks, with isometric quadriceps exercises in the cast, then with
  —physiotherapy and active quadriceps exercises with progressive weight-bearing on crutches;
  —no return to sport is allowed before rehabilitation is completed.

Ligamentous Injuries with Instability (Third Degree Sprain)

ETIOLOGY

• often the result of a sport's injury;
• the athlete's foot is fixed by his cleats or by a ski, so when he turns quickly on that leg or is tackled from the side or from behind, the knee goes into
  —flexion and valgus, with internal rotation of the femur on the tibia; this

mechanism injures the medial ligamentous structures and the anterior cruciate; or, less commonly,

—flexion, with varus and external rotation of the femur; this injures the lateral structures;

- other mechanisms are
  —hyperextension and
  —anteroposterior displacement;
- other major causes include
  —motor vehicle and
  —industrial accidents.
- ligament ruptures almost never occur in children while the growth plates are open because the growth plate is weaker than the ligament. So the child suffers a growth plate injury instead.

CLINICAL FEATURES

History

- is important because the
  —mechanism of injury is a clue to
  —which structures are likely to be damaged. So
- listen to the patient because he may
- tell you the diagnosis;
- swelling of the knee immediately after injury denotes a
- hemarthrosis due to synovial tear or fracture;
- swelling in the knee 6 to 24 hours after injury is due to excessive synovial fluid in the knee and denotes a
  —synovial reaction to trauma.

Clinical examination

General

- examine the normal knee first and compare it with the injured knee, since some knees are normally more lax than others.
- ask the patient to relax and conduct the examination gently.
- look at the limb for
  —swelling and
  —deformity.
- palpate the knee with a pencil for point tenderness.
- examine the range of movement (ROM), especially the last few degrees of extension and of flexion.

Stress tests

Medial and lateral instability

- with the knee extended, test collateral stability first in
  —valgus for the medial structures, then in

—varus for the lateral structures;

—gross instability denotes torn cruciate ligaments as well;

- repeat the test, with the knee flexed 30°, for less obvious degrees of instability.

AP instability

- the drawer sign, elicited with the knee flexed and the foot fixed in neutral, denotes
  —anterior cruciate tear, if the anterior excursion of the tibial condyles is abnormal, and
  —posterior cruciate tear, if the posterior excursion is abnormal with increase in the patellar tendon slope (sagging or dishing of the tibia). But an intact medial meniscus may limit the anterior drawer sign, so circumvent this by the
- Lachman test which repeats the maneuver with the knee in extension. Feel for AP laxity and a "soft" end point, and look for loss or increase of patellar tendon slope.

Combined AP and rotational instability

- repeat the drawer test:
  —first, with the leg in 30° of internal rotation to tighten the lateral ligament and capsule. If the lateral tibial condyle rotates forward or backward, the lateral structures and a cruciate are torn;
  —second, with the leg in 15° of external rotation to tighten the medial ligament and capsule. If the medial tibial condyle rotates forward or backward, the medial structures and a cruciate ligament are torn.
- the pivot shift or jerk test and the Noyes flexion rotation drawer test are used to evaluate
  —anterolateral instability.

Classification of instability

- is based on abnormal movement of the tibia in relation to the femur;
- always compare clinically the injured knee with the sound one;
- complete ligamentous rupture is not essential for the development of functional instability; this may occur with a partial tear or stretching, and the capsuloligamentous complex may appear normal on visual inspection.

One-plane instability

Medial instability

- tibial moves away from the femur on the medial side;
- instability with the knee in extension denotes rupture of the
  —medial collateral ligament,
  —medial and posteromedial capsuloligamentous complex,

—anterior cruciate ligament and

—maybe the posterior cruciate too. If the

- knee joint opens on the medial side when the knee is flexed to 30° but is stable in extension,
  - —torn medial collateral ligament and
  - —torn medial capsule are indicated. The degree of instability is based on the severity of the injury to the medial structures.

Lateral instability

- tibia moves away from the femur on the lateral side;
- instability with the knee in extension implies rupture of the
  - —lateral collateral ligament,
  - —lateral and posterolateral capsuloligamentous complex,
  - —biceps tendon,
  - —iliotibial band,
  - —anterior cruciate and often the
  - —posterior cruciate ligament.
- stability with the knee in extension but opening with the knee flexed to 30° suggests rupture of the
  - —lateral ligament and
  - —capsule, with the degree varying with the severity of the injury.

Anterior instability

- a positive anterior drawer sign with the knee in neutral rotation signifies
  - —partial or complete rupture of the anterior cruciate ligament with damage to the
  - —medial and lateral capsule.

Posterior instability

- a positive posterior drawer sign and "dishing" of the anterior tibial profile indicate a
  - —torn posterior cruciate ligament with damage to the
  - —posteromedial and posterolateral capsular ligamentous complexes.

Rotary instability (Fig. 20.2)

- denotes injury to a combination of structures.

Anteromedial and posteromedial instability

- the joint opens on the medial side and the medial tibial condyle slides forward (anteromedial instability) and/or backward (anterolateral instability) on the medial femoral condyle;
- instability is secondary to rupture of the

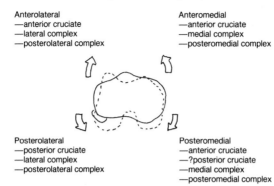

Anterolateral
—anterior cruciate
—lateral complex
—posterolateral complex

Anteromedial
—anterior cruciate
—medial complex
—posteromedial complex

Posterolateral
—posterior cruciate
—lateral complex
—posterolateral complex

Posteromedial
—anterior cruciate
—?posterior cruciate
—medial complex
—posteromedial complex

Figure 20.2. Rotary instability of the knee and the structures which are damaged. (Modified from Nicholas JA: The five-one reconstruction for anterior instability of the knee. *J Bone Joint Surg* 55A:899–922, 1973.)

—medial collateral ligament,
—medial and posteromedial capsuloligamentous complex and
—anterior cruciate ligament, and perhaps
—partial rupture of the posterior cruciate ligament with postero-medial instability.

Anterolateral instability

- the joint opens on the lateral side and the lateral tibial condyle slides forward on the femur. This is the
- pivot shift or jerk test;
- due to a torn
  —lateral and posterolateral capsuloligamentous complex and
  —anterior cruciate.

Posterolateral instability

- the joint opens on the lateral side and the lateral tibial condyle slides backward on the femur;
- caused by rupture of the
  —lateral and posterolateral capsuloligamentous complex,
  —biceps tendon and
  —sometimes the posterior cruciate.

RADIOLOGICAL FEATURES

- always order AP and lateral x-rays, and look for
  —fractures and
  —osteochondral fragments. Oblique and tunnel views may be of help.
- stress films in valgus and varus may be helpful especially in the

—adolescent, to differentiate ligament rupture from epiphyseal plate injury, and

—adult, to determine the degree of abnormal joint mobility.

- instability may be graded on stress films:
    —one plus when the opening of the joint is 5 mm or less in relation to normal side,
    —two plus when the opening is between 5 and 10 mm, and
    —three plus when the opening is 10 mm or more.

TREATMENT OF RECENT INJURIES

One plus instability

- can usually be treated satisfactorily without surgery by a
    —long leg cast for 6 weeks with the knee flexed 45° and
    —isometric quadriceps exercises;
- after cast removal
    —progressive knee mobilization and vigorous isotonic exercises for the quadriceps, hamstrings and triceps;
    —no sport is allowed until rehabilitation is complete. There
- may be a little residual ligamentous laxity.

Two and three plus instability

- require prompt surgical repair;
- if delay is more than 4 or 5 days, it would be better to
    —treat the instability with a plaster cast initially and
    —plan reconstructive surgery later for residual instability.

One-plane medial and medial rotary instability

- through a long, curved medial approach
- test stability under direct vision and examine
- medial support structures for injury to the
    —medial collateral ligament,
    —anterior, medial and posterior capsule,
    —semimembranosus tendon expansions to the posteromedial corner and to the
    —medial meniscus, and
    —cruciates.
- repair structures as necessary, paying particular attention to the posteromedial corner which is the key to a successful repair;
- excise the meniscus if it is torn in its substance, or suture it if it is detached from the capsule peripherally;
- if necessary, reinforce the
    —anteromedial capsule by vastus medialis or capsular advancement,
    —medial collateral ligament by sartorius advancement or pes ancerinus transfer, and

—posteromedial capsule by semimembranosus advancement or transfer of part of the tendon of the medial head of the gastrocnemius;

- pes anserinus transfer can be performed if further reinforcement of the medial structures and anterior cruciate is required and rotary instability is anteromedial.
- postoperatively, apply a
  —long leg cast with the knee flexed 40° and start the patient on
  —isometric quadriceps and hamstring exercises, NWB with crutches;
  —remove the cast 6 weeks later and
  —start the patient on active knee mobilization and isotonic quadriceps exercises, with the knee protected in a
  —brace and NWB until the quadriceps and knee are strong enough to take the patient's full weight;
- for return to sports, protect the knee with a derotational brace.

One-plane lateral and lateral rotary instability

- less common than medial injuries;
- through a long recurved lateral incision,
- test stability and examine
- lateral support structures for tears of the
  —biceps tendon and iliotibial tract,
  —lateral collateral ligament,
  —capsule anteriorly, laterally and posteriorly,
  —popliteus muscle and tendon (arcuate ligament complex) at the posterolateral corner and the
  —lateral meniscus, and
  —cruciate ligaments;
- examine the lateral popliteal nerve if signs of nerve damage were present before surgery;
- repair all torn or damaged structures, starting with the cruciates, and
- remove the lateral meniscus if it is torn in its substance, or reattach it if it is torn peripherally;
- structures to be used for reinforcement of lateral repair if necessary are the
  —lateral part of the tendinous origin of the lateral head of the gastrocnemius,
  —transplantation of part or all of the biceps tendon, or
  —part of the iliotibial band.
- postoperative care is similar to that for medial repair.

One-plane AP instability

- isolated rupture of a cruciate ligament is unusual;
- recent, complete rupture which is clinically evident requires surgical repair.

Anterior cruciate

- long anteromedial incision;
- examine the medial meniscus, and if it is torn in its substance, perform partial or complete meniscectomy;
- examine other structures for stability;
- the cruciate ligament may be torn, even though its synovial sheath remains intact, so incise this longitudinally and examine the ligament;
- if the ligament is torn in its midportion, suture it and reinforce this repair by the MacIntosh "over-the-top" method, using a strip of the patelloquadriceps tendon or the iliotibial band.
- if it is torn from bone or torn with a tibial flake, reattach it;
- repair other torn structures as necessary;
- then test for AP and rotary stability. If the anterior drawer sign is still present, reinforce the repair by the
- MacIntosh "over-the-top" method.

Posterior cruciate

- longitudinal curved, medial incision as for medial collateral ligament repair (see previous discussion);
- examine other structures for stability and repair them as necessary;
- suture the cruciate ligament or reattach it to bone;
- if the knee is still unstable after repair or the ligament was torn through its substance, reinforce it with the medial third of the tendon of the medial head of the gastrocnemius, a dynamic reconstruction.

Postoperative care

- similar to that for collateral ligament repair (see previous discussion).

COMPLICATIONS AND PROGNOSIS

Complications

- avoid a hematoma by
  —deflating the tourniquet before closure,
  —tying bleeders and
  —draining the wound.
- vigorous retraction by an enthusiastic assistant or cast pressure over the fibular neck may compress the peroneal nerve;
- knee stiffness may occur with severe ligamentous injury. A little stiffness is better than too much laxity. Return of normal mobility may take 6 months. If the return to normal mobility takes a long time, treat with exercises, wedged casts, traction or surgical release.
- instability! The surgery should have cured this!

- progressive degenerative arthrosis and meniscus wear occur in an unstable knee. This complication is less likely after repair. Severity and speed of development of degenerative changes depend on the
  —residual degree of laxity and on the
  —amount that the patient uses the knee.

Prognosis

- good after early repair,
- poorer after late repair;
- poor results are caused by
  —failure to repair some of the injured tissues,
  —poor healing of repaired tissues,
  —poor muscle power and
  —postoperative complications.

Old Untreated Ligament Ruptures

GENERAL

- at 3 months or more after injury the diagnosis is easier because the inflammatory reaction has subsided and the knee is relatively painless. Before definitive surgical treatment,
- reinforce the musculature by a concentrated program of exercises, then
- reexamine the knee and judge every injury on its own merits.
- late surgical repair is not indicated for a
  —debilitated patient, an
  —isolated cruciate ligament rupture, a
  —relatively stable knee or a knee with
  —degenerative and symptomatic arthrosis.
- there are many methods of treating chronic instability of the knee. The following are merely guidelines.

MEDIAL ROTARY INSTABILITY

- reconstruct the anterior cruciate ligament by either a MacIntosh "over-the-top" reconstruction (see the previous discussion) or the Jones technique;
- tighten the medial collateral ligament or reattach it more proximally under tension and reinforce it as necessary;
- tighten the posteromedial corner and reinforce it with the medial head of the gastrocnemius;
- transplant the pes anserinus as indicated.

LATERAL ROTARY INSTABILITY

- reconstruct the
  —cruciate ligaments as described previously and the

—lateral collateral ligament with use of a rolled strip of fascia lata or biceps tendon;

- the posterolateral corner and lateral collateral ligament can be reinforced by the Losee modification of MacIntosh's technique, i.e., threading a strip of
  —fascia lata through the
  —lateral femoral condyle,
  —lateral head of the gastrocnemius,
  —posterolateral capsule and
  —lateral ligament and suturing it to itself at Gerdy's tubercle.

Dislocation of Knee

ETIOPATHOLOGY

- uncommon in adults and rare in children and young adolescents who usually have growth plate injuries instead. Dislocation is
- usually caused by a
  —motor vehicle or
  —sport's accident;
- 50% are anterior dislocations, i.e., the tibia dislocates anteriorly, and are caused by a
  —hyperextension injury, first with a
  —posterior capsular tear, followed by a
  —partial or complete tear of the posterior cruciate, then with a partial or complete tear of the anterior cruciate and one or both collateral ligaments.
- other dislocations are caused by severe
  —varus or
  —valgus stress, often with a rotary component, and are associated with varying degrees of ligament injury;
- one third of knee dislocations are associated with a popliteal artery injury which may be a
  —complete rupture,
  —intimal tear, or
  —contusion with thrombosis. The
- popliteal artery, traveling distally down the center of the popliteal fossa, is very vulnerable because proximally it is
  —fixed to the distal femur as it passes through the adductor canal in the adductor magnus just above the adductor tubercle and because distally it is
  —fixed to the tibia where it passes under the tendinous arch of the soleus, just below the joint;

—so the artery lies taut in the popliteal fossa like a bowstring;
- 25% to 30% of dislocations involve neurological injury, especially
    —posterolateral dislocation which injures the peroneal nerve because this is fixed as it enters the peroneal muscles.

CLINICAL AND RADIOLOGICAL FEATURES
- deformity is usually obvious unless the patient is fat or the dislocation is already reduced before you see the patient;
- examine the vascular and neurological status of the leg;
- when you examine the knee for laxity, do so carefully and gently to avoid further risk of artery or nerve damage;
- take AP and lateral x-rays of the knee to rule out associated fractures.

TREATMENT
- reduction is urgent to avoid risk of further soft tissue damage and alleviate tension on the neurovascular structures;
- closed reduction with the patient under general anesthesia is usually successful and is all that is required for a child or adolescent;
- reduce by
    —traction on the leg with countertraction on the thigh, then
    —gentle manipulation of the femur and tibia, avoiding hyperextension and varus because these may injure the popliteal artery or peroneal nerve.
- examine the blood supply to the leg again after reduction, the
    —dorsalis pedis and posterior tibial pulses, and the
    —color, temperature and capillary return, and if you are still in doubt, perform an
    —arteriogram and, if necessary,
    —explore the popliteal artery without delay;
- if an x-ray shows good reduction and the circulation is satisfactory, apply a posterior backslab cast with the knee flexed 15° and assess circulation regularly;
- if the circulation is normal after 1 week of observation in the hospital,
- reexamine the knee and
- repair torn structures surgically. Then
    —apply a long leg cast with the knee flexed 25° and teach the patient to perform
    —isometric quadriceps and straight leg raising exercises in the cast;
- remove the cast at 6 weeks, protect the knee with a brace, and mobilize the knee with isotonic quadriceps exercises.
- indications for immediate surgery include
    —open dislocation,
    —arterial injury or insufficiency or

—failed or incomplete reduction due to a femoral condyle, which may buttonhole through the capsule, or a collateral ligament or the capsule which may be inverted into the knee joint.

COMPLICATIONS AND PROGNOSIS

- usually there is some remaining ligamentous instability which may cause early degenerative changes in the joint;
- residual vascular insufficiency may cause
  —intermittent claudication,
  —trophic ulcers and
  —Volkmann's ischemic contracture of the foot and toes;
- nerve injuries are usually traction injuries with neuropraxia or axonotmesis; the nerve may heal in time. If the
- nerve does not heal, residual problems will include
  —drop foot and
  —anesthesia along the outside of the leg if the peroneal nerve is injured, or
  —calcaneus deformity of the foot and
  —anesthesia of the sole if the tibial nerve is injured. Treat by
  —exploration and neurolysis or repair of the nerve and/or
  —bony stabilizing procedures, followed by tendon transfers about the foot if nerve healing is unlikely.

chapter 21

Meniscal Injuries
of the Knee

ETIOPATHOLOGY (Fig. 21.1)

- for surgical and functional anatomy, see Chapter 20.
- during flexion and rotary knee movements, menisci are stretched and displaced; they return to their normal position because of their elasticity and peripheral attachments;
- femoral rotation on a loaded, flexed knee may
  —force the meniscus toward the center of the joint and
  —trap it between the condyles. Then, when the knee
  —moves into extension, the condyles
  —tear the meniscus. The
- medial meniscus, especially the posterior horn, is injured more often than the lateral meniscus because the medial meniscus
  —is attached to the deep part of the medial collateral ligament and is less mobile than the lateral meniscus and because the
  —popliteus muscle is partly inserted into the posterior horn of the lateral meniscus and pulls this backward away from condyles during flexion, thus protecting the meniscus;
- the menisci are more vulnerable to injury if the
  —knee is unstable from an old ligament injury, or the
  —meniscus is degenerating, or the patient has a
  —congenital discoid meniscus which is oval instead of semilunar.
- a meniscal tear may be
  —partial, usually on the inferior surface of the meniscus, or
  —complete. Tears are
- classified as
  —longitudinal, in the body of the meniscus, and the free margin may be displaced into the intercondylar region, a "bucket-handle" tear; or
  —oblique, with the free fragment attached to the meniscus only at one end, a "parrot's beak" or pedunculated tear; or
  —peripheral, with the meniscus detached from the synovium and capsule

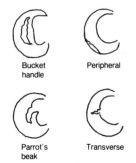

Figure 21.1. Meniscal tears.

at the periphery (do not mistake popliteal tendon hiatus for a peripheral tear of the lateral meniscus); or

—transverse, which is more common in the lateral meniscus because the inner concave border has a tight curve and the anterior and posterior segments are more easily separated. This tear also occurs in a degenerated meniscus.

- menisci may regenerate after removal, but the new meniscus is thin, narrow, fibrous and relatively insignificant.

Clinical and Radiological Features

HISTORY

- as with all knee injuries, the history is particularly important because you may sometimes make the diagnosis on this alone. In general, a
- young male adult with a twisting injury, often occurring at sport, may have an acute tear, whereas an
- older person with a mild injury, or even with a normal movement such as squatting, may tear a degenerated meniscus.

Acute stage

- patient may feel "something go" or snap in the joint while playing a sport, turning or squatting; he feels
- pain on one side of joint due to irritated or injured synovium or capsule;
- movement may be limited;
- the joint gradually swells over the succeeding hours.

Chronic stage

- over the ensuing months the untreated patient may have
  - —recurrent effusions (if the patient has never had an effusion, he is unlikely to have a torn meniscus);
  - —recurrent episodes of locking (30% of meniscal tears have this; the

patient may learn a trick movement to unlock the joint, usually rotation and passive extension);

—localized pain and tenderness;

—sensation of the knee "giving way," especially on rotary movements (if this occurs on flexion without rotation, it may be due to a weak quadriceps or an anterior cruciate tear, so beware!).

EXAMINATION

- the patient may have any of the following signs:
- quadriceps atrophy;
- intra-articular effusion;
- tenderness along the joint line (use the blunt end of a pencil for greater precision);
- limited movement, particularly loss of the last few degrees of extension or flexion, due either to the
  —effusion,
  —muscle spasm or a
  —meniscal tear blocking the joint;
- pain on forced, extreme flexion;
- positive McMurray test as the
  —rotated knee is brought from flexion to
  —full extension while the
  —tibial condyles are compressed against the femur;
  —if there is a tear, this test brings the torn fragment between the condyles, causing a painful click or even locking. A
  —painless click is not significant.
- Apley's test is based on a principle similar to that of the McMurray test, but the
  —patient is prone and tibiofemoral compression can be varied;
  —pain when the test is repeated without compression suggests a ligament injury;
- localized pain on squatting with the knees in
  —internal rotation suggests lateral meniscal pathology and with the knees in
  —external rotation implicates the medial meniscus. Location of pain in the medial or lateral compartment is also significant.
- 70% of torn menisci in young patients are associated with a torn anterior cruciate ligament with an anterior drawer sign because the
  —anterior cruciate is the guardian of the medial meniscus.

RADIOLOGICAL FEATURES

- take AP and lateral x-rays to rule out an
  —osteochondral fracture, a
  —loose body or other joint pathology;

- arthrography can be a useful diagnostic tool and may be of help in difficult diagnoses, showing
- in particular the popliteal fossa, the posteromedial and posterolateral meniscal attachments, and the anterior horns and the undersurface of the menisci, areas that cannot be well seen by arthroscopy.
- interpretation of the arthrogram depends on the experience of the arthrographer;
- arthrography is
  —not infallible, should
  —not be used routinely, and should
  —not be the sole criterion on which the treatment is based.

ARTHROSCOPY

- is a useful diagnostic adjunct, but
  —time and patience are needed to master the technique, and
  —accurate intepretation is proportional to the experience of the surgeon;
- it should be used only in
  —conjunction with a
  —good history and clinical examination,
  —x-rays and arthrography, and should not be the sole criterion on which the treatment is based.
- indications for arthroscopy include the
  —diagnostic problem knee,
  —synovial biopsy,
  —inspection of the patellar and femoral intercondylar articular surfaces, the lateral meniscus and the anterior cruciate ligament, all structures poorly shown by arthrography, and
  —visualization of the posterior meniscal horns, the compartment opposite the incision, and patellofemoral functional relationship, all areas difficult to see through an arthrotomy.
- through the operating arthroscope
  —multiple synovial biopsies can be made and
  —small loose bodies and
  —parts of a torn meniscus can be removed.

CHILDREN

- meniscal tears occur much less frequently in children, especially in girls, than they do in adults;
- you should be very cautious before making a definite diagnosis of meniscal tear and operating;
- most children's knee problems are solved with
  —rest and
  —time, so be patient.

Differential Diagnosis

- the knee is a difficult joint to evaluate and requires experience, so examine as many knee joints as you can;
- many conditions have similar signs and symptoms to meniscal tears, so
- never make a definitive diagnosis on the first examination. Reexamine the patient on several occasions and write down your findings each time.
- mimics of meniscal tears are:
- osteochondral fracture. Loose bodies in the joint may have a
  —history of injury with
  —recurrent effusions and
  —locking;
  —the fragment can usually be seen on good x-rays or an arthrogram.
- chondromalacia is
  —more common in women than in men. The
  —pain is around the patella and is aggravated by walking up or down stairs and standing up from squatting. There is
  —pain on contraction of the quadriceps with the patella fixed by the examiner's hand and
  —painful patellofemoral crepitus, although this is not a reliable sign. A
  —painful click and pseudolocking may also occur.
- subluxing patella is
  —more common in women than in men. There is
  —pain and tenderness along one side of patella, usually medially, and the
  —skyline patella x-ray of both knees shows eccentricity of the symptomatic patella with the patient supine and the knee flexed 30°.
- ligamentous instability. Careful examination should differentiate a meniscal tear from a ligament injury, but do not forget that an
  —abnormal meniscus makes the knee more vulnerable to ligament injury and
  —vice versa, and therefore
  —both may coexist in the same knee;
- traumatic synovitis usually abates with time, rest and symptomatic treatment; do not operate on a knee that is getting better.
- a woman's knee may frequently mimic a meniscal tear. False positive diagnosis is 3 or 4 times higher in women than in men, so be very cautious with a woman's knee!

Treatment
NONOPERATIVE
- the injury must be a
  —small, recent peripheral tear proven by arthrography and/or arthroscopy in a

—previously uninjured knee with a
—full range of movement and
—no associated fracture or instability;
- inform the patient that the
  —tear may not heal and that
  —surgery may be necessary later;
- immobilize the knee in extension with a
  —cylinder cast and teach the patient
  —daily isometric exercises;
- remove the cast at 4 or 5 weeks,
  —mobilize the knee and start the patient on
  —intensive exercises for all muscle groups of the limb.
- if the tear does not heal and symptoms persist,
  —reevaluate the knee and
  —consider surgery.

OPERATIVE

Rationale

- the functional disability caused by leaving an unhealed torn meniscus is usually greater than the probability of developing degenerative changes after meniscectomy. This is the rationale of surgery.

Arthrotomy

- through a parapatellar incision
- examine the
  —synovium,
  —synovial fluid for quantity, color and consistency,
  —articular cartilage,
  —cruciate ligaments and as much of the
  —opposite compartment as is visible, including the
  —other meniscus;
- always perform this general examination first, so that you do not forget it;
- then examine the meniscus in question. If the meniscus is
- not torn, look for another cause of the patient's problem;
- do not remove a normal meniscus.

Meniscectomy

Partial excision

- if the torn fragment is
  —small,
  —confined to the concave edge and
  —easily removed and the

- rest of the meniscus is normal and stable, the
- torn portion only may be removed. The
- advantages of partial meniscectomy are a
  —single incision,
  —less traumatic surgery and
  —faster rehabilitation. The
- disadvantages are that the portion of the meniscus left in the knee may have
  —occult tears or
  —degenerated areas making it more vulnerable to injury later on.

Total excision

- in general, a meniscus which is
  —torn in its substance, or has a
  —large peripheral tear or
  —multiple tears, or causes
  —recurrent locking or effusions, or has been
  —repeatedly injured should be
  —excised in its entirety.
- two incisions, anteromedial and posteromedial or anterolateral and posterolateral, are preferred to allow
  —better visualization of the posterior horn and other posterior structures in the joint and to permit
  —repair or tightening of the capsular structures as necessary.

Postoperative care

- bulky dressing or a cast, with isometric quadriceps and straight leg raising exercises;
- at 14 days, remove the cast and dressing and
  —mobilize the knee. When this flexes to 90°, start the patient on
  —isotonic quadriceps exercises unless there is patellofemoral chondromalacia;
- start the patient on progressive weight-bearing (WB) when muscle strength around the knee has been regained.

Complications

- operating on the
  —wrong side or the wrong patient is a mistake which can be
  —avoided by
  —asking the patient before surgery which side it is and
  —checking his chart;
- technical errors are easy to make. The careful surgeon

—makes fewer mistakes,
—recognizes them at the time and
—treats them immediately and, if he is wise,
—talks to the patient about the problem afterward. This way he may
—retain the patient's confidence and cooperation.
- hemarthrosis can be
  —prevented by careful hemostasis before closing and by draining the knee for 48 hours after surgery;
  —treat it by aspiration, rest and immobilization of the limb.
- synovitis and effusion are often caused by mobilization or WB started too early. Treat by immobilization. If a synovial sinus develops, treat by immobilization, and if it is unclosed at 2 weeks, excise it and close it with nonreactive sutures.
- infection may
  —destroy the articular cartilage and
  —stiffen the joint. Need one say more?
- retained posterior horn can be avoided by making two incisions.
- degenerative arthritis may be caused by an
  —untreated, torn meniscus, especially if it is the source of instability, recurrent locking and effusions;
  —total and even partial meniscectomy may also produce degenerative changes because the underlying cartilage is no longer protected and removal of the meniscus may produce or increase instability. Finally, the
  —initial injury may also be implicated in causing degenerative changes.

Prognosis

- with the
  —correct diagnosis,
  —appropriate treatment and
  —no complications,
  —early results are good. But
- many of these patients will develop early degenerative arthrosis.
- late results may be affected by the
  —sex of the patient (the results are worse in women than in men),
  —side of the injury (results are worse with lateral meniscectomy than with medial meniscectomy),
  —delay between injury and treatment,
  —frequency and severity of symptoms and
  —associated ligament injury or instability.

Meniscal Cysts

- cysts are more common on the lateral meniscus than on the medial meniscus and are
- associated with degenerative changes in the meniscus or may
- develop after injury;
- a cyst is filled with a gelatinous substance;
- clinical features include
    —a loud snap or click on flexion and extension of knee; the snap is usually painful;
    —no locking or effusion unless the meniscus is torn also; a
    —small, hard palpable mass in the joint line just in front of the fibular head with the knee in extension;
    —the mass becomes smaller or disappears into the joint on flexion.
- differential diagnosis includes a
    —discoid meniscus, which may cause a loud painless snap or an effusion even if it is not torn, or an
    —abnormal popliteus tendon slipping over the margin of lateral femoral condyle.
- treatment is excision of the meniscus as well as of the cyst because the meniscus usually has degenerative changes which predispose it to a tear.

chapter 22

Proximal Tibial Fractures

Articular Fractures of Proximal Tibia

ETIOPATHOLOGY

- mechanism is a
  - —varus or, more commonly, a
  - —valgus stress on the knee while the leg is supporting body weight, sometimes with a
  - —rotational component;
- femoral condyle breaks into the tibial plateau, with the collateral ligament on the opposite side acting as a fulcrum, or
- both femoral condyles together may fracture both tibial condyles, as in vertical compression due to a fall from a height;
- type of fracture, location and degree of displacement and comminution depend on the
  - —force and its angle of impact, the degree of
  - —knee flexion at the moment of impact, and
  - —whether body weight is on the leg or not. The opposite
- collateral and the cruciate ligaments may be torn.

CLASSIFICATION (Fig. 22.1)

- there are many classifications. The following, which is modified from Hohl, is practical and simple.

  #### Split fracture
  - a tibial condyle or part of a condyle is split off in one piece;
  - cortex and the articular cartilage of the fragment may be intact;
  - fracture line may be
    - —vertical, fracturing part of the condyle, or
    - —oblique, fracturing the whole condyle. The
  - fragment may be
    - —anterior, posterior, or lateral, and it may be
    - —undisplaced,
    - —displaced laterally, displaced distally or tilted.

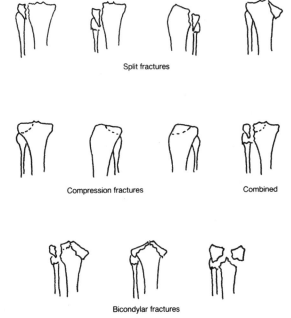

Figure 22.1.   Tibial plateau fractures. (Modified from Hohl M: Tibial condylar fractures. *J Bone Joint Surg* 49A:1455–1467, 1967.)

Compression fracture

- part of the tibial condylar articular surface is pushed down into the tibial metaphysis;
- articular surface is usually comminuted with multiple fractures through the cartilage.

Combined split-compression fracture

- is a combination of the first two types of fracture;
- either part may be displaced;
- comminution is common.

Bicondylar fracture

- both tibial condyles are fractured;
- fractures may be any combination of above three types with
- any combination of displacement and comminution.

RADIOLOGICAL FEATURES (Fig. 22.2)

- anteroposterior (AP) and lateral x-rays are essential. If there is a compression fracture, ask for another AP x-ray angled 10° downward and backward to parallel the
  —normal tilt of the tibial plateau. An
  —ordinary horizontal AP x-ray would exaggerate displacement of a compression fracture in the posterior part of the condyle;
- oblique x-rays and tomograms may also be of help.
- with the knee in extension, stress it in varus or valgus holding your thumb on the joint line opposite the fracture. If this line opens, repeat with x-ray to see whether the collateral ligament is torn.

TREATMENT

Undisplaced fractures

- includes all fractures displaced less than ½ cm;
- if the patient is elderly, or the skin over the knee is in poor condition, or surgery is inadvisable for other reasons, a displacement of up to 1 cm can be treated by closed methods too;
- long leg cast with the knee in 5° of flexion for 3 weeks, non-weight-bearing (NWB), and isometric quadriceps exercises. The leg must be properly aligned to avoid varus or valgus;
- knee mobilization exercises after cast removal;
- if the patient is in the hospital for other reasons, treatment with 1 or 2 kg of skin traction is better than treatment with a cast because traction allows knee mobilization from the beginning;
- patient starts weight-bearing (WB) when x-rays show that the fracture has united, usually at 8 weeks.

Displaced fractures

Split fracture

Vertical partial condylar fracture

- a displacement of more than ½ cm should have open reduction and internal fixation. Use an
- appropriate incision according to the position of the fracture, usually anteromedial or anterolateral, curving posteriorly at the distal end;

Figure 22.2. Tibial condyles slope back.

- for open reduction of all types of tibial condylar fractures, the following general principles apply:
  —open the knee joint to aid in accurate reduction;
  —it may be necessary to divide the peripheral attachment of the meniscus to the tibia and elevate the meniscus with the femoral condyle to see clearly the tibial articular surface. Resuture the periphery of the meniscus after surgery. Do not remove the meniscus unless it is torn;
  —do not remove soft tissue attachments from the fragment. Dissect along the fracture line, reduce the fracture (not as easy as it looks), and fix it firmly with bolts, screws or a buttress plate;
  —repair associated cruciate and contralateral capsular and ligamentous tears concurrently through appropriate incisions;
  —irrigate the joint and remove loose fragments of bone and cartilage;
  —AP and lateral x-rays before closing are important. If the reduction is inadequate, try again.
- postoperatively, treatment consists of
  —mobilization in skin traction for 10 days, then a
  —long leg cast for 4 weeks and isometric quadriceps exercises; and
  —NWB for 8 weeks after surgery.

Oblique total condylar fracture

- articular surface is often not comminuted;
- fracture fragment is angulated and impacted onto the metaphysis;
- if there is a varus or valgus deformity of more than 5° (i.e., 5° more than that on the normal side), try
  —closed reduction by manipulation with the patient under anesthesia and a
  —molded long leg cast;
  —verify the position after 5 days, and if the fracture has redisplaced, treat by
- open reduction and internal fixation with a plate.
- postoperative care is the same as that discussed previously.

Compression fracture

Posterior

- cast or traction, then mobilization, as discussed previously.

Middle or anterior

- if the displacement is less than ½ cm, treat with a cast or traction. If
- displacement is more than ½ cm, treat by
  —open reduction through a tibial window just distal to the fracture. use a

—buttress bone graft beneath the depressed condyle, if necessary, and

—internal fixation with a plate, with the screws used to hold the graft in place;

—the articular surface may be very comminuted, resembling crazy paving, so

—irrigate the joint before closing;

—preserve the meniscus unless it is torn;

- postoperative care is the same as that discussed previously.

Combined split-compression fracture

- if the

—split fragment is displaced laterally and no longer supports the femoral condyle, try

—closed reduction and percutaneous pinning. If this

—fails or the

—compressed fragment is large and depressed more than ½ cm, perform

—open reduction and internal fixation, supporting the compression fragment with a bone graft beneath it if necessary.

- postoperative care is the same as that discussed previously.

Bicondylar fracture

- vessels are particularly vulnerable in bicondylar injuries, so check repeatedly the blood supply to the foot;
- accurate open reduction and internal fixation may be ideal but are very difficult to perform. Unless there are intra-articular fragments, it is better to use
- skeletal traction through the distal tibia. Closed manipulation with the patient under anesthesia may be necessary to reduce the fragments;

—start the patient on early passive and active mobilization of the knee in traction and on quadriceps exercises;

—remove the traction at 4 weeks and apply a

—long leg cast for another 4 weeks. Then

—start WB if the fractures have healed and

—continue physiotherapy (for knee mobilization) and quadriceps exercises.

COMPLICATIONS

- ischemia of the leg due to a vessel injury or a compartment syndrome;
- peroneal nerve injury, particularly in varus injuries;
- poor reduction or loss of reduction, with varus or valgus angulation of the tibia;

- instability of the knee;
- limited motion of the knee;
- degenerative arthritis, which is particularly likely with a comminuted fracture, instability or axial deformity.

MALUNITED FRACTURES

- if angulation is less than 8° valgus or 5° varus and the knee is stable, treat symptomatically;
- if angulation is greater than this, perform
  —corrective high tibial closing wedge osteotomy and, if necessary, a fibular osteotomy. This usually
- corrects instability too. If it does not, late ligamentous repair may be necessary.

Nonarticular Fractures of Proximal Tibia

TIBIAL SPINES AND INTERCONDYLAR EMINENCE (Fig. 22.3)

- the fragment is usually pulled off by the cruciate ligaments, the anterior ligament in adolescents and the posterior ligament in adults. So
- test ligamentous stability of the knee, if necessary with the patient under general anesthesia and with x-ray control. If the fracture is
- undisplaced or is
- elevated less than 20° at one end and the knee is
- stable,
- treat with a cast and isotonic quadriceps exercises;
- remove the cast at 6 weeks and mobilize the knee. If the fragment is
- displaced or
- elevated more than 20° at one end or the fragment is
- blocking full extension, try
- closed reduction with the patient under anesthesia and take x-rays. If the fracture reduces and the knee regains full extension, treat with a cast for 6 weeks. If
- closed reduction fails or the joint is
- unstable, perform
- open reduction and internal fixation with a screw or nonabsorbable sutures

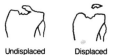

Undisplaced   Displaced

Figure 22.3.   Intercondylar tibial fractures.

and repair other capsular and ligamentous structures as necessary. Treat with a long leg cast for 4 weeks and quadriceps exercises, then apply a protective brace.

TIBIAL TUBERCLE FRACTURES

- the patellar tendon inserts here, so the tubercle is part of the extensor mechanism of the knee;
- fracture of the tubercle occurs mainly in adolescents. The tubercle may be
  —avulsed completely or
  —lifted off with part of the adjacent tibial epiphysis. In the
  —adult the injury is usually associated with a condylar fracture. If the fragment is
- undisplaced or can be
- reduced closed, treat by
  —immobilization in a cast with the knee in extension for 6 weeks. If the fragment is
- displaced more than 5 mm and
- cannot be reduced closed, perform
- open reduction and
  —internal fixation with a screw or nonabsorbable sutures through bone, not across the growth plate, and apply a
  —cast for 4 weeks;
- start the patient on resistive quadriceps exercises when the fragment has united.

PROXIMAL METAPHYSEAL FRACTURES (Fig. 22.4)

- usually a transverse fracture,
- often comminuted, and may have an
- intra-articular component;
- the fibula is usually fractured too. The tibial
- fracture occurs at or just above the
  —upper border of the interosseous membrane where the
  —anterior tibial artery passes forward between the tibia and the fibula to reach the anterior muscular compartment of leg. So the fracture easily

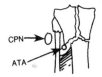

Figure 22.4. Fractures endangering the common peroneal nerve (*CPN*) and anterior tibial artery (*ATA*).

- injures either the
  —popliteal artery at its bifurcation into anterior and posterior tibial arteries
    or injures the
  —anterior tibial artery. For treatment of this complication, see Chapter
    32. With no vascular injury,
- treat by
  —closed reduction to align the tibia, then a
  —long leg cast for 6 weeks and isometric quadriceps exercises, followed by
    a
  —cast brace until the fracture is healed and the quadriceps has regained
    its strength.

Specific Children's Fractures

PROXIMAL TIBIAL EPIPHYSEAL PLATE INJURIES (Fig. 22.5)

- much less common than distal femoral growth plate injuries because the
  collateral ligaments are attached
  —proximally to the distal femoral epiphysis and can pull it off, whereas
  —distally the medial ligament bypasses the tibial epiphysis to reach the
    metaphysis, and the lateral ligament is not attached to the tibia at all.
- nearly always a Type I or II injury;
- stress x-rays may be required to differentiate this injury from a ligamentous
  injury;
- may be associated with vascular injury to the popliteal artery;
- treatment for Types I and II consists of
  —closed reduction and a
  —cast for 6 weeks. If this is unsatisfactory, perform
  —open reduction and internal fixation;
- Types III and IV usually need open reduction and internal fixation.

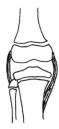

Figure 22.5. Collateral knee ligaments are not attached to the proximal tibial epiphysis.

Figure 22.6.   Valgus greenstick fracture of the proximal tibia.

PROXIMAL METAPHYSEAL FRACTURES

Greenstick fracture (Fig. 22.6)

- occurs usually in children under 7 years of age. The fracture
- angulates in valgus, opening on the medial side;
- the fibula is intact;
- treatment consists of
  —closed reduction with the patient under general anesthesia, with
  —correction of valgus by completion of the fracture and
  —application of a long leg cast molded in slight varus;
- if this is not done, even though the fracture looks undisplaced, the leg may develop a
  —valgus deformity.

Complete fracture

- occurs in older children;
- usually of both bones;
- the popliteal artery and its branches are in danger, so check the
  —blood supply and
  —pulses both
  —before and after reduction;
- treat by
  —closed reduction and a
  —long leg cast in slight varus.

chapter 23

Fractures of the Tibial Shaft

Surgical Anatomy

- the medial surface and anterior border of the tibia are subcutaneous;
- muscle groups lie in four compartments;
- each compartment, especially the anterior compartment, is bounded by strong, inelastic fascia, so that increased fluid in a compartment, e.g., blood from a fracture, immediately increases the pressure and may compress capillaries and vessels with resultant ischemia;
- the anterior compartment contains the
  - —tibialis anterior (TA), extensor hallucis longus (EHL) and extensor digitorum longus (EDL) muscles,
  - —deep peroneal nerve (anterior tibial) and
  - —anterior tibial artery. The
- lateral compartment contains the
  - —peroneus brevis (PB) and peroneus longus (PL) muscles and the
  - —superficial peroneal nerve (musculocutaneous). The
- superficial posterior compartment contains the
  - —soleus and gastrocnemius muscles which form the triceps. In the
- deep posterior compartment are the
  - —tibialis posterior (TP), flexor hallucis longus (FHL) and flexor digitorum longus (FDL) muscles,
  - —posterior tibial nerve,
  - —posterior tibial artery and
  - —peroneal artery (branch of posterior tibial).

Etiopathology and Clinical Features (Figs. 2.2, 2.3 and 22.4)

INDIRECT VIOLENCE

- a low-energy rotational injury causes an
- oblique or spiral fracture. The
- fibula may not be fractured,

- comminution is rare, and there is
- little soft tissue damage.

DIRECT VIOLENCE

- motor vehicle or industrial accidents and high-velocity
- missile wounds cause
- high-energy injuries. The
- fracture is usually
  —transverse,
  —comminuted or segmental and the
- fibula is usually fractured. The
- soft tissue injury to
  —skin and
  —muscle is often severe.

CLASSIFICATION

- classify the fracture by
  —association of the skin lesion (the tibia is subcutaneous, so the skin is easily damaged or broken by displaced or angulated fracture);
  —presence of comminution;
  —degree of displacement and angulation;
  —anatomical position of the fracture and whether the
  —fibula is fractured or not;
  —associated nerve or arterial damage, which is not common except in fractures of the proximal metaphysis at its junction with shaft. Nevertheless, always examine the neurovascular status of the leg and foot.
- for example, describe a fracture as a
  —closed, simple, undisplaced spiral fracture at the junction of the middle and distal thirds of right tibia with an intact fibula or as a
  —Type II open, comminuted, displaced, segmental fracture of the shaft of the left tibia with fracture of the fibula;
- this descriptive classification helps you to
  —evaluate the injury and
  —plan the treatment.

Treatment

GENERAL PRINCIPLES

- the tibia is one of the most frequently injured bones in the body;
- tibial fractures are
  —easy to treat badly but
  —difficult to treat well. The

- treatment of tibial fractures is very simple. Leave a
    —closed fracture closed and an
    —open fracture open,
    —elevate a very swollen leg before casting, and treat an associated
    —vascular injury as an emergency. The
- subcutaneous position of the tibia makes surgery very tempting, but
- open reduction with internal fixation has few advantages over closed reduction and a long leg cast. Open reduction should be employed only after failure of closed methods;
- anatomical reduction is not necessary. You can accept
    —10° posterior angulation, but more than 5° anterior angulation is not permissible because bone may cause pressure necrosis of overlying skin;
    —5° varus or 8° valgus;
    —8° external rotation or 5° internal rotation; and
    —1.5 cm of shortening;
- pad the cast over the
    —malleoli,
    —Achilles tendon, and
    —neck of the fibula.
- correct
    —rotation or excessive
    —shortening by a second reduction, and correct
    —angulation by a cast change or an open wedge. A closing wedge is dangerous because you may injure the skin. The
- technique of open wedging is performed as follows (Fig. 23.1):
    —the cast must be dry and well padded;
    —measure the angulation accurately on x-ray and
    —place the wedge where the long axes of the two shaft fragments intersect;
    —cut the cast three quarters of the way around, leaving the cast uncut over the apex of the angulation;
    —make a small, vertical cut at each end of the wedge to prevent the plaster from splitting right around;
    —then open the wedge until angulation is corrected. The angle of the wedge should then equal the original angle of the deformity;
    —hold the wedge open with small pieces of cork, wood or plaster,
    —take x-rays to confirm correction, and
    —roll plaster around the wedge to maintain the new position;
- angulation in two planes, AP and lateral, can be corrected by placing the center of the wedge between the apices of the two angular deformities.
- fracture healing in an adult takes from
    —16 to 26 weeks or more, depending on
    —degree of bony and soft tissue damage;

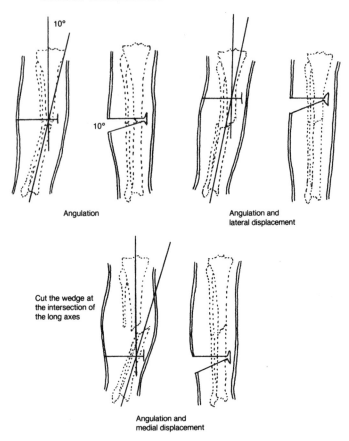

10°

10°

Angulation

Angulation and
lateral displacement

Cut the wedge at
the intersection of
the long axes

Angulation and
medial displacement

Figure 23.1.   Wedging a tibial cast.

- healing and rehabilitation are accelerated by early weight-bearing. A patient
  can walk with a long leg cast if the knee is not flexed more than 10°. A
- patellar tendon-bearing (PTB) cast allows knee flexion, but in tibial fractures the knee is less of a problem than are the ankle and subtalar joints.

CLOSED FRACTURES

Spiral, oblique and simple transverse fractures

Fibula intact

- fracture is stable but may angulate into varus;
- apply a long leg cast, with the patient under general anesthesia if
  necessary;

—mold the cast around the tibial and femoral condyles and

—slightly flatten the cast from side to side over the distal femur with the knee flexed 10° for comfort and for prevention of rotation at the fracture site; put the

—ankle at 90° and the

—foot plantigrade;

—molding in valgus may prevent varus tendency. A

- Sarmiento PTB cast can be applied when the fracture is "sticky." If the
- fracture is in the distal tibia, leave the ankle in 20° equinus for 4 weeks to avoid posterior angulation of the fracture, and when this is "sticky," change the cast and put the ankle at right angle.

Fibula fractured

- less stable;
- reduce the fracture, with patient under general anesthesia, by hanging the patient's leg over the end of the table and applying traction. Then apply a
- short leg cast and mold it around the ankle and leg to maintain reduction. When the cast is dry, lift the leg, complete the
- long leg cast with the knee flexed 10°, and take
- AP and lateral x-rays to verify reduction. If the fracture is
- angulated anteriorly, the tibia may
  —erode through the skin. Beware of this because it will convert a
  —closed fracture into an
  —open fracture. This is
  —particularly likely with fracture of the proximal third because the quadriceps pulls the proximal fragment forward.
- apply a PTB cast once the fracture is stable, usually at 4 to 6 weeks.

Follow-up

- teach the patient to use crutches and to perform
- isometric quadriceps exercises in the cast;
- the patient can start progressive weight-bearing (WB) at 3 weeks;
- take x-rays weekly for the first month to see that the reduction is not lost;
- change the cast at 3 months and evaluate the fracture
  —clinically and
  —radiologically.
- apply a new cast if the fracture is not completely healed and
- change it every 6 weeks until union is complete. Then treat with
- physiotherapy for mobilization of the
  —subtalar, ankle and knee joints and
  —muscle strengthening exercises for all muscle groups of the limb.

Comminuted fractures (Fig. 23.2)

- if gross swelling and fracture blisters are present, treat the limb by
    —skeletal traction with 3 or 4 kg through the distal tibia (best) or calcaneus and by
    —elevation on a Böhler-braun frame with a
    —posterior plaster splint.
- when the swelling has subsided, treat the fracture with a
    —long leg cast or
    —pins and plaster if you cannot maintain the reduction in a cast. Use
    —two Steinmann pins transversely in the proximal tibia and one in the distal tibia;
    —align the leg as it hangs over the end of the table,
    —apply a short leg cast to incorporate the pins in the plaster, complete the cast to the root of thigh as discussed previously, and take
    —AP and lateral x-rays to verify reduction;
- remove the pins at 4 weeks and apply a new cast to avoid delayed union or nonunion due to distraction of the fracture by the pins.
- follow-up care is the same as that discussed previously.
- if pins and plaster do not maintain good alignment,
    —continue treatment with
    —skeletal traction, with a posterior plaster splint used for comfort and for prevention of rotational movements.

Segmental fractures

- the middle fragment is difficult to control by closed methods. If the
- reduction is unsatisfactory, use an
- intramedullary nail with closed or open reduction. A
- plate is contraindicated because disturbance of the periosteum would
    —further jeopardize the blood supply of the middle segment, which is already

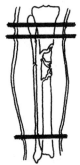

Figure 23.2.   Pins and plaster technique.

—relatively ischemic. If the
- nail controls rotation, a short leg Sarmiento walking cast will suffice for added protection.

Ipsilateral tibial and femoral shaft fractures

- best results are obtained by
    —open reduction and internal fixation of the femoral fracture and
    —closed reduction and a plaster cast for the tibial fracture, followed as soon as possible by
    —muscle strengthening exercises and later by
    —cast bracing and mobilization of the knee;
- open reduction of both fractures has a high complication rate, especially infection;
- closed reduction of both fractures with use of
    —pins and a short leg cast for the tibia and
    —traction through the most proximal tibial pin for the femur, with early isometric exercises followed by a spica or, better still, by a cast brace, is a
- safe method, but the pseudarthrosis rate is high.
- always examine the knee because these combined injuries may be
    —associated with ligamentous injury of the knee.

OPEN FRACTURES

- see Chapter 4 for general principles.
- prompt and adequate surgical debridement of the bone and surrounding soft tissues is of
- cardinal importance.
- external fixation with a
    —windowed cast is adequate for stable fractures and a small wound, whereas the
    —Hoffmann or Roger Anderson external skeletal fixation apparatus is ideal for unstable fracture or a large wound requiring daily care. The
- initial goal is a clean, closed wound. Once this is achieved, the
- secondary goal is union of the fracture.

Complications

- see Chapters 6 and 7

VESSELS (Fig. 22.4)

- injury to the anterior tibial artery is most likely with a high, comminuted fracture, and injury to either tibial vessel is most likely with fracture of the distal tibia and posterior displacement of the distal fragment. If
- arterial repair is indicated,

- internal fixation may be necessary to stabilize the fracture, but usually this can be managed by closed reduction and cast or pins and plaster or by external fixation after arterial repair.
- see Chapter 32.

COMPARTMENT SYNDROME

- see Chapter 32.
- is an ischemic syndrome, usually of the anterior muscular compartment of the leg, and is most common in closed fractures without displacement;
- occurs usually within 48 hours of fracture;
- clinical features are particularly
  —increasing pain and tenderness over the muscles with progressive development of
  —anesthesia and paralysis;
- intramuscular pressure readings with use of the Wick catheter and a manometer are helpful in
  —confirming the diagnosis and
  —guiding the treatment. At the first suspicion of muscle ischemia,
- cut all dressings down to the skin and elevate the leg. If there is no improvement after 30 minutes and the intramuscular pressure is more than 30 mm Hg, perform a
- complete fasciotomy and elevate the leg without a circular cast.
- there may be ischemia of more than one compartment, so examine all of them.

NERVE INJURY (Fig. 22.4)

- due to a
  —high fibular fracture or
  —badly molded cast around the neck of the fibula. The common peroneal nerve
- usually heals with time if the cast is split over the nerve. If there is
- no recovery at 3 months, explore the nerve.

DELAYED UNION AND NONUNION (Fig. 6.3)

- delayed union is defined as the
- absence of signs of union in a fracture at 16 weeks;
- the fracture will probably unite in time if the patient bears weight on it in a cast, but
- cancellous, autologous bone grafting will expedite healing and is therefore justified at this time.
- nonunion is defined as
- the absence of signs of union in a fracture at 26 weeks.
- nonunion is most likely when the fracture is
  —open and particularly when it is infected also, or when the fracture is

    —distracted, comminuted or segmental, or the fracture is in the

    —distal third of the tibia, or the

    —treatment has been inadequate.

- treatment of established nonunion consists of an
    - —autologous cancellous bone graft with
    - —internal or external immobilization;
- if the skin anteriorly is scarred or of poor quality, use a posterolateral or posteromedial approach for the graft. If the
- nonunion is infected,
    - —attain union first and
    - —then try for definitive treatment of the infection.

POSTTRAUMATIC DYSTROPHY

- also called Sudeck's atrophy;
- more common with prolonged immobilization in a cast and/or prolonged non-weight-bearing (NWB). The
- mechanism is unknown, but it is an exaggerated autonomic nervous system response to the injury and to subsequent inactivity.
- clinical features include a
    - —painful and
    - —edematous foot with
    - —stiff joints;
- radiologically the bones of the foot and distal tibia are very osteoporotic with spotty areas of decalcification.
- treatment is long and difficult;
- reduce swelling by
    - —elevation,
    - —elastic bandages and
    - —active muscle exercises. Then treat by
- physiotherapy with active joint movements;
- lumbar sympathetic blocks may help.

CLAW TOES

- due to a
    - —poorly molded cast beneath the forefoot,
    - —ischemic contracture of posterior compartment or plantar muscles, or
    - —adherence of long flexor tendons at the fracture site;
- prevent by
    - —proper molding of the cast which extends beneath the toes to their tips as a platform,
    - —early recognition and treatment of an ischemic syndrome, and
    - —active and passive mobilization in the cast;
- if clawing is severe, interphalangeal (IP) fusion or proximal resection of

proximal phalanges, particularly of the great toe may be necessary, as stiffness and deformity at the metatarsophalangeal (MP) joint may prevent normal rollover of the foot in walking.

Fractures of Fibular Shaft

- usually accompany tibial fractures, in which case treatment of the fibula is of secondary importance.
- when the fibular fracture is apparently isolated, verify the medial malleolus and the medial collateral ligament of the ankle to be sure that this is not a combination injury (Fig. 2.4);
- isolated fracture usually has little or no displacement and heals well;
- treatment is
  —symptomatic, with
  —crutches used until pain has subsided sufficiently to start WB. A
  —cast is not usually necessary.

Fractures in Children

TREATMENT

Isolated tibial fracture (Fig. 3.1)

- a child's fibula bends, so many tibial fractures have a bowed but intact fibula and are stable. However, the
- intact fibula pulls the fracture into varus. So
- treat with a long leg cast molded into slight valgus to prevent varus deformity, and x-ray the tibia through the cast at regular intervals.
- for an infant, flex the knee to 90° and remove the cast at 3 to 4 weeks;
- for a child 4 to 10 years old, bend the patient's knee to 15° and allow WB with a walking heel after 1 week. Remove the cast at 8 weeks;
- for a child older than 10 years, treat with a cast for 10 to 12 weeks.

Fractured tibia and fibula

- most simple fractures are stable after reduction and are well treated by closed reduction and a long leg cast;
- take care to reduce rotation and angulation;
- early WB is not necessary.
- comminuted and segmental fractures are rare in children;
- treat with a
  —long leg cast or
  —pins and plaster technique;
- always re-x-ray at regular intervals, and if the position of fracture has

slipped, repeat the reduction and apply a new cast. Do not delay remanipulation because children's fractures become "sticky" very fast.

Ipsilateral tibia and femur

- treat both by closed methods.

COMPLICATIONS (Fig. 6.1)

- neurovascular problems are less common and have a better prognosis in children than in adults. Peroneal nerve palsy is usually due to poor plaster technique. The treatment is similar to that outlined for adults.
- 1 cm of shortening may correct with overgrowth, depending on the child's age, but
- rotation and varus or valgus angulation do not, so avoid these by careful reduction; otherwise, corrective osteotomy may be required later.

chapter 24
Ankle Injuries

Surgical and Functional Anatomy

STABILITY OF ANKLE JOINT

- medial and lateral malleoli and the distal tibial articular surface form a mortise for the talus. The
- tibia and fibula are stabilized just above the ankle joint by the
  - —interosseous ligament, the strongest bond between the bones, and the
  - —anterior and
  - —posterior inferior tibiofibular ligaments. The latter deepens the mortise posteriorly. These ligaments are collectively called the distal tibiofibular ligament complex. The
- talus is held in mortise by two ligaments. The
- medial (deltoid) ligament is attached to the medial malleolus and divides into the
  - —deep part to the talus and
  - —superficial, triangular part to the navicular tuberosity, plantar calcaneo-navicular (spring) ligament, sustentaculum tali and posterior talus. The second is the
- lateral collateral ligament from the lateral malleolus in three bands to the
  - —talar neck,
  - —calcaneus and
  - —posterior talar tubercle.

FUNCTION

- in weight-bearing (WB) the tibia receives 85% of the force, but the
- lateral malleolus is the key to stability of the ankle joint because at
  - —heel strike the lateral malleolus
  - —prevents the talus from subluxing laterally and rotating externally;
- the fibula normally moves a little during walking, adapting itself to and controlling the movement of the talus.

Etiopathology and Classification

- this classification is based on that of Lauge-Hansen.

LIGAMENT INJURIES

Isolated collateral ligament injuries

- see Chapter 5.
- rupture of the lateral collateral ligament, particularly of the anterior talofibular band and capsule, may be an isolated injury. The
- ligament may rupture
  —in its middle or
  —at its junction with bone, or it
  —may avulse a fragment of bone;
- differentiate between partial and complete tears by use of stress x-rays. The injury is occasionally associated with an
- osteochondral fracture of the lateral margin of the talar dome. If this fragment is
  —displaced or later becomes
  —symptomatic with pain, swelling and locking,
  —excise it.
- complete rupture of medial collateral ligament is associated with either
  —fracture of lateral malleolus or
  —fibular fracture with tibiofibular diastasis. It
  —rarely occurs in isolation.

Dislocation of ankle

- rare without associated fractures;
- often an open injury;
- the talus with the foot dislocates anteriorly or posteriorly, due to a blow on the leg with the foot fixed;
- collateral ligaments and the capsule are torn, and the
- anterior or posterior vessels are endangered;
- for other types of talar dislocation, see Chapter 25.

FRACTURES AND COMBINED INJURIES

General remarks

- the key to these injuries is the fibular fracture because from this fracture one can deduce the nature of associated ligament injuries, particularly injuries of the distal tibiofibular ligament complex.
- thus, fibular fractures fall into one of two major groups:
  —fractures at the level of or distal to the distal tibiofibular ligament complex, i.e., the lateral malleolus, and

—fractures proximal to this ligament complex, i.e., the fibular shaft. In the context of this chapter,

- external (lateral) and internal (medial) rotation around the vertical axis refers to the movement of the talus relative to the tibia;
- supination and pronation are synonymous with inversion and eversion;
- adduction and abduction refer to the lateral movement of the talus in the mortise.
- double injuries, e.g., a bimalleolar fracture or a torn ligament with a contralateral fracture, are generally unstable, whereas an isolated undisplaced fracture may be relatively stable.
- severe ankle injuries are often open, usually from within without on the lateral side, so there is little contamination or tissue devitalization.

Lateral malleolar fracture

- the distal tibiofibular ligament complex is
  —intact, the distal
  —tibiofibular joint is stable, and there is
  —no diastasis.

Oblique or spiral fracture (Figs. 24.1 and 24.2)

- abduction causes an
  —oblique fracture upward and outward, frequently with comminution of lateral cortex. With the foot in
- supination, there is a torque conversion effect on the
  —talus which rotates backward and externally around the relaxed and intact medial (internal) collateral ligament and
  —pushes the lateral malleolus posteriorly. The malleolus breaks with an
  —oblique or spiral fracture line extending upward and backward, often with a fracture of the
  —posterior tibial lip which remains attached to the lateral malleolus by the intact posterior tibiofibular ligament. If the
  —force continues, there is medial failure with a
  —medial ligament rupture or an

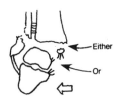

Figure 24.1. Abduction injury of the ankle. (Modifed from Lauge-Hansen U: Fractures of the ankle. *Arch Surg* 60:957, 1950.)

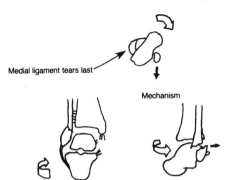

Medial ligament tears last

Mechanism

Figure 24.2. Supination and external rotation injury. (Modified from Lauge-Hansen U: Fractures of the ankle. *Arch Surg* 60:957, 1950.)

—avulsion fracture of the medial malleolus. In a
- double malleolar injury the talus may displace laterally. Note that an
- isolated avulsion fracture of the medial malleolus or an isolated tear of the medial collateral ligament is uncommon, so look for an associated bony or ligamentous injury on the lateral side.

Transverse avulsion fracture of lateral malleolus or rupture of lateral collateral ligament (Figs. 24.3 and 24.4)

- both these injuries are caused by
  —internal rotation and/or
  —supination;
- lateral cortex of the lateral malleolus is not comminuted;
- may be associated with
  —oblique or nearly vertical fracture of the medial malleolus, with the fracture line extending from the
  —angle between the distal tibia and medial malleolus, upward and medially above the ankle joint; the
  —medial part of the distal tibial articular surface at the angle between the tibia and malleolus may be compressed by the talus and comminuted. The prognosis is worse with this injury than with external rotation and pronation injuries;
- medial malleolar fracture may include a
  —posteromedial or anteromedial fragment of tibia, or there may be a separate fragment. This trimalleolar fracture is caused by compression as well as internal rotation and supination. In a
- double malleolar injury the talus may be displaced medially.

Fibular shaft fracture (Figs. 24.5 and 24.6)

- external rotation and pronation stresses the medial side first and produces either an

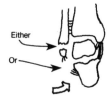

Figure 24.3. Supination injury. (Modifed from Lauge-Hansen U: Fractures of the ankle. *Arch Surg* 60:957, 1950.)

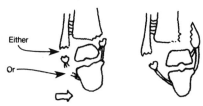

Figure 24.4. Adduction injury. (Modified from Lauge-Hansen U: Fractures of the ankle. *Arch Surg* 60:957, 1950.)

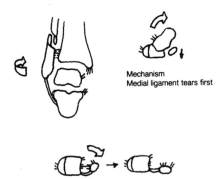

Mechanism
Medial ligament tears first

Figure 24.5. Pronation and external rotation injury. The posterior tibiofibular ligament is intact, but there is partial diastasis. (Modified from Lauge-Hansen U: Fractures of the ankle. *Arch Surg* 60:957, 1950.)

—avulsion fracture of the medial malleolus with the fracture line being distal to the ankle joint, or a
—tear of the medial ligament. The
—talus then rotates forward and laterally around the intertibiofibular ligament and
—twists the fibula,

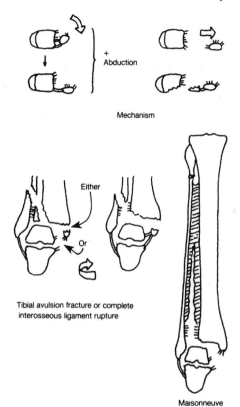

Figure 24.6. Pronation, external rotation, and abduction. Complete tibiofibular diastasis. (Modified from Lauge-Hansen U: Fractures of the ankle. *Arch Surg* 60:957, 1950.)

> —rupturing first the anterior tibiofibular and then the interosseous ligament, and then causing a
> —spiral fracture of the fibular shaft. There is
> —partial tibiofibular diastasis. When an
- abduction force is added, this
  > —ruptures the posterior tibiofibular ligament also or avulses the posterior tibial lip and then causes an
  > —oblique, transverse or comminuted fibular shaft fracture with
  > —complete tibiofibular diastasis;
- lateral border of the distal tibia may have a comminuted fracture;

- fibular shaft may fracture anywhere in its length;
- soft tissue damage is considerable because the interosseous membrane is usually torn as far proximally as the fracture of the fibula.

Medial malleolar fracture (Figs. 24.1, 24.4 and 24.6)

- isolated fracture of the medial malleolus is uncommon;
- transverse avulsion fracture or medial ligament rupture is usually associated with
    —external rotation or pronation fracture of the lateral malleolus or
    —fibular shaft;
- high, oblique fracture of the medial malleolus is usually accompanied by
    —transverse avulsion fracture of lateral malleolus or
    —rupture of the lateral ligament.
- see the previous discussion for etiopathology and later dicussion for treatment.

Anterior and posterior tibial lip fractures

Anterior lip fracture (Fig. 24.7)

- caused by vertical compression with forced dorsiflexion of the foot, as in a head-on car collision with the break pedal being driven up into the driver's foot;
- the anterior lip may be crushed or sheared off by the talus and may be
- associated with fracture of the neck of the talus, so look for this.
- anteromedial margin of the distal tibia may be fractured with the medial malleolus.

Posterior lip fracture

- may be caused by
    —vertical compression, with the talus being driven upward and backward, shearing off the posterior tibial margin or crushing it. Or it may be due to
    —avulsion by the posterior tibiofibular ligament in an external rotation injury.

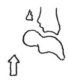

Figure 24.7. Forced dorsiflexion. (Modified from Lauge-Hansen U: Fractures of the ankle. *Arch Surg* 60:957, 1950.)

Vertical compression fractures of tibia

- localized tibial articular cartilage fractures may accompany pronation or supination injuries of the ankle and are confined to one small area of the distal tibial surface. They are often comminuted.
- vertical compression injury, as in a fall from a height, drives the talus up into the tibia with resultant
    —multiple tibial intra-articular fractures and
    —articular fragments impacted into the distal tibial epiphysis. Fracture lines may
    —extend proximally into the tibial shaft;
    —the talar articular surface is frequently damaged too. This is the
    —Humpty Dumpty fracture of the ankle.

Clinical and Radiological Features and Diagnosis

GENERAL REMARKS

- fractures around the ankle joint are generally easy to diagnose, but
- ligamentous injuries are not.
- ligament does not heal as well as bone, so a ligament injury must be
    —diagnosed early and
    —treated properly.
- the alert surgeon (you?) can suspect the presence of a ligament injury by taking a
    —detailed history of the mechanism of injury, by making a
    —thorough clinical examination of both ankles, looking particularly for localized tenderness over the collateral and interosseous ligaments, and by
    —thoughtfully studying the x-ray films, including stress views if necessary;
- in general, a
    —displaced fracture of only one malleolus means rupture of the opposite collateral ligament, and a
    —fibular shaft fracture with lateral displacement of the talus suggests rupture of the tibiofibular interosseous ligament and of the medial collateral ligament if the medial malleolus is intact.

CLINICAL FEATURES

- the mechanism of injury is usually a twisting fall with the foot fixed on the ground or trapped in something, so that the body and leg rotate around the foot;
- always examine the neurovascular status of the foot first. If the ankle is obviously deformed and the foot is cold and pale or blue, reduce the deformity and splint the leg before examining further;

- point tenderness with localized swelling over a ligament or the capsule is significant, particularly if there is no fracture in that area;
- always examine the whole length of fibula shaft for tenderness in order not to miss a high fracture.

RADIOLOGICAL EXAMINATION

Plain views

- anteroposterior (AP) and lateral x-rays are obligatory. An
- undisplaced malleolar fracture may be visible in only one view, so examine both films carefully. If you are still in doubt, take oblique x-rays;
- on the routine AP x-ray the fibula is a little behind the tibia, and the distal tibiofibular joint is hidden. To see the tibiofibular joint clearly, for evaluation of integrity of the interosseous ligament, rotate the leg internally 10° and take another AP x-ray. If the
  —smallest distance between the tibia and fibula is more than 4 mm,
  —diastasis exists and the distal tibiofibular ligament complex is probably ruptured;
- x-rays of the leg may reveal a high fibular shaft fracture.

Stress views

- for evaluation of ligament injury, stress x-rays of the ankle are very important;
- use local or general anesthesia,
- rotate the leg 10° internally, and
- stress the ankle in inversion for the lateral ligament and in eversion for the medial ligament, holding the hindfoot, not the forefoot;
- stressing the ankle joint in the sagittal plane evaluates the anterior and posterior parts of the collateral ligaments;
- stress the normal side for comparison.

Arthrography

- difficult to interpret and
- adds very little to the foregoing examinations.

Treatment

GENERAL

- vascular injury is an emergency. The
- prognosis for an open fracture is good if it is treated promptly by
  —careful surgical debridement and reduction and
  —stabilization of the fracture. The
- principles of treatment for all ankle injuries are

—anatomical reduction of malleoli,

—accurate repositioning and stabilization of the talus in the ankle mortise, and reconstitution of

—smooth articular surfaces;

- if these aims are not achieved, degenerative arthritis will ensue;
- reduction is attained by following in reverse order the mechanism of injury. This is why Lauge-Hansen's classification is useful;
- during surgery, inspect all articular surfaces that are visible and note their condition in the operating note, as comminution also leads to degenerative changes.

LIGAMENT INJURIES

Isolated collateral ligament injuries

- see Chapter 5.
- with a stable ankle, treat with strapping and WB for 4 weeks;
- but if there is a lot of swelling and pain or you are in doubt as to stability, treat with a below-knee walking cast (BKWC);
- with talar instability on stress films, treat by
  —positioning the foot to appose the ligament ends, e.g., pronation for a lateral collateral ligament tear, and a
  —BKWC in this position for 6 weeks. Then treat with an
  —elastic bandage with the foot in the same position for 4 weeks;
- if perfect repositioning of the talus in the ankle mortise is prevented by interposition of the torn ligament, perform
  —open reduction and
  —suture the ligament. Treat with a cast for 6 weeks, as discussed previously.

Dislocation of ankle joint

- vessels are very vulnerable in this injury, so the
- treatment is
  —immediate closed reduction by longitudinal traction and manipulation, then
  —x-rays to verify reduction and to see that there are no associated fractures. If the injury is a simple dislocation and it is well reduced, apply a
  —long leg cast, with non-weight-bearing (NWB) for 8 weeks.
- prognosis is fair.

FRACTURES AND COMBINED INJURIES

Undisplaced fractures

- solitary undisplaced fractures are usually stable and can be
  —treated by a BKWC for 6 weeks. But apparently undisplaced fractures of

- both malleoli may be unstable and should be treated by a
  —long leg cast and NWB.
- if reduction of a malleolus is not perfect, the periosteum may be interposed in the fracture, especially in a medial malleolar fracture. This requires open reduction and internal fixation.
- x-ray all fractures at 1 and 2 weeks to see that they have not displaced in the cast.

Displaced fractures

- if an apparently isolated malleolar fracture is displaced, suspect a tear of the contralateral ligament;
- unstable ankle injuries in the adult are best treated surgically.

Bimalleolar fractures

Open reduction

- do not operate on a very swollen ankle because
  —skin closure will be difficult and
  —infection may follow. If the
- swelling is marked, reduce the displacement and apply a
  —compression dressing,
  —elevate the leg, and
  —wait until the swelling subsides. At surgery
- accurate anatomical reduction is important, so verify this visually and with x-rays during surgery. If the malleolar fragments are
- too small or too comminuted for screw fixation, use pins and figure-of-8 tension wiring or a Rush pin up the fibula after reaming;
- always fix both malleoli, not just one.
- postoperatively, if fixation is firm,
  —elevate the leg in a posterior splint and start the patient on exercises for 7 days, then
  —apply a below-knee (BK) cast, with NWB for 8 to 10 weeks. But if the fixation is not very stable,
  —apply the cast immediately.
- physiotherapy for muscle strengthening and joint mobilization is important after cast removal.

Closed reduction

- if surgery is contraindicated, attain the
- best position possible by closed manipulation with the patient under anesthesia and apply a
- well-molded long leg cast with the
  —knee flexed 25° and the ankle in
  —slight varus for a pronation and external rotation injury and in

—slight valgus for a supination injury. If there is a
- posterior lip fragment, reduce it as best you can by
  —lifting the heel forward and then
  —dorsiflexing the foot.
- verify radiologically the reduction and take
- x-rays at weekly intervals for 4 weeks. If the cast becomes loose and the reduction is lost, change the cast and remanipulate. At 6 weeks, change the cast and, if the fractures have stabilized, apply a BKWC for 4 weeks.

Malleolar fracture with ligament rupture

- indications and treatment for this type of fracture are similar to those for bimalleolar fractures;
- when operating, fix the malleolus first, then suture the ligament.
- note that closed reduction may be prevented by interposition of the
  —ligament or
  —peroneal tendon laterally or the
  —tibialis posterior tendon medially between the talus and malleolus. This obstruction can only be removed at operation.

Tibiofibular diastasis

- partial tear of the tibiofibular interosseous ligament can be treated by accurate
  —closed reduction and a long leg cast for 8 to 10 weeks or
  —open reduction and internal fixation if closed methods fail.
- complete rupture of the ligament requires surgery;
- stabilize the medial side of joint first, as discussed previously;
- if the distal interosseous ligament complex has avulsed a large fragment from the tibia, reduce this and fix it with a screw. If the
- ligament itself is ruptured, stabilize the tibiofibular joint with a transverse screw or bolt, holding the ankle in dorsiflexion to bring the widest part of the talus into the mortise. Then treat with a
- long leg cast for 8 weeks and with a BK cast and NWB for 4 weeks;
- remove the transverse screw or bolt before the patient starts WB on the injured ankle, otherwise the screw will break.

Anterior and posterior tibial lip fractures

- anatomical reduction by closed methods rarely succeeds;
- if the fracture involves more than one third of the articular surface of the distal tibia and is displaced, reduce and stabilize it with a screw in the sagittal plane through an
- extension of the malleolar incision or through a separate incision. If a

- large fragment is not reduced, the talus subluxes with resultant
  —instability and
  —degenerative arthritis. If the fracture is
- comminuted, reduction and fixation are impossible. In this case, the best treatment is early motion but with NWB for 3 months.

Vertical compression fractures of tibia

- treat an undisplaced fracture with a cast, as for tibial shaft fractures, but with NWB until the bones are united.
- displaced or comminuted fractures ideally should be treated by
  —open reduction, bone grafting and internal fixation. This is technically difficult and requires an experienced surgeon. It may be better to treat by
- closed methods, using
  —traction with transcalcaneal pin on a Böhler-Braun frame and with
  —early motion of the ankle while in traction. At
- 3 weeks, apply a long leg cast with NWB until the fracture has healed.
- ankle fusion is often required for these fractures.

Complications

VASCULAR DAMAGE

- anterior and posterior tibial vessels lie on the distal tibia and are easily compressed by subluxation or dislocation of the talus;
- severely displaced ankle injury should be reduced immediately and splinted before patient is sent for x-rays.

NONUNION

- 5% to 10% of medial malleolar fractures unite with fibrous tissue. If the
- fracture fragment is small, the ankle is usually stable and asymptomatic and needs no treatment. But
- pseudarthrosis of a fracture at the level of the joint line or proximal to it may be painful or may allow abnormal lateral movement of the talus. In this case, graft the malleolus with an iliac bone peg.

MALUNION

- if the talus is stable in normal position, no treatment is required. If the talus is
- subluxed but posttraumatic arthritis is not evident, correct the malunion by osteotomy and internal fixation to stabilize the ankle joint. If
- symptomatic degenerative arthritis is present and is disabling, fuse the ankle.

SYMPATHETIC DYSTROPHY

- this is Sudeck's atrophy, characterized by rapid development of
  —marked, spotty osteoporosis of the bones of the foot,
  —burning pain and
  —trophic skin changes.
- treatment is
  —early and aggressive physiotherapy with
  —progressive WB;
  —sympathetic lumbar blocks may also be of help.

POSTTRAUMATIC DEGENERATIVE ARTHROSIS

- predisposing factors are
  —comminution of the fracture,
  —malunion and
  —instability;
- treat symptomatically;
- if pain and disability are severe, fuse the ankle.

TALAR INSTABILITY

- recurrent sprains of the ankle joint are a complication of rupture of the lateral collateral ligament, especially if the initial treatment was inadequate;
- confirm the diagnosis by stress x-rays of both ankles for comparison;
- treat by
  —physiotherapy to strengthen peroneal muscles for mild instability and by
  —ligamentous reconstruction, using the Watson-Jones or Evans technique, for severe talar instability.

Fractures in Children

EPIPHYSEAL PLATE INJURIES (Fig. 24.8)

- in children, injuries about the ankle joint are usually epiphyseal growth plate injuries;
- the ankle joint itself is disrupted less often in children than in adults, and ligaments are almost never torn;
- accurate reduction is usually achieved by closed manipulation.

Type I

- these injuries show no fracture on x-rays and may not be diagnosed if
  —displacment is minimal or
  —spontaneous reduction has occurred;
  —oblique x-rays may help;

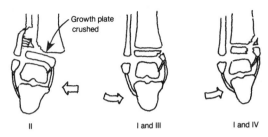

Growth plate
crushed

II   I and III   I and IV

Figure 24.8.   Growth plate injuries.

- common in the fibula;
- make the diagnosis on
  —point tenderness over the growth plate and
  —localized swelling;
- treat on suspicion with a
  —long leg cast for 3 weeks.

Type II

- common in the tibia. If it is
- undisplaced, apply a cast for 6 weeks. When it is
- displaced, it may be accompanied by a
  —bent or fractured fibular shaft, and the
  —center of the tibial growth plate may be crushed by the corner of the
  tibial metaphysis;
- treat a displaced tibial fracture by
  —closed reduction with the knee flexed and
  —long leg walking cast for 6 weeks.

Type III

Medial malleolus

- if the malleolus is undisplaced, apply a long leg cast for 6 weeks with
  NWB. But when the fracture is
- displaced, treat by
  —closed reduction or, if this fails,
  —open reduction and internal fixation with Kirschner (K) wires or a
  transverse screw, then a
  —long leg cast and NWB for 6 weeks;
- remove the K wires once the malleolus has united.

Anterolateral part of distal tibial epiphysis

- the Tillaux fracture;
- occurs in adolescents when the medial half of growth plate has closed
  but the lateral half is still open. The anterolateral epiphyseal

- fragment is pulled off by the anterior inferior tibiofibular ligament in external rotation injury and is the equivalent of distal anterior tibiofibular ligament rupture with partial diastasis in the adult;
- treatment is
  —reduction by full internal rotation of the foot and a
  —long leg cast for 6 weeks;
- a few fractures require open reduction and internal fixation if closed reduction fails.

Type IV

- some medial malleolar fractures are Type IV;
- accurate reduction is essential to prevent growth problems, so perform
  —open reduction and
  —fix the fragment with K wires, then treat with a
  —long leg cast and NWB for 6 weeks;
- remove K wires after union.

Type V

- uncommon; the diagnosis is made on clinical grounds alone;
- treat on suspicion with a protective cast for 3 weeks;
- warn parents of possible growth plate damage and
- review the patient regularly for 2 years after treatment in case deformity develops.

COMMINUTED FRACTURES

- unusual in children;
- anatomic reduction can only be achieved by surgery, but this is usually difficult. It may be more prudent to treat the fracture
- closed with a long leg cast and NWB for 6 weeks.

COMPLICATIONS

- premature closure of the growth plate with progressive deformity and shortening, especially with Types IV and V injuries, may occur;
- stiff joints are rare and
- nonunion is very rare;
- malunion occurs and may require surgical correction;
- degenerative arthrosis is rare because the tibiotalar relationship is usually undisturbed;
- progressive angular deformity may require
  —serial osteotomies or
  —excision of the bar and its replacement with methyl methacrylate or a free fat graft.

chapter 25

Fractures and Dislocations of the Hindfoot

Talus

SURGICAL ANATOMY (Fig. 25.1)

- almost entirely covered with articular cartilage and has
- no muscular or tendinous attachments;
- the superior, domed surface of the body is
  —wider anteriorly than posteriorly and
  —articulates with the tibia;
- inferiorly, the body articulates with the calcaneus through two facets separated by the sulcus tali;
- laterally and medially, the body carries the malleolar facets, triangular and comma-shaped, respectively; and posteriorly, it carries the posterior tubercle (os trigonum when separate) for the posterior talofibular ligament. Medial to this is the flexor hallucis longus (FHL) tendon groove.
- the talar head articulates with the
  —navicular anteriorly and the
  —calcaneonavicular spring ligament inferiorly.
- the neck has no articular cartilage and receives most of the blood vessels of the talus
  —superiorly from the anterior tibial artery and
  —inferiorly through the sinus tarsi from posterior tibial and peroneal arteries. Other vessels from the posterior tibial artery enter the body beneath the medial ligament and through the posterior tubercle. The talus
- distributes body weight
  —posteriorly to the calcaneus and
  —anteriorly to the heads of the metatarsals;
- the angle between the longitudinal axes of the talus and calcaneus, in line with the first and fifth metatarsals (MTs), respectively, is 20° to 40° open distally on the anteroposterior (AP) x-ray. This angle is
  —reduced in varus and

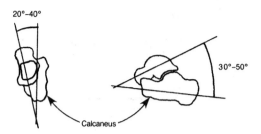

Figure 25.1. Talocalcaneal angles.

—increased in valgus. On the lateral x-ray, the
• talocalcaneal angle is 30° to 50° open posteriorly.

RADIOLOGICAL FEATURES

• if there is pain and swelling around the hindfoot or midfoot after an
  accident, there must be an injury there, so
  —take good x-rays,
  —examine them carefully, and
  —compare them with x-rays of the noninjured side, if necessary, as injuries
    of the talus and its articulations are sometimes hard to recognize.
• AP x-rays of the
  —ankle with the leg in 10° of internal rotation will show the talotibial
    joint, talar dome and malleolar facets, and AP x-rays of the
  —foot will show the head and neck of the talus and talonavicular joint;
• lateral x-ray of the ankle shows a
  —profile of the talus and its
  —relationships with the tibia, calcaneus and navicular bones;
• oblique x-ray of the foot shows clearly the midtarsal joint. The
• talus is the second most frequently fractured tarsal (the calcaneus is the
  first).
• talar fractures are rare in children. The treatment is similar to that for
  adults.

CHIP FRACTURES

Osteochondral dome fracture (Fig. 25.2)

  • a chip of bone and articular cartilage is sheared off the lateral edge of
    the dome when the talus subluxes after lateral collateral ligament rupture.
    As the talus
  • subluxes medially, the edge of the dome is levered against the articular
    surface of the lateral malleolus and the chip is prized up;
  • less common on the medial edge of dome;

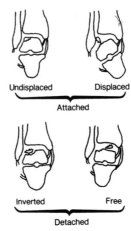

Figure 25.2. Osteochondral talar fractures.

- the fragment may be
  - —undisplaced,
  - —elevated, but still attached at one end,
  - —inverted in its bed, or
  - —completely displaced, becoming a loose body in the joint.
- an undisplaced fracture may heal, so treat the patient with a below knee (BK) cast and non-weight-bearing (NWB) for 6 weeks;
- remove a displaced fragment or an undisplaced but symptomatic fragment through an anterolateral or anteromedial approach and drill the bed.

Avulsion fractures

- a small piece of bone may be pulled off the talus by a ligament or capsule. The
- problem is not the fracture but the associated ligamentous instability. So
- evaluate the stability and treat this.
- do not confuse the os trigonum with a fracture. Compare an x-ray of it with an x-ray of the uninjured talus if you are in doubt.

FRACTURES OF HEAD OF TALUS

- uncommon;
- caused by a fall on the foot in extreme dorsiflexion. The talar head hits the anterior lip of the tibia. There is
- tenderness over the talar head and talonavicular area;

- fracture is usually comminuted but not displaced;
- treatment consists of
  —elevation and a compression bandage if the foot is very swollen, then a
  —below knee walking cast (BKWC) for 6 weeks. If the
- talonavicular joint is disrupted and the patient later has degenerative arthrosis with marked pain on walking, fusion of the midtarsal joint may be necessary.

INJURIES OF NECK OF TALUS

Fractures of the neck (Fig. 25.3)

Clinical features

- caused by forced dorsiflexion of the foot, e.g., by a motorcycle foot rest, car brake pedeal or airplane rudder bar. The talar neck is fractured by the anterior lip of the tibia;
- study x-rays and look for other injuries;
- may have associated vascular insufficiency of the foot, so examine this carefully.

Treatment

- if the fracture is undisplaced, treat by
  —elevation with a compression bandage to reduce the swelling, then with a
  —BK cast and NWB for 12 weeks. For the more common
- displaced fracture with no vascular impairment,
  —elevate the foot to reduce swelling, then perform

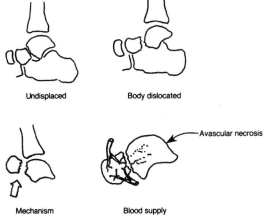

Undisplaced   Body dislocated

Mechanism   Blood supply

Avascular necrosis

Figure 25.3. Talar neck fracture.

—open reduction and internal fixation with a screw or Kirschner (K) wires through the anteromedial approach;

—do not injure the anterior tibial vessels or damage the soft tissue attachments of the talus; treat with a

—cast and NWB for 16 weeks, then remove the K wires and start

—mobilization and progressive weight-bearing (WB) if the fracture is healed. When the fracture is

- displaced with vascular impairment of the foot, perform
  —immediate open reduction and internal fixation and
  —explore the vessels if necessary;
  —postoperative care is the same as that discussed previously.
- avascular necrosis of the body may occur with any neck fracture, so x-ray at regular intervals for 2 years after the injury.

Fracture dislocation of neck (Fig. 25.3)

Etiopathology

- caused by forced dorsiflexion and rotation;
- the body of the talus may be subluxed or dislocated from the
  —ankle joint (rare without a medial malleolar fracture) and/or
  —subtalar joint with displacement and/or rotation of the body in any direction, though usually posteriorly. Posterior vessels may be compressed. Rarely, the
- head and neck fragment of the talus may be dislocated from the navicular and rotated in any direction. Anterior tibial vessels may be compressed.

Treatment

- subluxation of the body from the calcaneus is reduced by
  —plantar flexion and
  —inversion of the foot. Apply a BK cast in this position for 8 weeks, then change to the neutral position for 4 weeks. If
  —closed reduction fails, perform
  —open reduction and internal fixation. With
- complete dislocation, immediate reduction is mandatory because vessels and skin are endangered. Attempted
- closed reduction by manipulation and traction with a transcalcaneal pin with the patient under general anesthesia may fail, in which case perform
- immediate open reduction and fixation with K wires. Use the
  —posteromedial or posterolateral approach unless the body is dislocated anteriorly;
  —an associated medial malleolar fracture can be reduced and fixed through extensions of these incisions;

- BK cast and NWB for 16 weeks;
- then remove the K wires and, if the fracture has united, start the patient on partial weight-bearing (PWB)
- if it has not, apply a BK cast for 8 more weeks, with PWB afterward.
- complete displacement of the head and neck fragment usually necessitates open reduction and internal fixation.

Prognosis

- with subtalar subluxation of the calcaneus,
  —avascular necrosis of the body will occur in 20% to 30% and
  —subtalar arthrosis will occur in 60% to 70%;
- with posterior dislocation of the body,
  —avascular necrosis will occur in 90% to 100%.

FRACTURES OF BODY OF TALUS

Etiopathology

- caused by forced dorsiflexion with comminution by compression;
- the fracture is usually intra-articular and involves both the
  —ankle and
  —subtalar joints.

Treatment

- undisplaced, linear fracture requires a
  —BK cast and NWB for 8 weeks. Treat a
- displaced fracture by
  —immediate open reduction and fixation with a screw or K wires through the
  —anteromedial approach or the
  —transverse medial approach with an osteotomy of the medial malleolus. This latter approach exposes the whole length of the talar body. Screw the malleolus back at the end of the procedure. Postoperatively, apply a
- long leg cast for 16 weeks, with NWB, then remove the K wires. If the fracture has united, start the patient on PWB. If it has not, use a BK cast for 8 more weeks, then PWB. In
- comminuted fractures the treatment is difficult and the results are unsatisfactory. First
  —elevate the foot with a compression dressing until edema subsides. Then perform
  —primary tibiotalar fusion with the ankle in neutral position.

Prognosis

- if the body is not dislocated from the ankle mortise,
  —avascular necrosis will occur in 40% to 50%. But if the body is

- completely dislocated from the ankle and subtalar joints, the incidence of
  —avascular necrosis will be 90% to 100%.

DISLOCATIONS OF TALUS

Dislocation of tibiotalar joint

- see Chapter 24.

Subtalar dislocation

Clinical features

- forced inversion with a plantar-flexed foot;
- the calcaneus slides laterally or medially from beneath the talus, taking the whole of the foot, including the navicular, with it, and the
- talus is left sitting by itself in the ankle mortise;
- skin is stretched over the talar head.

Treatment

- immediate closed reduction with the patient under general anesthesia. For
- medial dislocation of the foot, plantar-flex and adduct it, then apply traction and abduct it. Push on the talar head to reduce the talonavicular joint. The calcaneus usually reduces without difficulty. For
- lateral dislocation of the foot, apply plantar flexion and abduction, then traction and adduction. If closed reduction
- fails, perform
- open reduction through
  —Ollier's lateral approach. The medial approach might cause skin slough;
- after reduction and before casting,
  —take good x-rays and look for associated osteochondral or avulsion fractures. Then place the foot in a
- BKWC for 6 weeks.
- less than 20% develop avascular necrosis.

Total dislocation of talus

- rare;
- an inversion and plantar flexion injury;
- the talus is usually in an anterolateral position and rotated;
- all ligaments and vascular and capsular attachments are torn.
- treatment by
  —immediate reduction is obligatory to reduce the risk of vascular and skin problems. Apply
  —traction through a calcaneal traction bow,

—hold the foot in plantar flexion and inversion, reproducing the mechanism of injury, and

—gently push the talus into position as you

—gradually dorsiflex the foot;

- avoid open reduction if possible because this almost always becomes infected.
- after reduction, apply a

—long leg cast for 3 months, with NWB; then after 3 months with

—progressive WB. The

- prognosis is poor because most develop avascular necrosis, and arthrodesis later may be difficult because of the dead talus. Nevertheless, closed reduction is better than excision and tibiocalcaneal fusion.

OPEN INJURIES OF TALUS

- apply occlusive dressing and a posterior plaster splint and elevate the leg.
- clean and debride the wound as soon as possible and irrigate it copiously with the patient under general anesthesia;
- reduce and fix the fracture or dislocation with K wires,
- close deep tissues over the joints, if possible, but
- leave the skin open. Consider
- delayed primary closure at 3 days if the wound is

—clean and the

—edges can be approximated without tension. If they cannot, leave the skin open and perform a

—skin graft later when it is covered with healthy granulation tissue, or

—let it close by itself secondarily;

- immobilize the ankle in a cast as for a closed fracture.

AVASCULAR NECROSIS AND DEGENERATIVE ARTHRITIS

- if avascular necrosis is likely, continue NWB to avoid crushing bone and cartilage and in hope that the bone will gradually be revascularized.
- if late symptoms are tolerable, treat symptomatically;
- if pain is severe and disabling,

—localize the origin of pain by intra-articular injections of local anesthetic and

—fuse the appropriate joints. Do not excise the talus.

Calcaneus

SURGICAL ANATOMY

Bony anatomy (Fig. 25.4)

- cortex is eggshell thin;
- trabeculae are arranged to distribute talar thrust

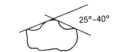

Figure 25.4. Böhler's angle.

—posteriorly to the floor and
—anterolaterally to the forefoot;
- the superior surface slopes up to the midpoint like a pitched roof slopes to a peak, forming
—Böhler's angle, normally 25° to 40° on a lateral x-ray.

Articular facets

- the superior surface of the middle third has a convex facet, the long axis of which runs obliquely forward and laterally. This is the posterior facet for the talus;
- sustentaculm tali, a broad process projecting medially from the anterior third of the calcaneus, carries the anterior concave talar facet on its superior surface;
- between these two facets is the calcaneal sulcus. This along with the talar sulcus forms the sinus tarsi. The
- anterior end of calcaneus is saddle-shaped and articulates with the cuboid bone. The
- prominent anterosuperior angle of the calcaneus is called the anterior process.

Ligaments

- strong, Y-shaped, bifurcate ligament from the anterior process of the calcaneus to the cuboid and navicular bones;
- strong interosseous ligament in the sinus tarsi;
- plantar aponeurosis attached on the undersurface of the calcaneus to the medial and lateral processes of calcaneal tuberosity.

Muscle attachments

- the tendo achillis is attached to the tuberosity at the posterior extremity of the calcaneus. Bursa and fat pad lie in the angle between the tendon and the posterosuperior margin of the bone;
- abductor hallucis (abd H), flexor digitorum brevis (FDB) and abductor digiti minimi (ADM) originate from medial and lateral processes beneath the calcaneus;
- extensor digitorum (EDB) originates from the anterolateral part of the superior surface of the calcaneus just anterior to the sinus tarsi.

Tendon sheath attachments

- tibialis posterior (TP) lies medial to the sustentaculum tali;
- flexor digitorum longus (FDL) lies just inferior to the TP, and
- flexor hallucis longus (FHL) lies in the groove beneath the sustentaculum tali. This groove is converted to a tunnel by fibrous sheath. The other two tendons lie in separate synovial sheaths;
- peroneus brevis (PB) (anterior) and peroneus longus (PL) tendons pass through fibrous sheaths, with one on each side of the peroneal tubercle on the lateral surface of the calcaneus 2 cm below the tip of the lateral malleolus.

GENERAL FEATURES OF CALCANEAL FRACTURES

- the calcaneus is fractured more often than any other tarsal bone and is
- usually injured by a fall from a height onto the heels with the foot in inversion, eversion or neutral position;
- 10% are accompanied by vertebral compression fractures, and
- 25% of the patients have other injuries of the limbs. So examine especially the hips and spine;
- compressive force of the fall acting on the thin cortex often produces
  —blowout fractures of the body of the calcaneus, with
  —hemorrhage and fracture fragments causing
  —gross swelling and enlargement of the heel in the coronal plane;
- intra-articular fracture lines cause
  —limited and painful subtalar or midtarsal movements.
- calcaneal fractures are uncommon in children but may occur through a bone cyst or infected bone. The classification, clinical features and treatment are similar to those in the adult.
- radiologically, three views of the heel are necessary:
- an AP view of the foot for the anterior end of calcaneus and calcaneocuboid joint;
- a lateral view to show the profile of the calcaneus and Böhler's angle; and
- an axial view of the heel to see the posterior half of calcaneus, both posterior and anterior facets of subtalar joint, and the sustentaculum tali.

EXTRA-ARTICULAR FRACTURES (Fig. 25.5)

- are fractures of the calcaneus which do not involve the subtalar joint;
- all are uncommon except those of the body and
- none require reduction, except displaced beak fractures of the tuberosity.

Tuberosity

Medial or lateral margin

- fracture is seen best on an axial x-ray;
- treatment consists of

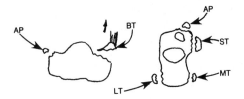

Figure 25.5. Extra-articular calcaneal fractures. *AP*, anterior process; *BT*, beak fracture of the tuberosity; *ST*, sustentaculm tali; *MT*, medial margin of the tuberosity; *LT*, lateral margin of the tuberosity.

—elevation of the limb, ice and a compression bandage. When the swelling has subsided, apply a
—BKWC for 4 weeks.

Superior margin

- a beak-shaped fragment is usually pulled off by the Achilles tendon;
- caused by a fall with acute dorsiflexion of the ankle joint and reflex contraction of the triceps surae;
- the patient walks with a calcaneal limp because he has no "push-off" on the injured side;
- fracture is well seen on the lateral x-ray;
- treatment for
  —undisplaced fracture is the same as that discussed previously, with a cast for 6 weeks. If the fracture is
  —displaced, perform open reduction and internal fixation with a screw or wire. Then treat with a
  —BK cast and NWB with the foot in 30° equinus for 4 weeks and in neutral position for 4 weeks.

Sustentaculum tali

- fracture is caused by a fall with the foot in extreme inversion. The patient has
- pain and tenderness just below the medial malleolus beneath the deltoid ligament;
- hyperextension of the great toe increases the pain;
- the axial x-ray shows the fracture;
- treat as for a tuberosity fracture, with a BKWC for 6 weeks.

Anterior process

- anterior process is avulsed by the bifurcate ligament when the foot is
- acutely flexed and adducted;

- lateral and oblique x-rays of the foot show the fracture, but this may be difficult to see if it is undisplaced;
- treatment consists of
  —elevation, then a
  —BKWC for 6 weeks.
- this fracture may enter the calcaneocuboid articular surface of the calcaneus and cause symptoms later. If this occurs, excise the fragment. If symptoms persist, calcaneocuboid fusion may be required.

Body

- fractures of the body are the most common type of calcaneal fracture;
- those that do not involve the subtalar joint are less common than those that do;
- fractures are produced by a fall from a height with the foot everted or inverted;
- look for a fracture on lateral and axial x-rays;
- treatment consists of immediate elevation, ice and a compression bandage. When the swelling has diminished, the patient should have
  —daily physiotherapy with active movements of ankle and subtalar joints and can start walking with crutches but must be
  —NWB for 12 weeks. He should elevate the foot whenever possible and wear an elastic bandage for several months;
- prognosis is usually good.

INTRA-ARTICULAR FRACTURES

- 75% of all calcaneal fractures involve the subtalar joint.

Etiopathology (Fig. 25.6)

- mechanism is a fall from a height onto the heel. The
- lateral process of the talus is shaped like an inverted triangle and acts as a wedge which is driven into the body of the calcaneus by impact, splitting the calcaneus.
- split fracture of the body occurs with the foot in neutral position;
- split-tongue fracture occurs with the foot in eversion, and
- central depression fracture occurs with the foot in dorsiflexion but neutral eversion and inversion;
- the degree of displacement, comminution and widening of bone depends on the height of the fall, the patient's weight and age, and the mineral content of the bone.
- when these fractures are displaced, the
  —tuberosity is elevated, with the effect that the
  —Achilles tendon is lengthened. If the tuberosity is not reduced, the patient will have a
  —flat-footed gait with diminished push-off.

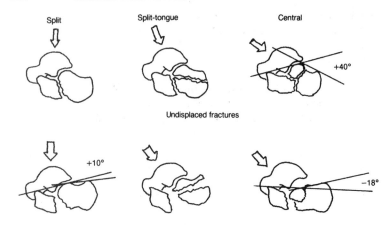

Figure 25.6. Intra-articular calcaneal fractures. (Modified from Essex-Lopresti P: The mechanism, reduction technique, and results in fractures of the os calcis. *Br J Surg* 39:395–419, 1952.)

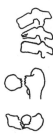

Figure 25.7. Triad.

Clinical and radiological features (Fig. 25.7)

- pain with exquisite tenderness on lateral compression of the heel;
- often gross swelling with enlargement of the heel from side to side;
- ankle movement is possible but the
- subtalar joint is blocked;
- look for an associated ipsilateral
  —fractured femoral neck or dislocation of hip and
  —compression fracture of any vertebra. Examine the
  —other calcaneus because these injuries are often bilateral.
- if the fracture is displaced, Böhler's angle is reduced and may even be reversed.

Treatment

Undisplaced

- elevate the leg in a compression bandage and encourage ankle, foot and toe movements. When the swelling subsides, apply a
- BK cast for 6 weeks, with NWB; then have the patient begin
- range of motion and muscle strengthening exercises.

Displaced (Fig. 25.8)

- in a young patient,
  —compress the heel from side to side with the patient under general anesthesia, to correct lateral spread of the calcaneus and valgus deformity, and
  —elevate the depressed subtalar articular surface and reduce the upward displacement of the tuberosity with its attached Achilles tendon. Reduction of articular surfaces must be accurate for a reasonable result. Perform
  —closed reduction with a Gissane spike or a Steinmann pin driven from the back of the calcaneus forward and downward until the tip is beneath the subtalar fragment. Then
  —lever this fragment up and the tuberosity down. If necessary
  —fill the cavity beneath the elevated fragment with a block of iliac cancellous bone. Incorporate the pin into a
  —plaster slipper to allow ankle motion for 6 weeks, with NWB for another 4 weeks in a BK cast after removal of the spike.
- in an older, less active patient or in a patient whose articular surfaces are very comminuted, treat nonoperatively by
  —manual compression with the patient under general anesthesia, to correct lateral spread and valgus deformity, then by
  —elevation of the limb in a compression dressing and
  —early, active toe and ankle movements. The patient can move about

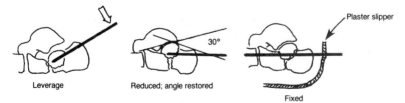

Leverage   Reduced; angle restored   30°   Plaster slipper   Fixed

Figure 25.8.   Reduction of central depressed fracture with a Steinmann pin. (Modified from Essex-Lopresti P: The mechanism, reduction technique, and results in fractures of the os calcis. *Br J Surg* 39:395–419, 1952.)

once the swelling has subsided, usually in 2 to 3 weeks, but must be

—NWB for 3 months.

COMPLICATIONS

Posttraumatic subtalar arthritis

- the most common complication of intra-articular fractures of the calcaneus;
- the patient has pain in the region of the sinus tarsi on eversion and inversion;
- differentiate this from other causes by
  —injection of local anesthetic into the subtalar joint through the sinus tarsi. If this relieves pain, inject 1 cc of
- corticosteroid. This may relieve the pain for some time, but if it only
  —partially relieves the pain, apply a
  —BK cast. If the cast relieves pain, consider a
  —triple arthrodesis. Subtalar arthrodesis by itself is less satisfactory.

Peroneal stenosing tenovaginitis

- peroneal tendons as they pass across the lateral face of calcaneus may be
  —squeezed against the fibula by a widened calcaneus or
  —trapped in callus;
- the patient has pain and tenderness along the tendon sheaths and pain on passive inversion of the foot;
- treat by
  —intrasynovial injection of local anesthetic and steroid;
- if symptoms recur after 2 or 3 injections,
  —explore and decompress the tendons and remove the offending bone fragments.

Tarsal tunnel syndrome

- bone fragments and callus may
  —compress the tibial nerve as it crosses the medial face of the calcaneus, causing
  —pain and paraesthesia or hypoesthesia in the sole of the foot.
- confirm the diagnosis by nerve conduction studies, and
- treat by surgical decompression.

Pain beneath heel

- the patient may have pain and tenderness beneath the heel, at and immediately distal to the medial and lateral processes, where the plantar aponeurosis originates from bone;
- infiltrate the bone-aponeurosis junction with local anesthetic and steroid and
- hollow out the heel of the shoe, filling this with soft material;
- operate only if a large fracture fragment beneath the heel or in sole of foot is causing pain on WB.

chapter 26
Injuries of the Midfoot and Forefoot

Surgical Anatomy

MIDFOOT

- the navicular articulates with the talus proximally, with the cuboid laterally, and with the three cuneiforms distally. The tendon of the tibialis posterior (TP) and the spring ligament are attached to the tuberosity;
- the cuboid articulates with the calcaneus proximally, with the navicular and third cuneiform medially, and with the fourth and fifth metatarsals (MTs) distally. The undersurface is grooved for the peroneus longus (PL) tendon. Calcaneocuboid and talonavicular joints form the midtarsal joint of Chopart;
- three cuneiforms articulate distally with the medial three MTs, with the second cuneiform being shorter and forming a recess for the base of the second MT.

FOREFOOT

- includes all the MTs and the toes;
- the central longitudinal axis of the foot lies along the second MT;
- the base of the second MT is locked into the cuneiforms;
- the tarsometatarsal joint is Lisfranc's joint.

ARCHES

- two longitudinal arches and one transverse arch of the foot form half a dome, with the apex being beneath the tibia, so that body weight is spread evenly to the three major weight-bearing (WB) areas, i.e., the inferior surface of the calcaneal tuberosity posteriorly and the heads of the first and fifth MTs anteriorly;
- arches are maintained by the
  —structure of the tarsals and by
  —extrinsic tendons and intrinsic muscles, ligaments and fascia;
- skin and the subcutaneous structure of the sole are unique and therefore irreplaceable.

ACCESSORY AND SESAMOID BONES

- the tuberosity of the navicular where the TP inserts and the
- styloid process of the fifth MT where the peroneus brevis (PB) inserts may have secondary ossification centers. If these remain separate after skeletal maturity, they are called
- accessory navicular and styloid bones.
- a sesamoid bone lies within the PL tendon where it lies in the groove beneath the cuboid, just proximal to the styloid of the fifth MT, and
- two sesamoids lie side by side in the tendon of the flexor hallucis brevis (FHB) beneath the first MT head. These latter may be bipartite.
- accessory and sesamoid bones are
  —round and smooth with
  —clearly defined margins, and are usually
  —bilateral;
- do not mistake them for chip fractures.

Midfoot Injuries

- isolated fractures of tarsals are rare. They are
- usually associated with other fractures and/or dislocations, so look carefully for these on good
  —anteroposterior (AP),
  —lateral and
  —oblique x-rays of the foot.

NAVICULAR FRACTURES

- navicular is the keystone of the medial longitudinal arch.

Body of navicular

- these fractures are rare;
- if they are undisplaced, treat with a below-knee walking cast (BKWC) for 6 weeks. If they are displaced, perform
  —open reduction and
  —fixation with K wires through a dorsomedial approach, and treat with a
  —below-knee (BK) cast and non-weight-bearing (NWB) for 8 weeks;
- if the articular surface is comminuted, fuse the talonavicular and naviculocuneiform joints.

Chip fractures

- fairly common;
- flakes of bone are usually avulsed by the
  —capsule or

—ligaments and are often associated with sprains or ligament injuries of the ankle or foot, particularly with a midtarsal injury, so look for these;

- treatment of a navicular chip fracture alone consists of a
    —bandage and elevation, then
    —partial weight-bearing (PWB) with crutches until pain subsides.
- if the chip is large and displaced, it may be palpable and interfere with the wearing of a shoe. In this case,
- excise the fragment.

NAVICULAR TUBEROSITY FRACTURE AND MIDTARSAL FRACTURE-SUBLUXATION

Clinical and radiological features (Fig. 26.1)

- fractures of the navicular tuberosity are relatively common and may be simply
- avulsed by the TP tendon or may be part of a
- midtarsal fracture-subluxation caused by
    —acute eversion of the forefoot on the midfoot, with the tuberosity and attached TP tendon being avulsed from the navicular. This injury is often misdiagnosed as a sprain. There is
    —localized pain and tenderness on the lateral as well as the medial side of the forefoot and pain on passive eversion. The fracture of the tuberosity is best seen on a
    —medial oblique x-ray of the foot and
    —may appear to be undisplaced because the foot usually reduces spontaneously. But initial displacement may have been considerable, with
    —subluxation of the talonavicular and calcaneocuboid joints or a
    —comminuted crushing injury of the calcaneocuboid joint. This latter injury is seen best on a lateral oblique x-ray. Look for these injuries

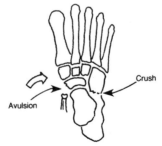

Figure 26.1. Occult midtarsal (Chopart) fracture-subluxation. (Modified from Dewar FP, Evans DC: Occult fracture-subluxation of the midtarsal joint. *J Bone Joint Surg* 50B:386–388, 1968.)

and take stress x-rays if you are in doubt.
- do not mistake tuberosity fracture for an accessory navicular; the
  —fracture margin is poorly defined, irregular, squared-off and painful, whereas the
  —accessory navicular has smooth, round, well-defined margins and is usually bilateral and painless. If you are in doubt, x-ray the noninjured side for comparison.

Treatment

Simple avulsion

- bandage and
- PWB until it is painless. If the fragment is
- displaced and the patient is an active person or has severe pain, treat with a BKWC molded beneath the longitudinal arch for 4 weeks;
- if the fragment is bothersome later, excise it.

Midtarsal fracture-subluxation

- treat this injury by
  —primary calcaneocuboid fusion, and
  —reattach the navicular tuberosity if this is displaced;
- improper treatment leads to
  —chronic pain and
  —disability.

TALONAVICULAR DISLOCATION

- without an associated fracture, reduce the dislocation closed by traction on the forefoot with countertraction at the ankle and gentle manipulation of the forefoot until the head of the talus slides back into the navicular socket;
- when a displaced navicular fracture is present,
  —open reduction may be necessary with
  —fixation of the fracture with K wires and with
  —stabilization of the dislocation with a K wire through the forefoot into the talus.

INJURIES OF CUNEIFORMS AND CUBOID

Fractures

- isolated fractures are uncommon. They are
- usually associated with other injuries of the foot, e.g.,
  —midtarsal fracture-subluxation or
  —tarsometatarsal fracture-dislocation;
- the foot is usually
  —crushed or
  —twisted;

- swelling may be considerable, with severe pain and tenderness;
- AP and oblique x-rays show the fractures best;
- treatment for
    —undisplaced chip fractures is symptomatic, but for
    —fractures of the bodies of these bones, apply a well-molded BKWC for 3 months, followed by a longitudinal arch support in the shoe.

Dislocations

- are not common and are
- difficult to diagnose. On looking at x-rays you have the feeling that
    —"something is wrong with this foot, but I don't know what it is!" So take
    —comparative x-rays of the normal foot and study all the x-rays carefully.
- treat immediately by
    —closed reduction, and
    —stabilize with percutaneous K wires because these are unstable injuries. Apply a
    —BK cast for 8 weeks, with NWB. Then
    —remove the wires and start the patient on
    —PWB with an arch support in the shoe. An
- old untreated injury may do well with open reduction and K wire fixation, but if the cartilage has deteriorated, fusion may be better.

TARSOMETATARSAL INJURIES

Fracture-dislocation (Fig. 26.2)

- involves Lisfranc's joint and
- occurs more frequently than reports suggest.

Etiopathology and clinical features

- caused by
    —acute plantar flexion with rotation, with the foot folding like a concertina, or
    —violent abduction or adduction injury of the forefoot, or a
    —crushing injury of foot. The
- key to the injury is the second MT because the base of this MT is recessed into the row of cuneiforms and must fracture or dislocate to allow other MTs to displace.
- all MTs may dislocate in the same direction,
    —usually laterally or,
    —less often, medially; or they may
    —diverge, with the first moving medially and the other four moving laterally;

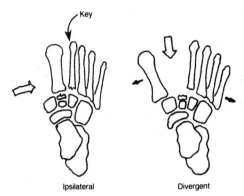

Figure 26.2. Tarsometatarsal (Lisfranc) fracture-dislocations.

- in all these injuries, there may be associated fractures of the
  —third or fourth MTs and/or
  —cuboid;
- the dorsalis pedis artery is often ruptured, causing
  —hemorrhage,
  —severe swelling, and sometimes
  —gangrene (for which Jacques Lisfranc amputated the forefoot through the tarsometatarsal (TMT) joint while traveling with Napoleon's Grande Armée).

Radiological features

- if spontaneous reduction has occurred, all you will see is a fracture of the second MT base. In this case,
  —examine the foot carefully and
  —take oblique x-rays and, if necessary,
  —stress views with the patient under general anesthesia, to confirm your suspicions.

Treatment

- with the patient under general anesthesia, apply traction on the forefoot, countertraction on the ankle, and manipulate the MTs into position;
- if the forefoot is unstable, pass K wires percutaneously, with
  —one through the first MT into the cuboid and with
  —the other through the fifth MT into the cuneiform. In both instances, apply a
- posterior splint for 1 week and elevate the leg. When swelling subsides, apply a

- BK cast for 6 weeks, with NWB;
- remove the K wires after cast removal. If
- closed reduction fails, perform
- open reduction through one or two dorsal incisions;
- do not operate through a swollen foot because this risks
  —skin necrosis and
  —infection;
- reduce the MTs and fix them with K wires. Postoperative care is the same as that discussed previously.

Dislocation

- one or several MTs may sublux or dislocate from the tarsals, usually dorsally;
- treatment consists of prompt closed reduction with K wire fixation if the reduction is unstable. If
- closed reduction fails, perform open reduction through appropriate incisions with K wire fixation;
- if the foot is too swollen for open reduction, wait until the edema subsides.

Forefoot Injuries

METATARSAL FRACTURES

Traumatic fractures

Etiopathology

- these fractures are caused by twisting or, more commonly, crushing injuries; if
- swelling and soft tissue damage are severe,
  —do not apply a complete cast and do not send the patient home because the foot may become ischemic.

Treatment

- undisplaced,
  —elevation and compression dressing, then
  —crutches with NWB until the pain subsides, then
  —progressive WB. If fractures are
- displaced, treat by closed reduction with the patient under general anesthesia. If the reduction is
  —stable, apply a BK cast, with NWB. Remove the cast at 4 weeks for

lateral MT fractures and at 6 weeks for first MT fractures. If the reduction is

—unstable, fix the fractures with percutaneous K wires passed

—longitudinally down the MT or

—transversely so that intact MTs splint the fractured ones. This is particularly helpful in comminuted or oblique fractures of the shaft when MTs are shortened. Some

- lateral displacement is acceptable, but
- dorsal or plantar displacement or angulation, especially of the MT heads, is not acceptable because it will cause

    —abnormal pressure areas in the sole and

    —deformity of the toes, with resultant pain, corns and inability to walk. If closed reduction fails,

- open reduction and K wire fixation may be required. In
- malunion of the MT necks with the MT heads in the sole preventing walking,

    —excision of the heads and an

    —MT bar fitted to the shoe will help.

Stress fractures

- called fatigue or "march" fractures.

Etiopathology

- repetitive and unaccustomed stress of increased magnitude on the foot causes
- microfractures which develop into
- complete fracture if the stress is continued;
- occurs commonly across the shaft of the second MT just proximal to neck and, less often, in other MTs.

Clinical and radiological features

- history of recent change in activity, e.g., basic training of a new military recruit or long or frequent walks in a citizen who is normally sedentary;
- increasing ache in the forefoot is relieved by elevation and rest;
- swelling over the dorsum of the foot may occur, and the
- patient will start to walk with a limp on the outside of foot. There is
- point tenderness over the involved bone, and the
- callus may be palpable if the fracture is several weeks old.
- x-rays are often normal for the first 2 weeks,
- then they may show a fine transverse line across the MT shaft with subperiosteal new bone formation around it;
- the fracture is never displaced.

Treatment

- union is not a problem;
- treat symptomatically with
  —elevation and analgesics, then
  —progressive WB; apply a
- BKWC if the pain is severe and prevents the patient from walking.

PHALANGEAL INJURIES

Fractures

- usually the result of direct trauma with a crushing injury. If the fracture is
- undisplaced, treat it symptomatically;
  —strapping an injured toe to its largest neighbor (buddy taping) helps reduce discomfort. Place gauze between the two toes to prevent maceration;
  —decompress a painful subungual hematoma. But if the fracture is
- displaced, with the intrinsic muscles angulating the fragments as they do in the fingers (see Chapter 14),
  —reduce the fracture and
  —immobilize the foot with a cast and
  —K wires if necessary.

Dislocations

- toes usually dislocate superiorly at the metatarsophalangeal (MP) joint;
- treatment for any of the four lateral MP joints is closed reduction with the use of local anesthesia. If the dislocation is
  —stable, strap the toe to its largest neighbor, but if the dislocation is
  —unstable, fix the toe with percutaneous K wires. When the
- first MP joint is dislocated, apply a BKWC right to the end of the great toe.
- interphalangeal joint dislocations are uncommon and are usually associated with other injuries. Treatment is the same as for the MP joints.

Injuries in Children

- are less frequent than the same injuries in adults;
- the pattern of injuries and their treatment are similar to those for adults, except for
- greenstick fractures and
- epiphyseal plate injuries. These can be treated closed unless the
  —articular surface is disrupted or

—growth plate damage is likely without anatomical reduction.
- do not confuse growth plates with fractures. The epiphyseal growth plate of the
  —first MT and
  —all the phalanges is at the base, but the plates of the
  —lateral four MTs are distal (similar to those in the hand).

chapter 27

Cervical Spine Injuries: General Features and Principles of Treatment

Introduction

- because the atlas and axis are unique vertebrae, some of the injuries in this area differ from those of the more typical cervical vertebrae, C3 to C7;
- vertebral injuries are like pelvic injuries in that injuries to the
  —bony ring are not as important as injuries to the contents because the
  —skeletal injury will not kill the patient but spinal cord damage might!
- treatment is influenced by two major factors,
  —spinal cord injury and
  —stability;
- if you suspect a neck injury, stabilize the head in the neutral position before you do anything else;
- a neck injury is often associated with a head injury, so keep this in mind.

Etiopathology

CLASSIFICATION OF INJURIES

Fractures (Figs. 27.1, 27.4 and 27.5)

- these may occur in the
  —body, articular processes,
  —pedicles, laminae or spinous process and
- may be
  —isolated,
  —multiple, or associated with
  —subluxation or dislocation.

Subluxation (Fig. 27.2)

- both facet joints may be subluxed, or
- one facet joint may be dislocated while the other is not, so that the vertebra above rotates forward around the intact facet joint, causing a rotational subluxation. In
- subluxation the vertebra above is displaced forward
  —less than 25% of the anteroposterior (AP) diameter of the vertebral body.

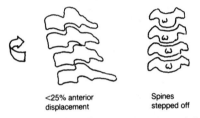

Figure 27.1.   Flexion compression fracture of C4.

<25% anterior
displacement

Spines
stepped off

Figure 27.2.   Unilateral rotary subluxation of C4-C5.

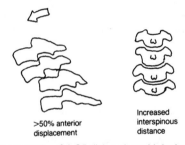

>50% anterior
displacement

Increased
interspinous
distance

Figure 27.3.   C4-C5 dislocation with locked facets.

Dislocation (Fig. 27.3)

- implies disruption of the
  —interbody disc joint and
  —both posterior facet joints. The
- superior vertebral body is usually dislocated
  —more than 50% on the lower one.

Neurological deficit

- the skeletal injury may be accompanied by a
- cord lesion, which may be
  —complete or
  —incomplete, or by a
- root lesion.

MECHANISM OF INJURIES

- neck injuries are nearly always caused by indirect violence transmitted through the head.

Flexion (Fig. 27.1)

- usually causes compression fracture of the body without rupture of the posterior ligaments and is generally
- stable.

Flexion-rotation (Figs. 27.2 and 27.3)

- produces unilateral or bilateral posterior facet dislocation with anterior subluxation or dislocation of the proximal vertebra. The
- injury may be accompanied by fracture of a facet, lamina or the body;
- posterior ligaments are torn, but the
- anterior longitudinal ligament is stripped up and not torn and, together with prevertebral muscles, is the only stabilizing structure remaining;
- incomplete cord injuries are more common than complete cord injuries.

Compression (Fig. 27.4)

- a heavy axial load on the head causes
- explosive, comminuted fracture of the body, usually of C5;
- bone fragments are frequently ejected posteriorly into the vertebral canal where they damage the cord;
- complete quadriplegia is common.

Extension (Fig. 27.5)

- causes either
  —compression fracture of the posterior arch or
  —disruption of the intervertebral disc with avulsion of the anterosuperior margin of the vertebra below by the anterior longitudinal ligament and annulus fibrosus. This little fragment may be the only radiological sign of a major injury.

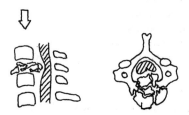

Figure 27.4. Compression burst fracture of C5 with cord compression by bone and disc.

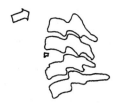

Figure 27.5.   Hyperextension injury with a "teardrop" avulsion fracture.

Lateral flexion
- causes unilateral fracture of a facet or pedicle and is
- stable. However, it may produce the
- Brown-Séquard syndrome or a nerve root injury.

Bullet wounds
- a low-velocity bullet may cause an incomplete or, more rarely, a complete cord injury if the bullet hits a vertebra;
- a high-velocity bullet smashes bone, and fracture fragments then act as secondary missiles. So
    —complete cord lesions are common;
    —shock waves from these high-energy bullets create a wide zone of necrosis and may cause quadriplegia even if the bullet only passes close to a vertebra and does not actually hit it.

Diagnosis

HISTORY
- description of the injury is important and may give you the clue that the patient has a neck injury;
- always suspect a cervical spine injury in a patient who has a
    —head injury or complains of
    —pain in the neck after an accident, and
- treat him as you would a patient with a neck injury until you have proved that his neck is normal;
- whether neurological involvement was immediate or appeared later is important for the treatment and prognosis.

GENERAL PHYSICAL EXAMINATION
- lay the patient on his back and immobilize his head temporarily with a sandbag on each side of it;
- on inspection, look for

—cranial or facial bruises, abrasions and lacerations;
—note the position of patient's head and
—voluntary movements of the head and limbs;
—sustained penile erection indicates severe cervical cord injury;
- palpate the neck without moving the patient, and note areas of
—tenderness, swelling, hematoma and deformity. The
- vital signs are obviously important. Traumatic paraplegia may cause hypotension, but pulse rate is usually normal and differentiates this from hemorrhagic shock.

NEUROLOGICAL EXAMINATION
Sensation (Fig. 27.6)

- correlate sensory changes with the dermatome pattern. If
- any sensation is present anywhere below the level of injury, the lesion is incomplete. The

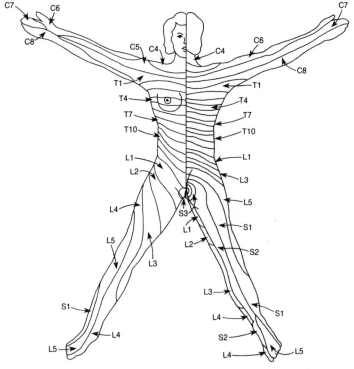

Figure 27.6. Dermatome pattern.

- most likely areas to be spared are the sacral dermatomes,
  —perianal, scrotal and labial skin and the skin
  —under the toes;
- always write down the results.

Voluntary motor function

- if the patient breathes spontaneously, C4 is intact (phrenic nerve). If the patient has
- deltoid and biceps function, C5 is intact. If the patient has
- extensor carpi radialis longus (ECRL) and brevis (ECRB) function, C6 is intact. If the patient has
- triceps or flexor carpi radialis (FCR) or extensor digitorum longus (EDL) function, C7 is intact. If the patient has
- flexor digitorum sublimis (FDS) or profundus (FDP) function, C8 is intact; and if the patient has
- intrinsic function, T1 is intact;
- examine both upper limbs. They will be different if the cord lesion is asymmetrical.
- examine voluntary muscles in the rest of body, particularly the
  —toe flexors and extensors and
  —rectal sphincter for sacral sparing;
- look for the
  —bulbocavernosus and
  —anal wink reflexes.

NEUROLOGICAL LESIONS

Spinal shock

- with spinal cord shock, there is complete absence of all neurological function below the lesion;
- shock usually lasts less than 24 hours. During this period you cannot differentiate a complete lesion from shock;
- anal wink (prick the perianal skin and see the anus contract) and the bulbocavernosus reflex (squeeze the glans penis or press on the clitoris and the anal sphincter will squeeze your finger) return when the cord recovers from spinal shock because these are normal cord-mediated reflexes. If
  —one or both reflexes are present but
  —anesthesia and motor paralysis are still total,
  —complete cord lesion is confirmed.

Nerve root injury

- usually due to a fractured or dislocated facet compressing the nerve at the neural foramen;

- this injury is a peripheral nerve lesion, and the patient may recover;
- root avulsion from the cord is rare.

Incomplete cord lesions (Fig. 27.7)

General remarks

- an incomplete cord lesion is signified by the presence of some
  —sensation and/or
  —voluntary muscle activity
  —distal to the spinal injury;
- the greater the
  —sensory and motor sparing and the
  —faster the recovery, the
  —better the prognosis;
- repeat the examination regularly and frequently to evaluate the progress of the lesion, and
- write down your findings every time.

Central cord syndrome

- the most common incomplete cord syndrome;
- due to hyperextension injury in a middle-aged person with an arthritic spine. The
- spinal cord is squeezed between osteophytes in front and infolding of the ligamentum flavum behind, but there may be
- no signs of spinal injury on x-ray;
- gray matter and spinothalamic and pyramidal tracts are damaged;

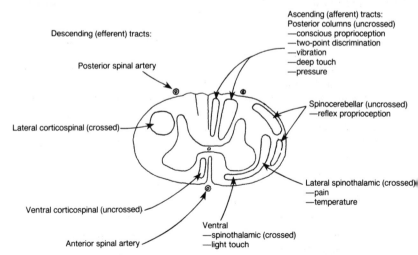

Figure 27.7. Tracts and sensory modalities of the spinal cord.

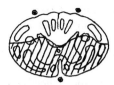

Figure 27.8. Spinal cord territory of the anterior spinal artery (*crosshatched area*, mainly motor) is affected in anterior cord syndrome.

- the patient has
  —flaccid, lower motor neuron paralysis of the upper limbs and
  —spastic, upper motor neuron paralysis of the lower limbs with
  —sacral sparing;
- prognosis is fair, with the likelihood of
  —return of bladder and bowel control and a
  —spastic gait, but the
  —upper limb paralysis is usually permanent.

Anterior cord syndrome (Fig. 27.8)

- similar to anterior spinal artery syndrome with damage to the
  —anterior horns and
  —pyramidal and
  —spinothalamic tracts;
- posterior columns are spared. The patient has
- complete anesthesia and paralysis distal to the lesion, except for
  —deep pressure and pain, vibration and
  —proprioception which are carried up the posterior columns.
- if recovery of sacral pain and temperature starts within 48 hours of the end of spinal shock, the prognosis is good. Usually the prognosis is poor.

Brown-Séquard syndrome

- occurs when one lateral half of the cord is injured. The
- patient has
  —ipsilateral motor paralysis and
  —contralateral hypoesthesia to pain and temperature below the lesion;
- partial recovery is likely, with return of
  —bladder and bowel control and the
  —ability to walk.

Complete cord lesion

- if there is total anesthesia and paralysis of voluntary muscles below the level of the lesion but the bulbocavernosus and anal wink reflexes are present, the
  —lesion is complete and

—recovery is impossible. For all complete quadriplegics a
- wheelchair is essential. With a lesion at
- C7 the patient
    —can become completely independent and may
    —live alone.
    —tendon transfers may improve hand function, e.g., the brachioradialis for thumb flexion, the flexor carpi radialis for finger flexion, and the pronator teres for thumb opposition. With a lesion
- above C7 the patient
    —requires help with most activities of daily living and
    —cannot live alone. An
    —electric wheelchair helps.

RADIOLOGICAL EXAMINATION
Lateral and anteroposterior views
- if you suspect a cervical spine injury,
    —stabilize the patient's head with sandbags or halter traction and
    —accompany him to the x-ray department;
- for a good lateral x-ray, pull gently downward on the patient's arms so that his shoulders do not hide C7 and T1. Then take a
- plain AP x-ray for C3 to T1 and an
- open mouth view to see the occiput, atlas and axis;
- examine soft tissue shadows as well as bone, especially the prevertebral soft tissue shadow which normally has a maximum width of 5 mm.

Obliques
- oblique views show the facet joints most clearly.
- pull gently on the head to stabilize the cervical spine and
- turn the whole patient 45°. If you turn the head by itself, you will only obtain a partial oblique view.

Swimmer's view
- if the cervicothoracic junction is difficult to see, take the swimmer's view, with
    —one arm abducted 180°,
    —the other arm by the side, and the
    —x-ray tube directed obliquely at 60° to the coronal plane.

Dynamic flexion and extension views (Fig. 27.9)
- lateral x-ray with the neck flexed and then extended. To
- avoid damage to the cord,
- hold the patient's head yourself and stop the movement immediately if

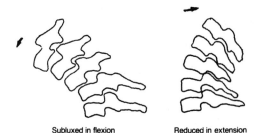

Subluxed in flexion   Reduced in extension

Figure 27.9. Flexion and extension radiographs showing unstable C5-C6 subluxation.

the patient complains of hyperesthesias;
- never do this under anesthetic. The x-rays will
- show AP instability and are of help
  —in making initial diagnosis and in evaluating
  —residual instability after treatment.

Tomogram and CAT scan

- are useful for delineating details of complex fractures and subluxations at one or more levels. The
- CAT scan in particular may show disc material or bone fragments lying in the vertebral canal.

Stability

- use White and Panjabi's chart to gauge the stability of the injury. This consigns
- two points each for
  —anterior element destruction,
  —posterior element destruction, sagittal
  —translation of more than 3.5 mm, sagittal
  —rotation of more than 11°,
  —positive stretch test, and
  —cord damage;
- one point each is awarded for
  —nerve root compression,
  —abnormal disc narrowing, anticipated
  —dangerous loading;
- five or more points signifies
  —instability.

Complications

EARLY

Neurological

- the major complication. Many of the following complications are secondary to this.

Pulmonary

- a quadriplegic patient has
  —vital capacity reduced by 75% because the intercostals are paralyzed, and he
  —cannot forcibly exhale because the adominal muscles are paralyzed. He
  —cannot cough either. So secretions collect in the lung with consequent
  —atelectasis and pneumonia;
- respiratory insufficiency is due to
  —paralysis and
  —recumbency, especially in the prone position;
  —prevent this by
  —respiratory physiotherapy and postural drainage,
  —turning the patient on his back and sides and
  —elevating the head of the bed to prevent diaphragmatic compression by intra-abdominal viscera;
- treat with
  —antibiotics and a
  —mechanical respirator when necessary.

Urological

- a urinary catheter is necessary but may cause a
- urinary infection which can develop into pyelonephritis;
- prevent infection by
  —strictly sterile technique,
  —closed drainage system,
  —urinary antiseptics and
  —removal of the catheter as soon as possible.

Skin

- sensitive skin breaks down over bony prominences with consequent
  —full-thickness ulcers which become
  —infected and act as
  —fluid and protein sinks, thus
  —prolonging the catabolic phase;

- prevent by
  —turning of the patient every 4 hours, night and day, and
  —skin care with oil and alcohol;
- treat by
  —debridement, dressing, antibiotics, skin grafts and flaps.

Gastrointestinal

- paralytic ileus is common, so treat by
  —nasogastric tube,
  —no food or fluid by mouth (NPO) and
  —adequate intravenous hydration;
- treat acute dilatation of the stomach similarly;
- gastrointestinal bleeding may occur from
  —diffuse, hemorrhage gastritis or an
  —acute duodenal stress ulcer (Curling's ulcer). Treat as for
  —gastric ulcer.

LATE

Joint contractures

- all jonts should be exercised through their
  —full range of motion by the physiotherapist every day to avoid contractures;
  —dynamic hand splints are of help too;
- if the patient is likely to walk, treat contractures by
  —serial cast wedging or
  —soft tissue releases;
  —osteotomy in the lower limb may be necessary if contractures are very severe. If the patient will be
- confined to a wheelchair all his life, correction of lower limb contractures is necessary only to facilitate sitting and hygiene.

Prolonged recumbency

- may cause many complications (see Chapter 6).

Psychological withdrawal

- becomes more important as time goes by.

Degenerative arthrosis

- commonly occurs in the intervertebral discs and the posterior facet joints of the vertebrae adjacent to the injury;
- symptoms include
  —pain in the neck which may radiate into one or both arms, to the occipital region and between the scapulae;

- nerve root compression may cause motor and sensory changes;
- treatment with
  —analgesics, anti-inflammatory drugs and
  —intermittent physiotherapy is usually sufficient.

Treatment

OBJECTIVES

- cervical spine injuries may be
  —stable or unstable,
  —with or without a partial or complete spinal cord or nerve root injury;
- objectives of treatment are to
  —provide best conditions for recovery from incomplete cord or root injury,
  —prevent more neurological damage by protecting the cord at all times and correcting hypotension and anoxia,
  —allow bone and ligaments to heal in satisfactory position by accurate reduction and adequate fixation in order to avoid late pain and to prevent redisplacement,
  —mobilize the patient early, and
  —rehabilitate him to the maximum degree of independence possible in society.

REDUCTION

- as with any other skeletal injury, reduction of a recent fracture or dislocation of the spine is important. It should be done as soon as possible, if a neurological deficit exists, in order to promote recovery;
- but if there is no neurological deficit or if quadriplegia is complete after 24 hours and recovery is impossible, a delay of 2 or 3 days will do no harm.
- reduce the spine gradually. Rapid reduction may increase soft tissue injury.

Cranial traction

- use a head halter, skull tongs or, best of all, the halo;
- in estimating the weight of traction, allow
  —5 kg for the head and
  —2 kg for each vertebral interspace above the lesion, to a
  —maximum of 15 to 18 kg;
  —greater pull than this will not improve reduction;
- sedate the patient with
  —analgesics and
  —muscle relaxants but do not anesthetize him;
- continue traction up to 48 hours and follow the patient's progress with lateral x-rays. If traction

- fails, gentle manipulative reduction with the patient under sedation may succeed;
- diminish the pull to about 3 kg after reduction.

Open reduction

- if cranial traction does not succeed, open reduction with internal fixation and grafting may be necessary, with skeletal traction used throughout the procedure.
- always take lateral x-ray after intubation but before skin incision, because the anesthetist may have reduced the injury during induction!

Old injury

- in general, if the lesion is more than 3 weeks old, reduction is difficult and dangerous. It is better to treat the patient with a
  —Minerva plaster if the lesion is stable or with
  —posterior fusion without reduction if the lesion is unstable.

IMMOBILIZATION

Traction

- light cranial traction will maintain the reduction until healing is sufficiently firm so that a Minerva plaster jacket or collar can be applied without risk of redisplacement;
- halter traction is uncomfortable and causes pressure sores when used for prolonged periods;
- cranial traction can be continued longer for a quadriplegic patient if surgery, jackets and collars are contraindicated.

Minerva cast (Fig. 27.10)

- a Minerva plaster jacket will not hold an unstable injury, but it does
- allow a moderate degree of immobilization, so that the

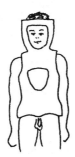

Figure 27.10.   Minerva cast.

- patient can walk and can be discharged home with the jacket if he has no paralysis. But the jacket
- cannot be used with quadriplegia because of the insensitive skin. A
- Minerva plaster collar encloses the head, rests on the shoulders, and extends anteriorly to the manubriosternal joint and posteriorly to the midscapula region. It can
- control rotation, flexion and extension;
- pad it well over the shoulders;
- useful for quadriplegic patient.

Halo cast

- gives excellent stability and can be
- continued for many months.

Final stability

- can be evaluated by
  —standard and
  —dynamic x-rays;
- intervertebral new bone formation anteriorly and the
- absence of abnormal movements indicate that the lesion is stable and that the collar or jacket can be removed;
- this is likely when the primary lesion is a fracture or reduction was difficult. But when the
- primary lesion is ligamentous or the reduction was easy, chronic instability may result and the spine may require internal fixation and fusion.

SURGERY

Decompression

Laminectomy

- indicated for
  —deterioration of a partial cord lesion due to hemorrhage. Do not confuse this with a complete cord lesion with ascending neurological loss of one or two root levels. This latter condition is usually due to edema and is not helped by laminectomy;
  —root compression by bone, disc or an articular facet can be approached and relieved by a partial laminectomy;
- laminectomy for an old untreated dislocation or for a fracture-dislocation with a partial cord lesion or a root lesion may be less dangerous than open reduction;
- identify the levels of cord compression by myelography and CAT scan before surgery;
- complications of laminectomy include
  —increased cord damage,
  —epidural hemorrhage,

—dural tear with CSF leak, and

—increased posterior instability of the cervical spine, which may require stabilization with wire and a posterior graft.

- laminectomy has
  —no place in the treatment of a
  —complete cord lesion.

Anterior decompression

- cord compression due to extruded disc or bone fragments is usually anterior, so for a
  —partial lesion which is
  —deteriorating due to anterior compression,
  —anterior decompression will be
  —more effective than will
  —laminectomy;
- assess the level preoperatively by myelography and CAT scan;
- graft the spine anteriorly after decompression and use rigid
- external fixation such as a halo cast, postoperatively.

Open reduction and internal fixation

- the posterior approach is indicated for a
  —subluxation or dislocation with locked facets, which cannot be reduced by closed means, or an
  —unstable injury which will not stabilize with nonoperative treatment, or a
  —quadriplegic patient with insensitive skin who cannot be treated easily in skull traction. Internal fixation may also prevent the complications of prolonged recumbency. Posterior fusion with autogenous iliac crest bone can be done simultaneously to ensure ultimate stability. The
- anterior approach is
  —rarely indicated because the remaining stable elements are usually anterior and this approach would
  —destabilize the spine even more;
- postoperatively, a well-padded jacket or collar is required for 3 months.

Spinal Injuries in Children

- everything stated in this and the next three chapters applies to children, with the following modifications:
- vertebral injuries are less common in children than in adults, but in children the
- cervical spine, especially at C1 and C2, is injured more often than the thoracolumbar spine;

- dislocations are rare in children because ligaments are stronger than bone and growth plates, but
- hypermmobility of the spine may mimic subluxation, especially at C2-C3 and C3-C4;
- x-rays are more difficult to interpret, so for spinal injuries in children the CAT scan may be particularly helpful;
- epiphyseal plate injuries affect the proximal plate more often than they affect the distal plate;
- growth plates and congenital and growth anomalies may simulate fractures;
- congenital malformations predispose the spine to injury.
- cord lesions without apparent vertebral injury are more frequent in children than in adults because a
  —child's spine is more flexible and
  —Type I epiphyseal plate injuries may reduce spontaneously without visible x-ray signs. These cord lesions may be due to
  —concussion, causing an incomplete transient lesion, or
  —contusion, leaving some permanent damage and spasticity, or
  —infarction, causing complete, permanent flaccid paraplegia.
- surgery for the injury is seldom necessary in children, and the immobilization time is shorter for children than for adults.
- late spinal deformity is particularly common in
  —complete thoracic paraplegia but may also be secondary to
  —epiphyseal plate damage.

chapter 28

Cervical Spine Injuries: Specific Injuries and Treatment

Fractures of Atlas

SINGLE ARCH FRACTURES

- arch fractures are uncommon;
- the posterior arch is fractured more often than the anterior arch;
- fractures are usually bilateral because a single fracture in a continuous ring is rare;
- caused by hyperextension with vertical compression;
- stable unless associated with other injuries, e.g., an
  —odontoid fracture or
  —fracture of the pedicles of the axis.
- treat a
  —stable injury with rest and a cervical collar for 6 weeks;
  —unstable injuries require posterior occipitoaxial fusion.

JEFFERSON'S FRACTURE OF BOTH ARCHES (Fig. 28.1)

Etiopathology

- is a fracture of the anterior and posterior arches, so that the lateral masses, which carry the articular facets, are displaced laterally away from the odontoid;
- may involve one or both lateral masses and may be comminuted;
- an open-mouth anteroposterior (AP) x-ray shows lateral displacement of one or both lateral masses relative to the odontoid and to the superior articular facets of the axis;
- caused by axial compression by the head on the spine;
- cord injury is not common but is usually fatal when it occurs;
- compression of the great occipital nerve of Arnold, C2, which supplies the posterior half of the scalp, may cause neuralgia;
- the vertebral artery is rarely injured.

Treatment (Fig. 27.10)

- union of an undisplaced fracture will occur with the patient in a Minerva jacket for 12 weeks. If the fracture is

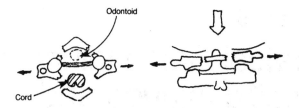

Figure 28.1.   Jefferson fracture of the atlas.

- displaced, use
    —traction for 2 weeks to reduce displacement, then a
    —Minerva or halo jacket for 10 weeks, with bed rest for first 4 weeks and ambulation for the remaining 6 weeks. Then
    —remove the cast and take dynamic x-rays in flexion and extension. If it is
    —still unstable, perform posterior occipitoaxial fusion.

Fractures of Axis

FRACTURES OF BODY

- are usually compression fractures due to forced flexion or are
- vertical or oblique fractures and are
- stable unless associated with other lesions;
- treat
    —stable fractures with a Minerva jacket for 12 weeks;
    —unstable fractures require traction for 2 weeks, then posterior C1-C2 fusion.

ODONTOID FRACTURES (Fig. 28.2)

Etiopathology

- caused by violent
    —hyperflexion, with the transverse ligament acting as a fulcrum, or
    —hyperextension, with the anterior arch of the atlas acting as a fulcrum and snapping the odontoid at its base or through its waist;
- odontoid and atlas may be
    —undisplaced or
    —displaced anteriorly or posteriorly.
- Type I fracture through the tip is stable and heals well. Differentiate this from an os odontoideum;
- Type II fracture through the waist may be slow to heal. The rate of pseudarthrosis is high;
- Type III fracture through the upper body of the axis heals well.

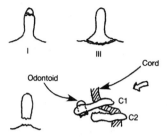

II. Unstable; nonunion likely

Figure 28.2. Odontoid fractures. (Modified from Anderson LD, D'Alonzo RT: Fractures of the odontoid process of the axis. *J Bone Joint Surg* 56A:1663–1674, 1974.)

- in children the fracture may be through the
  - —epiphyseal plate, and
  - —avascular necrosis and resorption of the central or basilar portion of the odontoid may follow;
  - —retropharyngeal swelling may be the only sign of injury on the original x-rays.

Diagnosis

- diagnosis is based on
- open-mouth and lateral x-rays centered on the atlas;
- dynamic lateral x-rays with the patient's head in flexion and extension will show instability. Hold the patients's head to avoid creating or aggravating a spinal cord injury.
- differentiate a fracture from
  - —congenital pseudarthrosis, which may look like a fracture but has rounded sclerotic margins, and
  - —congenital absence of the odontoid. Look for other congenital deformities of vertebrae, which may be associated.

Complications

- a cord lesion is especially likely with a posterior fracture-dislocation of C1 on C2, with the fractured odontoid being driven backward and compressing the anterior cord;
- vertebral artery insufficiency due to kinking;
- pseudarthrosis is common with both nonoperative and operative treatment.

Treatment

Recent fracture

- undisplaced fracture is treated by use of a Minerva or halo jacket for 12 weeks, then by evaluation for stability. If the spine is

—unstable or there is
—pseudarthrosis, perform
—posterior atlantoaxial fusion;
- displaced fracture is usually associated with atlantoaxial dislocation. See below for management.

Pseudarthrosis

- stable pseudarthrosis shown on dynamic x-rays does not require treatment. For an
- unstable injury with atlantoaxial dislocation, see below.

FRACTURE OF POSTERIOR ARCH (Fig. 28.3)

Etiopathology

- called "hangman's fracture" or traumatic spondylolisthesis of C2.
- caused by hyperextension from a
  —car collision during which the car is brought to a sudden halt, with the forehead and face of the patient striking the windshield and forcing the head back, or by hyperextension and distraction when the
  —knot of the hangman's noose is beneath the chin;
- neurological deficit is
  —rare in patients seen in hospital because cord damage is almost always
  —immediately fatal, especially from a hanging in which distraction tears the cord apart. This fracture accounts for 16% of deaths associated with head injuries,
- is bilateral, and usually passes through the
  —arch just posterior to the articular facet, or through the
  —facets, or through the
  —pedicles between the superior and inferior articular facets;
  —the disc between C2 and C3 is
  —partially or completely ruptured, sometimes with
  —avulsion of the anteroinferior corner of the body of C2, the teardrop fracture;
- the fracture is unstable in extension;
- when due to a car accident, it may be accompanied by compression fracture of the body of C2, as the neck flexes and extends violently.

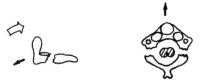

Figure 28.3. Traumatic spondylolisthesis of the axis. A hyperextension injury.

- diagnosis is based on
  —lateral and open-mouth x-rays, with
  —dynamic x-rays taken in flexion and extension to evaluate instability.

Treatment

- 95% of these fractures heal regardless of the method of treatment. Reduction is unnecessary;
- immobilize the head and neck in a
  —Minerva jacket for 12 weeks. Treat
- nonunion with residual instability at 3 months by anterior C2-C3 fusion because posterior C1-C3 fusion blocks rotation.

Dislocation and Fracture-Dislocation of Atlas and Axis

ATLANTOOCCIPITAL DISLOCATION

- caused by violent twisting force on the head or on the body with the head fixed;
- all atlantooccipital ligaments are torn and the joint is
- very unstable. Most patients die immediately from respiratory failure.
- immobilize the head and neck as soon as possible in a Minerva jacket and fuse the occiput to the axis through a posterior window in the cast;
- do not use traction because this will stretch the cord and kill the patient!

ATLANTOAXIAL DISLOCATION (Fig. 28.4)

Etiopathology and diagnosis

- this injury is always associated with either
  —odontoid fracture (anterior or posterior dislocation of C1) or with
  —rupture of the transverse ligament (anterior dislocation), which is usually fatal because the odontoid squashes the cord;
- diagnosis is based on lateral x-rays centered on the atlas with flexion and extension views, with the doctor holding the patient's head;
- the distance between the

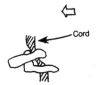

Figure 28.4. Dislocation of C1 on C2 after transverse ligament rupture. Cord compression.

—anterior arch of the atlas and the
—odontoid is normally
—less than 3 mm in the adult and less than 4 mm in the child;
—a distance greater than this suggests instability;
- differential diagnosis includes
  —congenital absence or pseudarthrosis of the odontoid,
  —pyogenic infection or tuberculosis with destruction of the odontoid or transverse ligament, or
  —rheumatoid disease with destruction of the transverse ligament.

Treatment

Recent dislocation

- reduce a recent injury by
  —traction for 10 days, then
  —posterior fusion of C1 and C2;
- open reduction is indicated only if closed reduction is incomplete.

Old untreated dislocation

- without neurological signs, treat by
  —traction. If the atlas reduces, perform a
  —posterior C1-C2 fusion. If the atlas remains unreduced, fuse C1 and C2 in situ because open reduction is hazardous and unnecessary.
- with cord compression, try
  —closed reduction by traction, and if this relieves the compression,
  —fuse C1 and C2. If long tract signs persist,
  —resect the posterior arch of the atlas and
  —fuse the occiput to the axis. Do not attempt open reduction of the dislocation.

ATLANTOAXIAL ROTATIONAL SUBLUXATION

Diagnosis

- one lateral mass of the atlas is subluxed or dislocated on the axis and is usually locked, so that rotation is limited. The injury is
- stable;
- diagnosis may be difficult and is often missed.
- clinically the patient has a
  —wry neck with limited extension, and
  —rotation is reduced on the side of the subluxation;
- AP x-ray through the open mouth shows that the
  —lateral mass which is displaced forward is larger and nearer the midline than the other, and this
  —abnormal relationship is constant on dynamic rotational views, with the atlas and axis moving as a single unit. The

—joint space on the side of the posteriorly displaced facet is narrowed and the

—spinous process of the atlas may be displaced from midline;

- AP tomograms will show the lateral masses of the atlas in different planes.
- the cord is not in danger because the displacement of C1 on C2 is limited, but
- nerve roots may be compressed.

Treatment

- for a recent injury, treat with
  —traction for 3 weeks and then
  —atlantoaxial fusion;
  —open reduction is difficult and usually not necessary.
- for an old injury, treat
  —symptomatically. If
  —pain is severe and constant, correct the subluxation as much as possible with traction and then perform a posterior C1-C2 fusion;
- nerve root compression may require partial laminectomy and decompression.

Injuries of Third to Seventh Cervical Vertebrae

WHIPLASH INJURY

- is a flexion and extension injury of the cervical spine without fracture or dislocation;
- is usually caused by rear-end car collision. The passenger's head
  —snaps back into hyperextension and then
  —recoils in flexion;
- paravertebral muscles, the anterior longitudinal ligament and the posterior ligamentous complex are stretched. There is
- pain around the neck, radiating into the occiput and shoulders, and sometimes dysphagia due to retropharyngeal hematoma;
- exclude fracture or subluxation by x-rays.
- treat
  —symptomatically and with a cervical collar;
- if symptoms persist after 2 weeks, physiotherapy may help;
- symptoms may linger for several months.

ANTERIOR WEDGE COMPRESSION FRACTURE OF BODY (Fig. 27.1)

- due to acute flexion without rotation;
- the lateral x-ray shows a crush fracture of the anterosuperior corner of the

body or of the superior border of the body which becomes wedge-shaped;
- if the posterior ligamentous complex is intact, there is
  —usually no cord damage and the
  —fracture is stable;
- treatment is a Minerva cast or halo jacket for 3 months.

BURSTING FRACTURE OF BODY (Fig. 27.4)

- due to axial compression on the head with the cervical spine slightly flexed;
- usually unstable;
- high incidence of associated quadriplegia, usually complete and permanent.
- x-rays show
  —comminuted fracture of the body with
  —outward displacement of the fragments and, sometimes,
  —displacement of the posterior cortex into the vertebral canal. If there is
- no neurological deficit, treat by
  —halo traction for 2 to 3 months, followed by a
  —halo or Minerva jacket for 2 months, then
  —dynamic x-rays to assess stability. If there is residual instability, anterior fusion will be required. If there
- is a neurological deficit, treat by
  —skull traction for 6 to 8 weeks and a
  —Minerva collar for 10 weeks or by
  —anterior fusion with external fixation if nursing is too difficult in traction.

SUBLUXATION (Fig. 27.9)

- a flexion-rotation injury with partial rupture of the posterior ligaments. The proximal vertebra
- may reduce spontaneously;
- dynamic flexion and extension x-rays will reveal the diagnosis.
- treat the patient with a
- Minerva jacket for 16 weeks, then take
- dynamic flexion and extension x-rays. If these show
- instability, proceed with
- posterior fusion and internal fixation.

ANTERIOR DISLOCATION AND FRACTURE-DISLOCATION (Fig. 27.3)

Etiopathology

- usually a rotation and flexion injury. There is
- disruption of the
  —posterior ligament complex and the
  —intervertebral disc. With

- anterior dislocation the articular facets of the superior vertebra may be locked in front of the facets of the inferior vertebra;
- one or both articular facets may be fractured, allowing rotational or lateral as well as anterior displacement;
- fracture of the body may be associated;
- a cord lesion is very common and is often complete.

Diagnosis

- lateral x-ray shows
  —anterior displacement of the superior vertebral body by more than 50% of its width with
  —dislocation of the facet joints. An associated
  —fracture of the body is usually obvious. On
- AP x-ray there is an
  —increased distance between the spinous processes of the two involved vertebrae, a key sign of disruption of the posterior ligaments. If the
- fracture-dislocation has reduced spontaneously, you may miss the diagnosis. If you are in doubt, take
- flexion-extension stress x-rays while you control the head.

Treatment

- reduce immediately by
  —skeletal traction and
  —verify the reduction with x-rays. It may be necessary to increase the weight progressively with use of fluoroscopic control or serial x-rays. As soon as the
- dislocation is reduced, diminish the traction and continue for 3 weeks, then use a
  —Minerva jacket or halo cast if there is no sensory deficit over the trunk or shoulders. If a sensory deficit is present, perform
  —posterior fusion with internal fixation; if surgery is contraindicated, continue traction for 12 more weeks. If
- closed reduction fails, usually due to locked facets, perform
  —open reduction, internal fixation and fusion through the posterior approach. This should be done
  —immediately if the cord is compressed or
  —within 5 days if no neurological lesion present.

UNILATERAL ROTATIONAL SUBLUXATION (Fig. 27.2)

Etiopathology

- rotational injury;
- one posterior facet joint is dislocated, with the superior facet being locked in front of the inferior facet;

- posterior ligaments are partially torn. This is a
- stable lesion;
- cord damage is uncommon, but the neural canal on one side is narrowed and may compress the nerve root.

Diagnosis

- is difficult and often missed;
- the patient has a wry neck, with head turned to one side and tilted to the other with limited rotation of the head to the side opposite the subluxation;
- AP x-ray shows lateral displacement of the proximal spinous processes toward the side of the dislocation;
- lateral x-ray shows
  —overlap of the articular processes at the level of injury with
  —anterior displacement of the body of the superior vertebra of less than 25% of its width. On
- oblique x-ray there is
  —dislocation of the articular facets on one side, with
  —deformity and narrowing of one neural canal.

Treatment

Recent injury

- reduce the lesion with skull traction and apply a
- Minerva jacket for 12 weeks, then assess stability. If it is unstable, perform posterior fusion with internal fixation and a graft;
- if traction fails, treat by early open reduction and posterior fusion.

Old injury

- closed reduction may be dangerous and is likely to fail. With
- no symptoms or neurological signs and a
- stable spine, no treatment is necessary. But if the neck is
- symptomatic or unstable or there are
- neurological signs, perform
- open reduction, internal fixation and fusion through the posterior approach.
- partial laminectomy may be required to decompress a nerve root.

HYPEREXTENSION INJURY (Fig. 27.5)

Etiopathology

- caused by violent hyperextension of the neck;
- anterior and posterior longitudinal ligaments and the intervertebral disc are ruptured;
- the anteroinferior corner of the superior vertebra may be avulsed by the

anterior longitudinal ligament, the "teardrop" fracture, and if spontaneous reduction occurs, this fracture may be the only clue;

- the cord may be squeezed by infolding ligamentum flavum causing
  —complete quadriplegia or the
  —central cord syndrome.

Diagnosis

- history is important. Look for
- abrasions on the face or forehead;
- the x-ray may appear normal, or
  —retropharyngeal hematoma or a
  —teardrop fracture may be present;
- dynamic flexion and extension x-rays will show instability on extension.

Treatment

- if vertebrae are undisplaced with
  —no cord lesion, immobilize with a halo cast or Minerva jacket for 16 weeks with the neck in mild flexion. But if a
  —cord lesion is present, treat with skull traction for 4 weeks with the neck in mild flexion, then immobilize as indicated previously for 12 weeks. If the vertebrae are
- displaced, reduce with skull traction and continue treatment as indicated previously.
- surgery is contraindicated because the
  —posterior approach would destroy the only intact ligaments remaining and
  —anterior fixation is difficult and unsatisfactory.

SPINOUS PROCESS AVULSION

- called "clay shoveler's" fracture;
- the spine is avulsed by a violent muscle contraction. This is
- stable and not associated with neurological injury.
- treat symptomatically.

chapter 29

Injuries of the Thoracic and Lumbar Spine and Spinal Cord

General Remarks

- half of all thoracic and lumbar spine and spinal cord injuries occur between T12 and L2 because this is the junction between the relatively
  —immobile thoracic spine and the
  —mobile lumbar spine;
- the spinal cord ends opposite the body of L1. So neurological deficit
  —above T10 is almost entirely due to cord damage,
  —between T10 and L1 is due to cord and nerve root (cauda equina) damage,
  —below L1 is due entirely to root damage.
- the blood supply of the spinal cord is just adequate for function of the cord and comes from the
  —anterior spinal artery, a branch of the two vertebral arteries, and from
  —two posterior spinal arteries, branches of the posterior inferior cerebellar arteries or of the vertebral arteries. All these arteries are small and are
  —reinforced at irregular intervals by small segmental arteries, the largest of which is the
  —artery of Adamkiewicz, usually on the left side between T4 and T12;
  —injury to this blood supply may cause permanent damage to the cord.
- ascending and descending nerve tracts in the spinal cord have no potential for repair if anatomic disruption occurs, e.g., division of axons or cell destruction. But patients with
- cauda equina injuries can recover from neurapraxia or axonotmesis because these nerves are anatomically and physiologically similar to peripheral nerves. Thus these injuries have a better prognosis than do spinal cord injuries.
- two or more vertebral levels may be injured with normal vertebrae in between, especially in high-speed accidents.

Etiopathology

- thoracolumbar (TL) spinal injuries are usually caused by
  —indirect violence to the vertebral column, and
  —only 5% are associated with neurological damage;
- direct violence, e.g., from a bullet or knife wound, is uncommon but is associated with a
  —high incidence of neurological deficit;
- 95% of injuries causing traumatic paraplegia occur in adults.

FLEXION INJURY (Fig. 29.1)

- commonest cause of vertebral injury;
- force applied to the
  —posterior thorax, e.g., from falling rocks, causes TL junction injury. Force applied to the
  —pelvis, e.g., from a fall from a height onto the buttocks, causes lumbosacral (LS) junction injury;
- the spine is acutely flexed forward;
- there is an anterior wedge compression fracture of the vertebral body. Rarely, the
- posterior cortex of the body may be comminuted and displaced into the vertebral canal, causing neurological damage;
- posterior elements and ligaments are usually intact, and the fracture is usually stable.

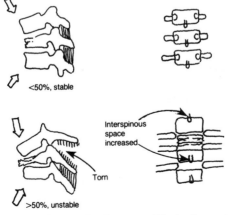

Figure 29.1. Flexion compression fractures of the lumbar and dorsal spine.

- during treatment the fracture may continue to angulate.
- neurological injury is uncommon.

HYPEREXTENSION INJURY (Fig. 29.2)

- rare (unlike in the cervical spine);
- usually in the midlumbar region;
- may cause
  —avulsion fracture of the anterior margin of the body or
  —fracture of the pars interarticularis, a traumatic spondylolysis;
- the injury is stable in flexion, and neurological damage is rare.

LATERAL FLEXION INJURY (Fig. 29.3)

- usually in the midlumbar region;
- causes lateral wedge compression fracture of the body;
- the injury is stable, and neurological damage is rare.

ROTATION AND FLEXION INJURY (Fig. 29.4)

- rotation injury alone is rare, but a
- rotation and flexion injury is
  —more common and causes
  —dislocations and fracture-dislocations which are usually unstable and, often,
  —cord and nerve root damage also;
- commonly occurs between T10 and L1;
- may include

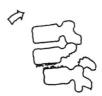

Figure 29.2. Acute, traumatic lumbar spondylolisthesis. A hyperextension injury.

Figure 29.3. Lumbar lateral wedge fracture.

—compression or slice (horizontal or oblique) fracture of the body or disruption of the intervertebral disc,

—rupture of the posterior ligamentous complex, and

—dislocation and/or fracture of the posterior articular facets with

—anterior, lateral or rotational displacement or a combination of all three. The

—disc may herniate posteriorly into the vertebral canal. Injuries in

- children usually occur without ligament rupture and heal well by bony union.

SHEAR INJURY

- causes horizontal displacement or dislocation of one vertebra on another without angulation or rotation;
- all joints and ligaments are disrupted;
- articular processes and/or the pars interarticularis may be fractured. The injury is
- very unstable, and
- neurological damage is common.

AXIAL COMPRESSION INJURY (Fig. 29.5)

- an axial or vertical compression load causes
  —central compression burst fracture of the vertebral body with
  —comminution but usually with
  —intact posterior elements;

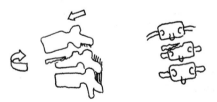

Figure 29.4. Rotational fracture-dislocation at D12-L1.

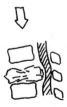

Figure 29.5. Compression burst fracture.

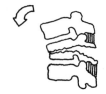

Figure 29.6.   Chance's lap belt fracture of the lumbar spine.

- the injury is stable, and
- neurological damage is uncommon;
- a milder form of this fracture occurs in the osteoporotic spine in which concave deformity of vertebral body and end plates is caused by pressure of the intervertebral discs.

DISTRACTION INJURY (Fig. 29.6)

- is the Chance lap belt fracture and is
- caused by an automobile collision in which the patient is wearing a lap seat belt without a diagonal band;
- the lower trunk is flexed acutely around the transverse belt, and the vertebra is pulled apart, with the
- fracture line running
    —horizontally through the body, pedicles, laminae and spine, or the
    —ligamentous structures are pulled apart with total distraction dislocation, or there is a
    —combination distraction fracture-dislocation;
- the injury occurs between L1 and L4;
- the fracture is stable, but the
- dislocation is unstable;
- neurological injury is uncommon.

MUSCLE CONTRACTION INJURY

- transverse processes may be pulled off by violent contraction of the psoas muscle, but spinous process fractures are rare.

Clinical and Radiological Features

HISTORY

- the patient usually has history of trauma, but
- pathological vertebral bone, e.g., due to metastasis or osteoporosis, may fracture after trivial trauma;
- the major symptom is mechanical pain.

PHYSICAL EXAMINATION

General

- if you suspect a spinal injury,
  —examine the patient briefly first in the position in which he lies because
  —moving him may cause or aggravate a spinal cord injury;
- remember your ABCs:
  —Airway,
  —Breathing and
  —Circulation have the first priority;
- examine the
  —chest for intrathoracic injury and the
  —abdomen for intraabdominal injury. Note that a lumbar vertebral injury may cause paralytic ileus. Then
- examine the vertebral column.

Inspection

- undress the patient by
  —cutting the clothes if moving him might endanger the cord;
- look at the entire trunk for
  —abrasions and bruises (an ecchymosis over one scapula suggests rotation and flexion fracture-dislocation at the TL junction, and a lap seat belt mark suggests a Chance fracture);
  —localized swelling or mass;
  —deformity., e.g., kyphosis.

Palpation

- paravertebral muscle spasm and
- localized tenderness over the injured spine are usually present;
- feel carefully the tips of the spinous process for two key signs of instability,
  —malalignment or step-off, i.e., lateral displacement of the upper spinous processes from the midline due to rotational or lateral displacement, or an
  —increased interspinous space with a palpable gap due to flexion-rotation injury with rupture of the posterior ligamentous structures.

Neurological examination (Figs. 27.6, 27.7, 27.8 and 29.7)

- see also Chapter 27.
- neurological examination is
  —essential, so
  —perform it for every back injury that you see and
- answer the following questions:

Does patient have neurological deficit?

- examination must include

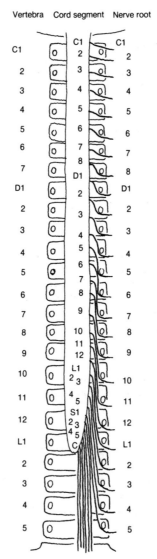

Figure 29.7. Relationship of vertebral bodies, spinal cord segments, and nerve roots.

—sensation,
—voluntary motor power, and
—reflexes including the anal sphincter reflex.

Is deficit complete or partial?

- the deficit is partial if the patient has some
  —voluntary muscle control distal to the vertebral lesion, e.g., toe flexors or extensors, or has some
  —sensation distal to lesion, e.g., around the anus (test this with a pin);
- remember that
  —spinal shock during the first 24 hours masks remaining neurological function. So
  —reexamine the patient at regular and frequent intervals, especially for the
  —anal wink and bulbocavernosus reflexes because these return before other reflexes. If
  —one or both of these reflexes return, signifying the end of spinal shock, but
  —motor paralysis and anesthesia are still total distal to the level of the vertebral injury, the cord lesion is
  —complete.

Is deficit due to injury of spinal cord, cauda equina, or both?

- paralyzed muscles with
  —tendon reflexes present indicate a
  —spinal cord or
  —upper motor neuron lesion (UMNL);
- paralyzed muscles with
  —tendon reflexes absent, even after recovery from spinal shock, indicate a
  —cauda equina or lower motor neuron lesion (LMNL);
- mixed lesions occur at the TL junction with
  —UMNL of the sacral segments and
  —LMNL of the lumbar nerve roots in the cauda equina. This "root escape" may make the difference between a patient who will eventually stand and walk and one who is permanently confined to a wheelchair.

Is deficit likely to recover?

- answer this question as soon as possible to benefit the patient and his family and to guide your treatment; the patient with a
- complete cord injury will not recover; the patient with a
- partial cord injury may recover partially or completely;
- cauda equina injury, whether partial or complete, may recover completely or partially;

- with a mixed cord and cauda equina lesion at T12 and L1, the
  —cord injury (sacral segments) may not recover, but the
  —cauda equina (lumbar nerve roots) injury may recover and some important muscular control of the hip and knee may be restored, with sensory return to the leg, thus enabling the patient to walk unaided.

RADIOLOGICAL EXAMINATION

X-rays

- do not roll the patient about to take the x-rays; move the tube instead!
- anteroposterior (AP) and lateral films may be sufficient, but if
- interpretation is difficult, take obliques, especially for the patient with an injury of the upper thoracic spine.
- tomography and CAT scanning may also be of help;
- with a neurological lesion and no apparent radiographic injury, x-ray the whole spine, and
- x-ray the cervical spine of every patient with a head injury.

Interpretation

- remember the "Playboy approach" (Chapter 2) and
- examine first the soft tissue shadows,
  —heart and lungs, mediastinum, diaphragmatic domes,
  —gastrointestinal gas shadows and spleen, liver and kidney shadows, because any of these may be abnormal and lead you to diagnose an
  —intrathoracic or
  —intra-abdominal injury and thus to save the patient's life;
- examine all of the bones which appear on the x-rays, including the
  —ribs and scapulae,
  —sacrum, iliac crests,
  —acetabula and femoral heads. Then
- look at the whole spine and note
  —alignment of the backs and fronts of the bodies on the lateral x-ray and of the sides of the bodies on the AP, for angulation or displacement, and
  —alignment of the spinous processes and the distance between these on the AP x-ray for rotation or distraction;
- examine carefully all the
  —bodies for change of shape and comminution or displacement of any part of the body, especially the posterior cortex into the vertebral canal,
  —pedicles for widening of one pair relative to the others,

—pars interarticularis for spondylolysis,
—posterior arches and
—transverse processes for fractures;
- do not forget that the injury may be
  —more severe than the x-rays show but is
  —never less severe.

Stability

- use White and Panjabi's charts to evaluate stability.

Dorsal spine

- two points each for
  —anterior element destruction,
  —posterior element destruction,
  —sagittal translation of more than 2.5 mm,
  —sagittal rotation of more than 5°,
  —cord or cauda equina compression, or
  —anticipated dangerous loading;
- one point for
  —costovertebral dislocation. A total of
- five or more points indicates
  —instability.

Lumbar spine

- three points for
  —cauda equina compression;
- two points each for
  —sagittal flexion of more than 8% or
  —extension of more than 9%,
  —sagittal rotation of more than 9°,
  —anterior element destruction, or
  —posterior element destruction;
- one point for anticipated
  —dangerous loading. A total of
- five or more points suggests
  —instability.

Myelography

- indicated only for
  —posttraumatic neurological deficit with no apparent vertebral injury or
  —neurological deficit which does not correlate with the known level of the vertebral injury.

Treatment

STABLE FRACTURES WITHOUT NEUROLOGICAL DEFICIT

- most of the following fractures are common and stable:
  - —avulsion fractures of the spines or transverse processes,
  - —anterior and lateral wedge-compression fractures of the body,
  - —central compression (burst) fractures of the body, and
  - —extension fractures (uncommon);
- pain at the level of the injury is the patient's main initial complaint.
- initial treatment is
- bed rest on a firm mattress;
- the patient should not sit up, but he may
- roll from side to side for eating, skin care and personal hygiene;
- watch for
  - —paralytic ileus. This may
  - —develop during the first 36 hours after injury, and
  - —lasts 3 to 5 days;
  - —treat this with a nasogastric tube, gastric suction, intravenous therapy, and nothing by mouth.
- the patient with avulsion fractures can be mobilized progressively after a few days. Start the patient on physiotherapy when pain has diminished.
- a plaster jacket for 3 months is indicated for
  - —compression or
  - —burst fractures;
- the jacket will not immobilize the spine, nor will it hold an unstable injury, but it
  - —helps prevent increase of the deformity and
  - —diminishes pain.

STABLE FRACTURES WITH NEUROLOGICAL DEFICIT

- the key to treatment of a patient with a cord injury is
- good nursing;
- skillful surgery cannot substitute for
- skillful nursing.
- initial treatment is
  - —bed rest with
  - —regular turning and
  - —routine skin care;
- give urinary antiseptics while the patient has a catheter;
- systemic steroids may reduce edema and prevent aggravation of a partial neurological lesion;

- surgical decompression of the cord or cauda equina is only justified if there is a
  —progressing neurological deficit. The
- dangers of laminectomy are
  —direct cord or cauda equina injury,
  —indirect injury by edema or hemorrhage, and
  —transformation of a stable injury into an unstable one with risk of further neurological damage.
- do not raise false hopes with the patient or his family;
- the major goal of treatment for a paraplegic patient should be
  —early rehabilitation as a paraplegic, with treatment
  —starting as soon as the diagnosis and prognosis are made (see Chapter 30).

UNSTABLE SPINAL INJURIES

General

- almost all dislocations and fracture-dislocations are unstable;
- only 10% of TL injuries are unstable, but half of these involve a neurological deficit;
- a patient with an unstable spine should not be transferred from stretcher to examining table to stretcher to x-ray table to stretcher to bed! Every movement increases the likelihood of neurological injury;
- physical examination, investigations and x-rays can be made with patient on one stretcher.
- use Harrington instrumentation for internal fixation, with
  —compression rods for Chance fractures and dislocations and
  —distraction rods for fracture-dislocations and burst fractures.

Without neurological deficit

Fracture-dislocation

Undisplaced

- displacement probably occurred at the time of the accident and has reduced spontaneously, but
- beware because the injury is
  —still unstable and can
  —redisplace with further
  —danger to the cord and nerve roots;
- fractures through the body heal better than disruption of the disc with posterior arch fractures and can be
  —treated without surgery. However,
  —posterior instrumentation and fusion followed by a body jacket for 4 months give more certain results.

Displaced

- treat by
  —closed or
  —open reduction,
  —posterior instrumentation and fusion;
- perfect reduction is not necessary, providing that neurological deficit does not develop;
- body jacket for 4 months.

Dislocation

- closed or open reduction,
- internal fixation and posterior fusion.

With neurological deficit

- treatment for dislocation and treatment for fracture-dislocation are the same.

Undisplaced

- treat initially with
  —bed rest and good nursing care,
  —turning the patient as you would roll a log to prevent displacement of the fracture-dislocation and aggravation of a neurological injury.
- when the physiological status of the patient is stable and before bed sores develop, perform
  —posterior fusion with internal fixation to
  —stabilize the spine, to
  —facilitate nursing and to
  —accelerate mobilization and rehabilitation of the patient.

Displaced

- reduction is urgent in order to
  —decompress the vertebral canal and its contents and should be done
  —within 12 hours of injury. If
  —more than 24 hours have elapsed, reduction is no longer urgent unless a partial deficit is becoming worse. If
- closed reduction fails, perform
  —open reduction with
  —internal fixation and posterior fusion;
- do not perform closed manipulation with the patient under anesthesia because this will increase the neurological deficit;
- laminectomy is indicated only for a progressive partial deficit or to facilitate decompression of a nerve root;
- nurse the patient postoperatively on a Stryker frame;
- a body jacket is contraindicated on insensitive skin.

COMPLICATIONS

Neurological injury

- the major early complication;
- see the previous discussion and Chapter 30.

Persistent pain

- is the most common long-term problem;
- of every 4 patients
  - 1 will have mild pain and
  - 1 will have severe, disabling pain. If the spinal injury is
- stable, the pain is felt in the
  - lumbar region below the fracture, where the lumbar spine is in hyperlordosis to compensate for kyphosis at the level of the fracture, or at the
  - L5 junction;
- treat symptomatically with physiotherapy and a LS brace if necessary. If the spine is
- unstable, consider surgery after a trial period in a body jacket.

Increasing deformity

- the incidence of spinal deformity is greatest when there is a
  - cord lesion in the high thoracic spine, or
  - there is muscle imbalance, or the
  - accident occurred in early childhood, or the patient had a
  - laminectomy;
- kyphosis is caused by chronic instability due to poor ligamentous or bony healing of the fracture;
- posterior fusion is only necessary if the deformity is
  - progressive,
  - likely to cause neurological deficit by angulation of the cord over the back of the vertebral body, or the
  - patient has intractable pain at the fracture site, which is uncontrolled by nonoperative treatment.
- lordosis is uncommon and can be managed by nonoperative methods;
- collapsing, paralytic scoliosis is usually due to muscle imbalance and is
- more common than one thinks. The
- curve eventually becomes fixed and may cause
  - fixed pelvic obliquity. The patient has
  - difficulty sitting and the
  - skin ulcerates over the ischial tuberosity;
- treatment consists of
  - support with a brace or

—posterior instrumentation and fusion with Harrington rods, or with the Luque system in a paraplegic patient. It may be necessary to operate anteriorly as well as posteriorly.

Summary

- is there a neurological injury? If so,
- is the injury
  —complete or
  —incomplete and
- which neurological structures are injured:
  —cord,
  —cauda equina, or
  —both?
- is the vertebral injury
  —stable or,
  —unstable?
- for the paraplegic patient,
  —good nursing is not an aid to surgery; it is
  —surgery that is the aid to good nursing.

chapter 30

Care and Rehabilitation of the Paraplegic Patient

Introduction

- the paraplegic patient compared with his healthy counterpart is at a great disadvantage;
- he requires
  —expert care in a spinal rehabilitation unit, if possible, for many months and
  —patience and understanding from his family and colleagues all his life;
- the aim of medical care and rehabilitation is the
  —total reintegration of the patient into his family, his social environment and his work. This treatment
  —starts with the transport of the injured patient and
  —really has no end.

Pathophysiology

- cord injury varies from
  —concussion with excellent prognosis to
  —complete transection;
- damage to the cord almost always
  —occurs at the moment of initial impact and causes
  —hemorrhagic infarcts in the cord; the
  —amount of hemorrhage depends on the degree of trauma;
  —edema follows hemorrhage;
- blood in the subarachnoid space causes
  —arachnoiditis with eventual
  —fibrosis and adhesions between the leptomeninges and the cord and, if bleeding is severe, can
  —obliterate the space.

Emergency Care

- if you suspect a spinal injury, move the patient
  —with great care and as
  —little as possible;
- transport the patient on something
  —flat and firm after
  —"log-rolling" or "log-lifting" him onto it with
  —helpers supporting the shoulders, trunk, hips and legs and
  —manual traction at the head and feet;
- immobilize the head by whatever means are available;
- similar rules concerning movement of the patient apply in the emergency room. Conduct activities related to the patient, including x-rays, without moving him from the stretcher;
- carelessness and ignorance in handling the patient can convert a partial lesion into a complete one!
- once the diagnosis is made, plan the treatment accordingly (see Chapters 27, 28 and 29 and below.).

Skin Care

- bed sores (decubitus ulcers) are preventable!
- their appearance is due to
  —ignorance,
  —neglect and
  —poor surgical and nursing care;
- even after healing the scar is always
  —thin,
  —fragile, and
  —poorly vascularized and can
  —easily break down again;
- prevent bed sores by
  —good surgical and nursing care, as
  —infected bed sores are a drain on the patient's resources and
  —treatment is long, difficult and expensive.

PREVENTION OF BED SORES

- the best treatment of bed sores is prevention;
- start skin care as soon as possible, even before the patient reaches the hospital;
- turn the patient regularly as you would roll a log and inspect the skin each time for

—redness or
—edema, the early signs of a pressure sore, especially over the
- pressure areas, i.e., the
  —occiput, chin, point of the shoulder and scapulae,
  —prominent vertebral spines, especially if there is a kyphosis,
  —sacrum, ischial tuberosities and greater trochanters,
  —pubis and anterior superior iliac spines,
  —patellae, fibula head, malleoli, heels and little toes;
- massage the pressure areas daily with soap and water, then gently dry them with a soft towel and powder them. Remember that
- turning and other special beds are not a substitute for good nursing care!
- position the patient on a thick, firm mattress with pillows
  —under each natural curve of the body and
  —between the knees and ankles. To
- prevent joint contractures, position the lower limbs with the
  —hips in extension and 10° abduction,
  —knees in extension,
  —ankles at 90° and
  —feet plantigrade;
- sheets must
  —not be stiff or starched, must
  —not have folds or creases in them, and must
  —not be covered with crumbs or any other objects which could cause localized skin pressure. Place a
- frame over the lower limbs to prevent the bed clothes from
  —pressing on or irritating the patient's skin or
  —pushing the feet into equinus;
- no plaster on anesthetic skin.
- teach the patient, once the fractured spine is stabilized, to
  —turn himself regularly, to
  —care for his skin and, with the help of his family, to
  —recognize the early signs of skin ischemia and know what to do about it;
- pad the wheelchair.

TREATMENT OF BED SORES

Erythema

- keep the patient off the area and
- keep it clean and aseptic with the use of diluted iodine solution if the patient is not sensitive to iodine.

Blister or abrasion

- similar to a second degree burn;
- epidermis is dead but dermis is alive;

- keep the patient off it;
- keep the area clean, dry and aseptic;
- use Mercurochrome in alcohol to dry the area and its periphery.

Full-thickness bed sore

- epidermis and dermis die, similar to a full-thickness burn;
- keep the patient off it.

Dressing

- clean the whole area with soap and water and debride it;
- culture and sensitivity (C & S) of the surface;
- start the use of wet dressings every 4 hours directly on the wound with
  —Eusol (sodium hypochloride) as general purpose solution. Change the dressing solution according to the results of C & S as follows:
  —for *Pseudomonas*, use ½% acetic acid (vinegar);
  —for *Staphylococcus aureus*, use Hibitane;
  —for hemolytic streptococci, give penicillin intramuscularly (IM).
- remove the dressing completely at each change to remove debris and pus.
- surround the dressing with a plastic sheet to prevent drying and then apply a bandage. Do not use sticky tape on anesthetic skin, as this may cause more skin damage;
- if infection persists, use 1% streptomycin solution on the dressing;
- when the wound is clean, excise sharp, bony prominences beneath the wound, e.g., sacral spines, because these will act as pressure areas and cause breakdown of new skin;
- the wound bed will start to granulate. When the
- skin at wound edges starts to grow, indicating that infection is controlled (as skin does not grow in the presence of infection), graft skin.

Grafting

- use split-thickness skin for the first grafting;
- the wound may later require full-thickness skin coverage to prevent recurrent breakdown of the skin, particularly over the sacrum and trochanter;
- this can be done by
  —swinging or advancing a local flap;
  —bilateral flaps can be used on the sacrum if the defect is large.

COMPLICATIONS OF BED SORES

- an infected bed sore
  —prolongs the catabolic phase and is a

—protein, fluid and electrolyte sink. The patient melts away! Prevention is better than cure, but if the ulcer is already infected,
—treat the infection vigorously and
—close the ulcer as soon as possible with skin grafts. If skin loss is over a joint,
- septic arthritis may result;
- osteomyelitis is frequent, especially when the ulcer is over the greater trochanter, sacrum or ischial tuberosities;
- recurrence of the bed sore is likely when the
  —skin coverage is thin and friable and is fixed to underlying bone,
  —nursing care is neglected, or the
  —patient returns home too soon.

Genitourinary System

ANATOMY AND PHYSIOLOGY OF BLADDER (Fig. 30.1)

Muscles and sphincters

- detrusor muscle lies in the
  —fundus of the bladder, consists of
  —smooth involuntary muscle fibers arranged at random, and is
  —innervated by parasympathetic nerves from the S2, S3 and S4 cord segments via pelvic nerves to the pelvic plexus, then to the bladder;
- the internal sphincter is a longitudinal prolongation of
  —smooth detrusor muscle fibers which surround the
  —posterior urethra. The sphincter also has a lot of elastic fibers,
  —is innervated by parasympathetic nerves, and is
  —necessary for urinary continence;

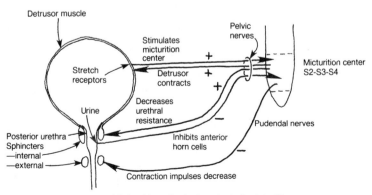

Figure 30.1. Neurological control of micturition.

- the external sphincter is a
  —striped, voluntary muscle which surrounds the
  —membranous urethra;
  —motor innervation is via the pudendal nerves from the S2, S3 and S4 segments; the external sphincter is
  —not necessary for continence if the internal sphincter is intact.

Sensory innervation

- pelvic parasympathetic nerves carry the sensations of
  —fullness, with desire to urinate, and
  —pain and temperature from the bladder and posterior urethra to the S2, S3 and S4 cord segments;
- pudendal nerves carry
  —superficial and
  —deep somatic sensation from the distal bladder and adjacent structures to S2, S3 and S4.

Central reflex centers

Spinal reflex center

- situated in the spinal cord at the S2, S3 and S4 levels, it serves two reflexes;
- as the bladder fills, stretch receptors in the bladder wall send afferent, proprioceptive impulses via pelvic nerves to a micturition center in the sacral cord;
- this sends efferent impulses via pelvic nerves to detrusor muscle which contracts, increasing intravesical pressure and shortening and widening the posterior urethra;
- urethral resistance is thus reduced and
- urine is forced into the posterior urethra, causing afferent impulses to return along the pelvic nerves to the micturition center which inhibits contraction of the external sphincter, and the
- patient urinates;
- this spinal center is under higher control.

Brainstem center

- pain and temperature (via crossed spinothalamic tracts) and proprioceptive impulses of fullness and the desire to urinate (via uncrossed funiculus gracilis in posterior columns) reach the pons (unconscious sensation) and cerebral cortex (conscious sensation);
- the brainstem center sustains
  —contraction of the detrusor muscle and
  —relaxation of the external sphincter muscle until the bladder is completely empty. It can also
  —inhibit a spinal micturition reflex at the unconscious level.

Cerebral cortical center

- receives afferent impulses of fullness, the desire to urinate, and the pain of muscle spasm;
- the cortex inhibits the spinal reflex center until a suitable time and place for urinating can be found. Then, by
- removal of cortical inhibition, the spinal center is activated and the patient urinates;
- the cortex can interrupt urination at any time.

Filling pressures of bladder

- as the bladder fills with urine, the bladder wall expands with very little increase in intravesical pressure due to adjustment in the tone of the detrusor muscle;
- the sensation of the bladder filling occurs first with 100 to 150 ml of urine in the bladder, and the
- first desire to urinate occurs with 150 to 250 ml of urine;
- urination normally occurs with 250 to 450 ml of urine, the maximum physiological limit;
- if micturition is inhibited by the cortex with more than this volume in the bladder, intravesical pressure greatly increases and the sensation is painful.

Physiology of micturition: summary

- when the bladder fills with 150 to 250 ml of urine,
  - —stretch receptors in the bladder wall are activated and cause
  - —contraction of the detrusor muscle and
  - —decrease in the posterior urethral resistance by
  - —reflex through the sacral cord;
- urine entering the posterior urethra causes
  - —relaxation of the external sphincter by a
  - —second reflex through the sacral cord;
- powerful contraction of
  - —detrusor, abdominal and diaphragmatic muscles occurs, and the
  - —bladder starts to empty;
- sphincters are kept open by impulses from the brainstem center until the bladder is empty;
- higher centers can inhibit micturition until the pressure becomes too great.

NEUROGENIC BLADDER

Pathophysiology

Early changes

- during the first 24 to 48 hours after spinal injury, the period of spinal shock, there is complete urinary retention. After this,

- urine dribbles away from the distended bladder, and the patient experiences overflow incontinence.

Periodic reflex micturition (Fig. 30.2)

- begins weeks or months after a complete cord lesion when the
- detrusor muscle gradually regains
  —tone, contractility and the
  —reflex of emptying;
- the type of bladder depends on the level of the cord injury;

Automatic bladder

- also called "cord," "reflex" or "upper motor neuron" (UMN) bladder.
- when the vertebral injury is above T12, the
- cord injury is above S2, so the
  —spinal micturition center and
  —neurological pathways between the bladder and the sacral cord are intact but
  —voluntary control from higher centers is cut off. So the
- bladder empties automatically when urine reaches a certain volume;
- the patient often knows when the bladder is about to empty because he may have
  —discomfort in the penis or suprapubic region,
  —sweating and
  —other strange feelings, mediated perhaps by sympathetic nerves through the hypogastric plexus;
- reflex emptying can often be started by the patient himself by stroking or stimulating the groin, lower abdomen or penis;
- the patient may void every 3 or 4 hours unless he has urinary infection.

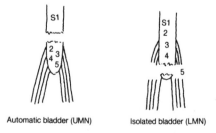

Automatic bladder (UMN)   Isolated bladder (LMN)

Figure 30.2. Spinal lesions with an upper motor neuron and a lower motor neuron (*UMN* and *LMN*) bladder.

Isolated bladder

- also called "autonomous," "atonic" or "lower motor neuron" (LMN) bladder. When the
- vertebral injury is at or below T12, the
- neurological injury may be through the
  —sacral cord, at or below S2, or through the
  —cauda equina including the S2, S3 and S4 roots;
- in both instances the bladder is completely isolated from all spinal cord control and
- periodic reflex micturition develops very slowly, usually after 6 months;
- the patient may have warning signs, as discussed previously;
- to start micturition the patient must strain and contract abdominal muscles to increase intra-abdominal pressure;
- the stream of urine is strong only while the patient continues to strain;
- some residual urine usually remains in the bladder after voiding. If this remains at more than 10% of bladder capacity, sphincterotomy may be required.

Management

Catheterization

- as soon as the patient reaches the hospital, insert a self-retaining catheter with strictly aseptic technique;
- in the male, bring the catheter up and tape it to the abdomen, not the thigh, to avoid urethral erosion. Allow
- free drainage;
- change the catheter every 48 hours,
- irrigate the catheter every 2 days with sterile physiological saline and aspirate debris with a syringe. Change to
- intermittent catheterization the day after intravenous therapy is stopped. This
  —allows the bladder to fill and empty regularly,
  —encourages establishment of the micturition reflex, and
  —helps the patient to appreciate warning signs of bladder filling. This technique also
  —diminishes the risk of infection and
  —helps the neurogenic bladder to start functioning early;
- pressure on the abdomen and 2 ml of carbachol IM may help the patient to void by himself after removal of the catheter;
- if he voids, replace the catheter immediately and measure the residual urine. This should be less than 25% before intermittent catheterization is discontinued.

Urinary antibiotics

- antibiotics are
  —not a substitute for strict sterile technique in catheterization and the patient's
  —personal hygiene;
- change the pH of urine with a
  —potassium citrate solution (alkalinization) or
  —Mandelamine (acidification) orally;
- reserve antibiotics for known urinary infection;
- in the case of urinary infection,
  —take a specimen for C & S and
  —give an antibiotic effective against Gram-negative organisms.
  —change the antibiotic if necessary according to the organisms' sensitivities.

Persistent incontinence

- when a male patient is still incontinent after catheter drainage has been discontinued he will need a
  —portable urinal with a penile sheath and he must be
  —taught how to change the apparatus and clean it.
- a female patient is more difficult to manage. For her there are three alternatives:
  —urinary dribble with the patient constantly wet,
  —a permanent indwelling catheter with urinary infection, or
  —urinary diversion with an ileal bladder.

Complications

Infection

- catheterization frequently results in infection which causes
  —cystitis, ascending infection and
  —pyelonephritis;
  —investigate and treat infection promptly and aggressively, and trace and eliminate the source of the organisms.

Stone formation

- both bladder (most frequent) and kidney stones are common due to
  —prolonged recumbency with disuse osteoporosis and increased urinary excretion of calcium,
  —urinary stasis with residual urine, and
  —urinary infection;
- prevent this by
  —plenty of oral fluids,
  —acidification of urine,
  —active muscle exercises for the trunk and arms, and

—early mobilization of the patient with a wheelchair or with braces and crutches.

Intestines

- a paralyzed bowel causes constipation, and a
- paralyzed anal sphincter causes incontinence;
- treat by
  —manual evacuation every 2 days until the patient is mobilized in a chair. An
  —enema helps severe constipation, whereas
  —laxatives encourage incontinence;
- too much fruit and spicy foods should be avoided;
- when the patient is mobilized, teach him a daily bowel routine including an
  —early morning hot drink to stimulate the gastrocolic reflex and a
  —bowel movement which can be started by
  —abdominal straining or
  —inserting a gloved finger into the anus;
  —this usually causes complete emptying of the rectum once a day and is satisfactory unless the patient has diarrhea. In this case, the patient should wear protective pads;
- LMN bowel may still require digital evacuation.

Mobilization of Patient

- includes
  —rehabilitation of muscles and joints, starting as soon after the injury as possible. Then, when the spinal column is stable,
  —teach sitting and standing balance and
  —a new gait pattern,
  —ordering and adjusting braces for the lower limbs and early involvement in
  —games and sports;
- it should be the concern of all the
  —nurses,
  —physiotherapists and
  —doctors who are involved in the care of the patient.

CONTRACTURES OF JOINTS

Soft tissue contractures

- contractures of hips, knees and ankles are avoidable and must be prevented if the patient is eventually to stand and walk;

- from the day of injury, all joints in the lower limbs should be put through a full range of gentle passive movement. Violent stretching will cause spasm, increased stiffness and periarticular bone formation. Between exercise periods
- position the limbs with the
  —hips and knees extended, or flexed no more than 10°, and the
  —ankles at right angles.
- treat established contractures by
  —soft tissue release and
  —osteotomy if necessary.

Para-articular ossification

- also called myositis ossificans;
- particularly common around the hips after a spinal injury. Causes
  —limitation of movement by mechanical block or an
  —extra-articular arthrodesis;
- wait until the new bone is mature, at least 6 months after onset of injury, and then excise it. This surgery is bloody and more difficult than it looks. Test the mobility of the joint to make sure that you have removed enough bone before closing the wound.

Spasticity

- after an UMN lesion the muscles may be in a spastic state, with greatly increased muscle tone and exaggerated stretch reflexes due to removal of inhibitory impulses from higher centers;
- spasticity may cause
  —pain and
  —dynamic joint contractures and may
  —prevent standing and gait training;
- this may be improved by
  —muscle relaxants, or
  —physiological peripheral neurectomy with the use of local infiltration of alcohol or phenol after a test with local anesthetic, or
  —surgical neurectomy of peripheral motor nerves after testing;
- contracted muscles can be lengthened.
- no treatment for spasticity is ensured of success.

SITTING, STANDING AND WALKING

- development of upper limb and trunk muscles is essential because the patient will depend on these for the rest of his life;

  ### Sitting up in bed

  - with paraplegia, sitting up is extremely difficult, so the patient must be taught this;

- the patient may have
  —one or two active muscles of the hips or thighs which will make sitting easier. If he does not, he can use
  —latissimus dorsi to balance the trunk on the pelvis;
- teach the patient sitting balance first with
  —arms at the side, then with
  —arms outstretched (more difficult), then with
  —sudden and unexpected movements of the arms, e.g., throwing a ball;
- this will enable him eventually to work with his hands while sitting.

Wheelchair

- if the patient is to have a wheelchair, he must be taught
  —how to transfer himself from bed to wheelchair and back again and
  —how to propel, stop and turn the chair without losing balance.

Standing and walking

Paraplegia above L3

- if the patient is paraplegic from the L3 spinal cord level or higher, he has no hip or knee control and will therefore need
  —two long leg braces with a
  —waist band and
  —two crutches in order to walk short distances;
- a wheelchair is essential. In
- thoracic paraplegia, the patient is wheelchair-bound and braces are unnecessary.

Paraplegia below L4

- the patient with paraplegia below the L4 spinal level has some muscle control of the
  —hips, through the psoas and adductors, and of the
  —knees, through the quadriceps. Although the patient may still require crutches, and even braces,
- walking will usually be possible.

Standing

- teach the patient first to stand in parallel bars and
- then with crutches. These must be correct length with 2 finger widths between the top of the crutch and the axilla to avoid brachial plexus palsy;
- the patient should stand and walk with his back straight. If he sags and droops on the crutches, the brachial plexus will be compressed.

Walking

- the type of gait depends on which muscles are intact;
- swing-through gait, with the patient swinging both legs together while using crutches as support, is taught first;

- if the patient has some hip and knee control, he can then be taught three-point gait, with the right crutch and left leg moving forward, then the left crutch and right leg moving forward;
- graduation from parallel bars to crutches must be slow and careful because
  —standing in the bars is easy, but
  —standing on crutches is more difficult and precarious and requires better balance.

Braces

- the below-knee brace provides
  —ankle stability;
  —the brace should have the ankle fixed at 90° and, if necessary, an
  —inside T strap to counteract varus deformity or an
  —outside T strap to counteract valgus deformity at the ankle.
- a long leg brace is required for
  —knee instability;
  —drop locks at the knee provide a fixed joint when the patient is walking but allow knee flexion when the patient is sitting;
  —a leather patella pad anteriorly with a thigh cuff prevents collapse of the knee when weight-bearing in the braces. A
- waist or pelvic band is necessary if the patient cannot control and balance the trunk on the pelvis. The band is joined to a long brace with a drop lock mechanism as described previously.

Sexual Activity

- "can I have intercourse?"
- "can I have children?" These are
- two questions on the mind of every cord-injured patient. Can you answer them?
- counseling in the psychological and physical aspects of sex is just as important as any other part of the rehabilitation program. This section deals with the physical aspects only.

MEN

- sexual activity is impaired by cord injury at any level, particularly in men. The
- average figures for all cord levels show that
  —erection and coitus are possible in 30% and
  —ejaculation and orgasm are possible in 10%, but that
  —less than 5% of men can sire a child. In fully rehabilitated
- athletes these figures may rise to 80%, 35% and 10%, respectively;

- sexual function is better when the
  - —cord lesion is low or partial, the patient is
  - —fully rehabilitated, and he was
  - —sexually active before the injury. It is
- worse when the paraplegia is flaccid, a LMN lesion;
- erection, when it is possible, can be attained by
  - —direct physical stimulation of the genitalia or, in some individuals, by
  - —psychic stimulation and can be maintained by a
  - —gentle constricting device around the base of the penis for not more than 30 minutes;
- quadriplegics may attain erection by reflex means;
- several positions for intercourse are possible for paraplegics, but the supine is the usual position for the quadriplegic;
- chronic urinary infection in the male is a risk to his partner. Careful attention to personal hygiene and voiding before coitus are important to avoid transmission;
- 50% of cord-injured men may be
  - —sterile due to
  - —spermatogenic dysfunction secondary to sympathetic denervation and poor testicular temperature control,
  - —hormonal changes or
  - —retrograde ejaculation. The
- divorce rate after injury is no higher than in the rest of the population.

WOMEN

- sexual intercourse is possible in
  - —several positions for the paraplegic but is usually performed in the
  - —supine position by the quadriplegic. The
- urinary catheter can be left in situ but
  - —cleanliness and attention to personal hygiene for
  - —both partners are important to avoid urinary infection;
- orgasm for a woman with a complete lesion is unlikely due to lack of genital sensation, but emotional and physical satisfaction may be attained in various other ways through real affection and stimulation of other erotogenic areas.

Reintegration into Society

- reintegration of the patient into his family and society is the final goal, and
- planning for it should start from the day the patient enters the hospital;
- multidisciplinary conferences between doctors, nurses, the social worker, physical and occupational therapists and the patient and his family are an essential part of this process;

- advice and help from a psychiatrist may also be necessary;
- the patient will probably not return to his old job, so he will need to
- learn a new one. The vocational rehabilitation therapist can help him in this;
- a sheltered workshop is an excellent institution and can solve many of the patient's problems;
- that the patient should either
  —earn his own living or at least
  —contribute to the family funds is important for his own pride and self-esteem.
- extended care after discharge must include regular multidisciplinary reviews for the
  —prevention, early diagnosis and prompt treatment of complications and for aiding the patient with
  —domestic, economic and legal problems.

chapter 31
Peripheral Nerve Injuries

Surgical Anatomy (Fig. 31.1)

- peripheral mixed nerve contains
  —sensory (both conscious and unconscious),
  —motor and
  —sympathetc fibers. These axons have their respective
- cell bodies in a
  —posterior root ganglion,
  —anterior horn of the cord, or a regional
  —sympathetic ganglion from which the sympathetic fibers reach the peripheral nerve by a gray ramus communicans;
- every axon is surrounded by a
  —Schwann cell sheath or neurolemma which secretes a layer of
  —myelin around those axons with a diameter greater than 1 μ. Around the Schwann cell sheath is
  —endoneurium, a thin layer of fibrous tissue. A
- group of these sheathed fibers forms a
  —fascicle, surrounded by
  —perineurium;
- several fascicles form the
  —peripheral nerve enclosed in the
  —epineurium. The
- myelin sheath is interrupted at 1-mm intervals by the
  —nodes of Ranvier which are
  —more permeable to ions than is the myelin sheath itself.
- nerve impulse is conducted by a transfer of ions, mainly K^+, Na^+, and Cl^-, across the membrane. This electrical impulse
  —travels faster in myelinated fibers where
  —saltatory conduction allows it to "leap" from node to node rather than travel continuously down the axon.

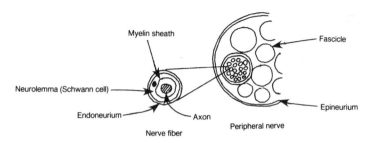

Figure 31.1.   Section of a peripheral nerve.

Etiopathology

ETIOLOGY

Closed injuries (Fig. 31.2)

- injury to a nerve may be
  —direct, from a blow or a fracture fragment, or
  —indirect, from traction as in a dislocation or a tardy ulnar nerve palsy due to long-standing cubitus valgus. The
- following nerves are vulnerable where they lie directly on or very near bones and joints:
  —brachial plexus with clavicle fracture;
  —axillary nerve with fracture of the surgical neck of the humerus or with dislocation of the shoulder;
  —radial nerve with midshaft or distal shaft fracture of the humerus;
  —median and radial nerves with extension type supracondylar fracture of the humerus and
  —ulnar nerve with flexion type supracondylar fracture or avulsion of the medial humeral epicondyle;
  —median nerve at the wrist with Colles' fracture or anterior lunate dislocation;
  —sciatic nerve with posterior dislocation or fracture-dislocation of the hip;
  —tibial nerve with dislocation of the knee;
  —common peroneal nerve with fracture of the fibula neck, varus injury of the knee, or posterolateral dislocation of the knee;
  —deep peroneal and tibial nerves with dislocation or fracture-dislocation of the ankle; and
  —cauda equina with injury of the lumbar spine and sacrum.

Open injuries

- penetrating injuries are usually due to an
  —open fracture or dislocation or a
  —bullet, knife or machete.

CLASSIFICATION OF INJURY

Neurapraxia

- is physiological interruption of the function of a nerve due to local demyelination of the nerve fibers without division of the axon and is caused by mild compression or traction;
- motor paralysis may or may not be accompanied by anesthesia;
- spontaneous recovery starts within a few days and is usually rapid and complete.

Axonotmesis

- is interruption of the axon but not of the endoneurial sheath. Recovery is slow but reasonably complete and depends on
  —which nerve is injured and
  —how far proximally the injury is located;

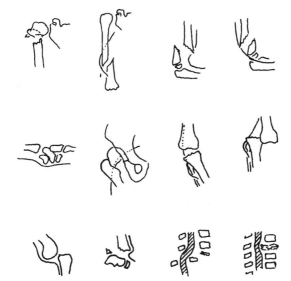

Figure 31.2. Peripheral nerves particularly vulnerable in fractures and dislocations.

- axon degenerates distal to the lesion, and paralysis and anesthesia are complete;
- most closed nerve injuries are either axonotmesis or neurapraxia.

Neurotmesis

- denotes section of the axons where spontaneous axonal regeneration is impossible. The nerve itself may be crushed or attenuated, in which case scarring prevents axonal growth, or the nerve might be partially or completely severed, thus preventing the regenerating axons from finding their proper distal endoneural tubes;
- most nerve injuries associated with an open wound are of this type.

FIBER DEGENERATION AND REGENERATION AFTER INJURY

Axonal degeneration

- when an axon is interrupted, that part distal to the division and for one or two segments proximal   to the division
- degenerates (wallerian degeneration), and it and its myelin sheath, if it has one, are
- phagocytosed;
- Schwann cells then multiply to fill the axonal space.
- changes also occur in the parent nerve cell which
  —swells and undergoes
  —chromatolysis. The
  —nucleus is eccentric. The
  —more proximal the injury, the
  —more marked the changes, and the
- cell may die.

Axonal regeneration

- if the nerve cell lives it will regenerate its axon;
- 4 to 6 weeks after injury the
  —intracellular edema subsides, the
  —nucleus is centralized, and the
  —Nissl granules, composed of ribonucleic acid (RNA) and polysomes, reappear. The
- proximal end of the injured axon then sends out several axonal sprouts;
- if endoneurium is
  —intact (axonotmesis) and there is no intraneural scarring, the sprouts, guided by the Schwann cells, grow down the
  —correct tube to the
  —correct end organ, and
  —normal nerve function is restored. If

- endoneurium is sectioned (neurotmesis) or there is a barrier of fibrous scar tissue, the sprouts may
  —grow down the wrong tubes or may
  —grow aimlessly to form a
  —neuroma, and normal nerve function is not restored.
- follow the progress of
  —axonal growth, by Tinel's sign and nerve conduction studies, and of
  —muscle reinnervation, by serial electromyograms (EMGs) and clinically.

CHANGES IN DENERVATED MUSCLE

- electrical excitability of denervated muscle is different because impulses no longer are transmitted by intramuscular nerve fibers but rather are transmitted by muscle fibers themselves. There is
- muscle wasting, and the muscle fibers are
- gradually replaced by fibrous tissue, an irreversible change;
- if regenerating axons have a long way to grow, the muscle may be irreversibly damaged before the axon sprouts reach it. These
- irreversible changes may be postponed by regular galvanic stimulation.

Clinical Features

SENSORY CHANGES

Anesthesia

- loss of sensation is not as reliable nor as constant as loss of motor power because the
  —test is subjective and the
  —autonomous zone supplied exclusively by a peripheral nerve is quite small. The remainder of the area supplied by that nerve is overlapped by adjacent nerves;
- the autonomous zone of the
  —ulnar nerve is the tip of the little finger, of the
  —median nerve is tip of the index finger, and of the
  —tibial nerve is the sole of the foot.
- sensory loss is most important in the
  —palmar surface of the hand and on the
  —sole of the foot.

Causalgia

- occurs in 3% of major nerve injuries;
- associated only with a nerve carrying sensory fibers, most often with
  —incomplete lesions of the median and sciatic nerves;

- its cause is unknown. Its syndrome is characterized by development of an
- exquisite burning pain, usually in the sensory territory of the injured nerve, within a week after injury. Pain is
- exacerbated by sudden changes in the patient's environment, such as loud noise and emotional upsets, and the patient resorts to
- fantastic remedies to relieve it;
- reflex osteodystrophies such as Sudeck's atrophy are much less acute and painful, and the patient's behavior is not as bizarre.
- treatment of causalgia includes
  —intensive physiotherapy,
  —local perineural anesthesia,
  —sympathetic ganglion blocks and
  —sympathectomy.

MOTOR LOSS

- motor testing is reliable if tendons and muscles are not damaged. You must
  —know the anatomy and
  —how to test each muscle by inspection, palpation and active joint movement;
- quick screening tests for the following nerves are:
  —accessory nerve, shrug the shoulder (trapezius muscle);
  —musculocutaneous nerve, flex the elbow (brachialis and biceps);
  —ulnar nerve, extension of the interphalangeal joints of the hand (intrinsic) and Froment's sign;
  —median nerve, opposition of the thumb (thenar muscles);
  —radial nerve, extension of the metacarpophalangeal joints and wrist (long extensors);
  —femoral nerve, knee extension (quadriceps);
  —tibial nerve, plantar flexion of the foot and toes (triceps surae);
  —common peroneal nerve, eversion of the foot (superficial peroneal nerve through peroneal muscles) and dorsiflexion of the foot and toes (deep peroneal nerve thorugh toe extensors and tibialis anterior).

TESTS

Sweat test

- skin supplied by an interrupted nerve does not sweat because the sympathetic fibers in the nerve are damaged;
- check for this by
  —looking for beads of sweat on the skin with an ophthalmoscope or
  —dusting the skin with quinizarin (iodine) powder. The denervated area will remain gray, but where there is sweat, the powder will turn purple.

Electrical studies

Electromyogram

- can only provide information on whether a muscle is
  —innervated or
  —not;
- immediately after denervation there is
  —no muscle response to
  —nerve stimulation proximal to the injury and
  —no motor unit potentials during attempted volitional contraction
  of the muscle;
- at 1 to 2 weeks
  —positive sharp waves appear, and spontaneous
  —denervation fibrillation potentials are seen a little later.
- reinnervation is heralded by
  —polyphasic motor unit potentials on attempted voluntary contraction. Initially these are of
  —low amplitude and short duration, but as
  —reinnervation progresses, the
  —number and amplitude of the potentials increase and approach
  normality.

Nerve conduction studies

- stimulation of the nerve proximal to the injury can
  —confirm physiological interruption and can
  —localize the site;
- failure of nerve conduction distal to the site of the lesion 1 to 3 days
  after injury indicates
  —wallerian degeneration and therefore
  —rules out neurapraxia.

Treatment

CLOSED INJURIES

Posttraumatic

- most closed nerve injuries resulting from direct trauma have an intact
  neural sheath and will
- heal spontaneously,
  —neurapraxia within a few days to weeks,
  —axonotmesis within a few weeks or months, depending on distance
  between the point of injury and the end of the organ;
- axon grows about
  —1 mm/day, so

  —measure the distance in millimeters from the point of injury to the
    most proximal muscle innervated and
  —allow that time in days plus 1 month for
  —start of recovery of contraction in that muscle;
- maintain flexibility of all joints affected by paralysis during the recovery
  period by
  —full range of movement exercises daily and
  —dynamic splinting to support joints, avoid contractures, and protect
    functioning muscles from overstretching;
- if joints become stiff or contractures develop (occurs very quickly in the
  adult hand), the final result will be poor no matter how complete the
  nerve recovery;
- if recovery does not start within the estimated time,
- explore the injured nerve. It is is in
  —continuity, perform neurolysis. If the nerve is
- divided, repair it (see below). An
- indirect, severe traction injury secondary to dislocation has a poor
  prognosis due to extensive intraneural scarring, e.g., injury of the common peroneal nerve at the knee;
- tardy ulnar nerve palsy responds to anterior transposition with neurolysis
  if there is intraneural scarring.

Iatrogenic

- when nerve injury appears after manipulation of a fracture, where there
  was no nerve injury before,
- wait 2 weeks, and if there are no signs of recovery,
- explore the nerve at the level of injury because the nerve may be caught
  in the fracture site with likelihood of
  —permanent neurological deficit and
  —pseudarthrosis;
- if nerve injury is the result of a poorly applied cast or of traction, e.g.,
  from a
  —long arm cast ending at the midarm level (radial nerve compression)
    or from the rim of a
  —below-knee cast or tight skin traction compressing the common
    peroneal nerve at the level of the fibula neck,
- change the cast or the traction materials, pad carefully over the compressed nerve, and wait. Function usually returns, but if it does not,
  consider exploration and neurolysis;
- peripheral neurological examination is important both
  —before and
  —after treatment.

OPEN INJURIES

- when nerve injury is associated with an open wound, explore the nerve at the same time that you debride the wound;
- if nerve ends are difficult to identify,
- extend the wound proximally and distally, find the nerve where the anatomy is undisturbed, and
- trace it from both ends of the incision toward the site of the injury. Tourniquet control helps identification;
- if the nerve is intact, make sure that reduction does not trap the nerve in the fracture or the joint!
- if the nerve is partly or completely severed, primary or secondary repair will be necessary. If you decide on secondary repair, tack the nerve ends together to prevent retraction.

NERVE REPAIR

Primary repair

Prerequisites for primary suture

- satisfactory general condition of the patient;
- adequate operative personnel, equipment and lighting. A
- clean, incised wound
- less than 6 hours old with
- minimal contamination;
- well-demarcated, clean bundles of nerve fibers present at both ends of the severed nerve;
- nerve ends capable of approximation without tension.

Contraindications

- absence of prerequisites;
- crushed skin or skin loss or
- crush injury of the nerve;
- fractured bone or section of tendons at the level of the nerve injury takes precedence over nerve repair;
- when extreme flexion of the wrist and fingers would be necessary to avoid tension on the suture line;
- nerve suture is a
  —long and
  —exacting procedure. Do not attempt it when you are
  —too tired or too busy.

Technique of primary suture

- most gaps in peripheral nerves can be closed by a combination of
  —mobilization of the nerve proximally and distally,

—transposition of the nerve, e.g., the ulnar nerve at the elbow, and

—moderate flexion of adjacent joints, e.g., knee and elbow to 90°, wrist and fingers to 45°;

—resect nerve ends to prevent intraneural fibrosis. After suture

- splint the appropriate joints (usually those nearest the injury) in moderate flexion to prevent tension on the suture line, and do not allow extension beyond this before 4 weeks for the arm or 6 weeks for the leg;
- then extend the joints by 20° weekly to allow sutured nerve to adapt by gradual lengthening. If joints are extended too fast, tension on the suture line will cause intraneural fibrosis and will jeopardize the result.

Regional injuries

- radial, median, ulnar and musculocutaneous nerves are mixed (sensory and motor), so accurate orientation of the cut ends is important to avoid motor fibers growing down sensory sheaths and sensory fibers growing down motor sheaths;
- median and ulnar nerves divide into motor and sensory branches at the wrist;
- the motor branch of the ulnar nerve and the sensory branch of the median nerve at the wrist are particularly important for hand function and must be sutured;
- digital nerve can be repaired when it is cut anywhere proximal to the distal interphalangeal joint. If the
    —palmar aspect of the hand and fingers is anesthetic, the patient will not use the hand until sensation is restored, no matter how good the motor function may be!
- do not repair nerves on the dorsum of hand.
- femoral nerve is mixed and
    —divides into several branches soon after entering the thigh;
    —suture at this point is difficult and unrewarding.
- sciatic nerve and its two terminal branches are mixed. Results are
    —poor after repair in the buttock or proximal thigh and
    —little better in the distal thigh and around the knee. A patient with
    —complete and permanent sciatic nerve paralysis
    —rarely has trophic ulcers unless there is a fixed deformity of the foot, causing excessive localized pressure.

Secondary repair

- 1% to 2% of potential motor fiber regeneration is lost for every week's delay between injury and repair;
- the optimum time for secondary repair is 2 to 6 weeks after injury; if the repair is not started until

- after 3 months after injury, the likelihood for motor reinnervation deteriorates rapidly, but
- sensory regeneration may occur even when several years have elapsed between injury and repair;
- use a large exposure (keyhole surgery is for keyhole surgeons!) and
- resect the neuroma and glioma with a sharp blade until normal axons pout from the nerve ends. If necessary,
- dissect and mobilize the nerve for not more than 20 cm proximally and distally to avoid tension on the suture line;
- the epineurium of older damaged nerve is thicker and holds sutures better than does freshly cut nerve;
- take care to orientate a mixed nerve properly.
- splint the limb as discussed previously;
- instruct the patient to protect the anesthetic areas of the skin;
- prevent contractures and stiff joints by dynamic splinting and active and passive range of motion exercises.

Nerve grafting

- where the gap is too long to close, a
  —nonessential nerve such as the saphenous can be used as a free graft to bridge the gap, with a
  —single strand used for a small nerve and multiple strands used as a
  —cable graft for a large nerve;
- a free graft depends on a good vascular bed for its viability.
- pedicle nerve grafting is possible where
  —two main nerves are damaged close together, e.g., the median and ulnar nerves in the forearm, and
  —direct suture of either is impossible. The
  —least important (the ulnar in this case) is sacrificed to graft the other.

Prognosis after repair

- sensation improves for 18 months, and although it may never be completely normal (e.g., two-point discrimination may still be impaired), it may be sufficient for most patients' needs. But the
- restoration of motor power is generally not as good, and depends on the following factors:
- patient's age,
  —the best results occur in children;
- time from injury to repair,
  —the likelihood for return of function (especially motor) deteriorates rapidly if the nerve is repaired 3 months or more after injury;
- level of injury,
  —the more proximal the lesion, the worse the results, with the

—brachial plexus and the sciatic nerve in the buttock being the least
amenable to repair;

- type of injury,
  —severe traction injury causes extensive damage over a large distance
  and has a poor prognosis no matter what the treatment, whereas a
  —clean cut has a good prognosis after repair;
- the nerve itself,
  —a mixed nerve has worse results than a purely sensory or motor nerve;
- tension on the suture line;
- surgical team and environment because an
  —experienced team working with
  —proper materials in a
  —good surgical environment achieves the
  —best results.

TENDON TRANSFERS*

- tendon transfers may restore hand function in
  —untreated nerve injuries 18 months old or more or in
  —failed nerve repair;
- test the strength of the muscles proposed for transfer before surgery because a
- transferred muscle loses one grade of strength (on a scale from 0 to 5).

Radial nerve paralysis in arm

- transfer the PT insertion to the ECRB for wrist extension;
- FCU tendon to EDC for MP joint extension;
- PL to EPL (releasing the EPL from around Lister's tubercle and trans-posing the EPL tendon to the radial side of the wrist to straighten the line of pull), or
- when the PL is absent, transfer the FCU to the EPL as well as to the EDC for thumb extension and abduction;
- leave the FCR intact to stabilize and prevent hyperextension of the wrist.

Radial nerve paralysis in forearm

- FCU to EDC for MP joint extension;

---

*The following abbreviations are used in this section: *AP*, adductor pollicis; *APB*, abductor pollicis brevis; *APL*, abductor pollicis longus; *BR*, brachioradialis; *DIP*, distal interphalangeal; *ECRB*, extensor carpi radialis brevis; *ECU*, extensor carpi ulnaris; *EDC*, extensor digitorum communis; *EIP*, extensor indicis proprius; *EPB*, extensor pollicis brevis; *EPL*, extensor pollicis longus; *FCR*, flexor carpi radialis; *FCU*, flexor carpi ulnaris; *FDP*, flexor digitorum profundus; *FDS*, flexor digitorum sublimis; *FPL*, flexor pollicis longus; *IP*, interphalangeal; *MP*, metacarpophalangeal; *PL*, palmaris longus; *PT*, pronator teres; *TP*, tibialis posterior.

- PL or BR to EPL for thumb extension and
- PT to APL for thumb abduction.

Ulnar nerve paralysis in arm

- EPB or the radial half of the EIP tendon to the insertion of the first dorsal interosseous muscle for abduction of the index finger;
- Zancolli capsuloplasty of the ring and little MP joints to prevent hyperextension if clawing of these joints is disabling;
- BR, by tendon graft (PL or plantaris tendon), through the third interosseous space between the third and fourth metacarpals and across the palm to tendon of the AP for adduction of the thumb;
- side-to-side suture of FDP tendons of ring and little fingers to the FDP tendon of the middle finger for flexion of the ring and little DIP joints. Test the function of the FDP tendon to the middle finger before transposition because it is sometimes innervated by ulnar nerve.

Ulnar nerve paralysis in forearm

- transfer as discussed previously but do not touch the FDP.

Median nerve paralysis in arm

- in median nerve injuries, a loss of sensation over two thirds of the anterior surface of the palm and fingers is a major disability, and
- no matter how well the tendon transfers may function, the patient may never use the hand if adequate sensation cannot be restored.
- for restoration of motor function the following procedures are available:
- side-to-side suture of FDP tendons of the index and middle fingers to FDP tendons of the ring and little fingers for flexion of the index and middle DIP joints;
- BR to FPL at the wrist for flexion of the thumb IP joint;
- EIP around the ulnar side of the wrist to the APB tendon, for thumb opposition.

Median nerve paralysis in forearm

- transfer the FDS tendon of the ring finger through a pulley made from the FCU, and suture it to the capsule of the MP joint of thumb and to the APB tendon for thumb opposition.

Combined median and ulnar nerve paralysis at wrist

- the anterior surface of the entire palm and all fingers is anesthetic, so
- tendon transfers are not likely to help unless sensation can be restored. An
- anesthetic hand is a functional amputation.
- success of transfers also depends on
  —correction of joint contractures and
  —passive mobility of the joints, especially MP flexion and IP extension, and the

—integrity of the flexor tendons to be transferred. To
- replace interosseous muscles, prolong the ECRB by a four-tailed graft, and pass the tails through the intermetacarpal spaces to the proximal phalanges of the fingers;
- FDS of the ring finger through the ECU pulley for thumb opposition;
- EIP through the third intermetacarpal space to the adductor tendon for thumb adduction.

Common peroneal nerve paralysis

- foot-drop is best corrected by a
  —brace or plastic orthosis or an
  —anterior transfer of the TP.

chapter 32
Peripheral Vascular Injuries

Introduction

- the amputation rate for limb injuries with major arterial division was
  - 50% in the Second World War,
  - 13% in the Vietnamese War;
- this marked improvement in results was due to
  - earlier diagnosis,
  - broader use of antibiotics, and
  - earlier and better resuscitation and vessel repair.
- amputation rates for closed and open injuries are similar (50% and 13%, respectively) because a
  - closed injury is diagnosed and treated late, whereas an
  - open injury requires prompt debridement, and from that point exploration of the artery is but a step.

Arterial Injuries

ETIOPATHOLOGY

Complete arterial section
- usually caused by penetrating wound from a
  - knife (sometimes the surgeon's!) or
  - bullet.

Hemorrhage
- bleeding usually stops due to
  - vasoconstriction by the muscular tunica media,
  - retraction of both ends of the severed artery with
  - compression by surrounding tissues and
  - clot formation which propagates proximally and distally. But
- bleeding may not stop, or may recur, if the patient is
  - arteriosclerotic or has a

—coagulation defect or if the injured artery is the

—internal iliac or an intercostal where surrounding structures prevent retraction or do not effectively compress it.

Ischemia

- ischemia usually affects tissues distal to the joint below the lesion;
- the degree of ischemia depends on
  —which artery is sectioned and where, on the
  —number, size and condition of collateral vessels, many of which may be destroyed by a severe injury, on the
  —duration of ischemia, and on the
  —sensitivity and metabolic demands of tissues distal to injury.
- peripheral nerves are most sensitive to ischemia with
  —paresthesias occurring within several minutes; then
  —touch, proprioception and temperature sense are lost; and lastly,
  —deep pain loss and motor paralysis occur;
  —recovery may be rapid, even after several hours;
- muscle is
  —more resistant to anoxia but
  —recovery is slower and
  —all contractility is lost at 4 to 6 hours. If ischemia persists for 12 hours or more, muscles will die. But even then, prompt restoration of circulation will improve the chance of some muscle regeneration;
- skin is less vulnerable and may survive ischemia for 24 hours. Ischemia prolonged beyond 24 hours causes gangrene, with no recovery possible;
- bone is the tissue least vulnerable to anoxia.

Partial arterial section

- usually due to a penetrating injury, including iatrogenic causes such as the point of a drill, screw, pin or needle, but it is
- occasionally due to a fracture fragment.

Hemorrhage

- bleeding is more severe in partial section than in complete section because
  —arterial ends cannot retract, so surrounding tissues cannot compress the artery,
  —contraction of the tunica media causes the ends to gape, and
  —continuous flow of blood prevents clot forming in the lumen.
- an open wound continues to bleed, but if the
- wound is closed, hematoma forms and gradually increases in size, pulsates, and may reopen the wound with resulting catastrophic hemorrhage;

- hematoma may organize with fibrous tissue replacement and gradual endothelialization of its central cavity, forming a "false" aneurysm which continues to expand because it has no elastic fibers in its wall. This may cause heart failure if large quantities of blood enter the aneurysm;
- an arteriovenous (AV) fistula may form if an adjacent vein is injured and blood flows from the artery to the vein throughout systole and diastole. This produces a
  —continuous "machinery" bruit (listen to arms and legs; you may learn something!) and a
  —thrill. High-output heart failure may occur with a large fistula, and pulsating varicosities of adjacent and distal veins may appear due to increased venous pressure.

Ischemia

- the distal part of a limb may be ischemic, but
- some blood may flow into the distal arterial lumen with the result that the
  —distal artery may pulsate, and if
  —collateral circulation is adequate, there may be
  —no immediate effects, though the patient may later suffer from
  —intermittent claudication in the leg or a
  —cold, painful hand on exercise. But if the
- partial ischemia is associated with increased compartmental pressure which is not relieved,
  —Volkmann's ischemic contracture may develop.

Arterial injury in continuity (Figs. 32.1 and 32.2)

- caused by
  —blunt force,
  —traction or a
  —high-velocity missile passing close to a vessel; or the artery may be
  —compressed by a tight cast or bandage or by massive swelling or hematoma which also compresses collaterals, or it may be
  —kinked or stretched by displaced fracture or dislocation;
- the tunica intima may be
  —torn and a flap lifted up (intimal roll-up) or an
  —intramural hematoma may push up the intima to block the vessel. Rarely, the
- tunica media may go into spasm, and this may spread to collaterals and occlude these also;
- thrombus forms at the site of the injury and may propagate proximally and distally to block the collaterals too.

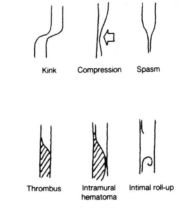

Figure 32.1.   Arterial injuries in continuity.

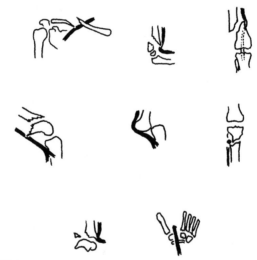

Figure 32.2.   Peripheral arteries vulnerable in fractures and dislocations.

CLINICAL FEATURES

General

History

- when and by what, e.g.,
  - —severity of blunt force,
  - —length and width of knife blade, direction and depth of penetration, and

—number of bullets fired and their direction. Bullets pass easily through the arm into the chest or through the thigh and into the abdomen; think of the whole patient!
- extent of blood loss;
- prior treatment;
- if a tourniquet has been applied, how long has it been applied?

Examination

- undress the patient to
  —examine all possible sites of injury,
  —compare one side with the other, and look for
- signs of ischemia. Examine the
  —distal pulse for strength and compare it with that of the normal side and with the proximal pulse (use a Doppler pulse meter if you are in doubt);
  —skin for color, temperature, venous distension and bruising (pressing the nail bed is not enough); alteration in
  —sensation, fine touch and pinprick, and its distribution (severed nerve causes hypoesthesia and anesthesia in a segmental pattern and ischemia in a glove or stocking distribution);
  —motor power. Look for
  —tender, swollen muscles and
  —flexion contracture of the fingers or toes with increase in pain on extending the digits;
- measure the circumference of the limb repeatedly for expanding hematoma,
- feel the limb for pulsation and
- listen to it;
- look for a fracture or dislocation and associated nerve and tendon injuries.

Specific

Complete arterial section

- if arterial flow is totally interrupted and collateral circulation is inadequate, e.g., a brachial artery in the midarm or a femoral artery in the midthigh, the result will be total ischemia;
- pulselessness is the earliest and most important sign because the
- four remaining Ps may not appear until later:
  —pallor changing later to mottled cyanosis,
  —paresthesia, hypoesthesia and anesthesia due to neural ischemia,
  —paralysis due to neural or muscle ischemia, and
  —pain.
- some major arteries do not normally have a palpable distal pulse, e.g.,

—carotids,

—internal iliac and profunda femoris, and

—renal and mesenteric vessels.

Partial arterial section

- clinical diagnosis is difficult because the distal pulse may still be present. On examination you may find a
    - large hematoma with systolic bruit and thrill, as blood is forced out through the arterial tear during systole, an
    - expanding hematoma or an
    - AV fistula with continuous bruit. If
- hematoma limits escape of blood from the artery, the patient may present after several days with a
    - warm, tender mass and red skin. If you think this is an abscess and you incise it, what a surprise you will have!
    - untreated, this may become a false aneurysm. An
- arteriogram will remove any doubts.

Closed arterial injury

- progressive signs of ischemia and loss of pulses with a
- history of trauma and
- no significant hemorrhage should alert you to this possibility.
- diagnosis may be certain only after arteriotomy.

Arteriography

- seldom necessary as vascular lesion is usually at the same level as the wound or skeletal injury and waiting for the arteriogram wastes valuable time;
- main indications for arteriography are
    - multiple missile injuries where the level of the arterial lesion is uncertain,
    - high-velocity missile wound near a major vessel, investigation of a suspected
    - false aneurysm or
    - AV fistula, or of a patient with
    - intermittent claudication, and in a
    - failed repair.

TREATMENT

Emergency procedures

- treat shock and respiratory or ventilatory insufficiency immediately because the resultant
    - hypotension, reduced perfusion, peripheral vasoconstriction and hypoxia

—compound the ischemia of a limb with an arterial injury. Application of

- firm, even compression over the site of the arterial bleeding is the best method of temporary control;
- do not use a tourniquet and
- do not fish blindly in the wound with artery forceps!
- correct severe deformity due to a fracture, reduce a dislocation, and
- splint the limb.

Surgery

General

- when the patient has been resuscitated and the limb is still ischemic,
- operate as soon as possible;
- a delay of more than 6 hours after injury increases the
  —probability of tissue death and the
  —likelihood of thrombus propagation and widespread intravascular clotting, thus
  —increasing ischemia and
  —vitiating attempts to reestablish the circulation.
- do not wait to confirm the diagnosis or you will be too late;
- operate on a high index of suspicion.
- in the operating room, use a pneumatic tourniquet, but inflate it only in case of uncontrollable hemorrhage;
- prepare the whole limb to palpate the distal pulses, the
- proximal torso to allow access to all major vessels, and a
- normal limb for access to a vein in case a vein graft is necessary;
- local heparinization and
- fasciotomy should accompany all vascular repairs;
- do not remove muscle at this stage, as it may recover in whole or in part.

Lacerated artery

- repair a divided artery by
  —end-to-end anastomosis or
  —vein graft (reverse the vein because of the valves), a
- partially divided artery by
  —transverse suture (to prevent narrowing of the lumen), a
  —vein patch, or
  —resection with end-to-end anastomosis or vein graft. A
- traumatic false aneurysm should be excised and the artery repaired;
- AV fistula should be resected after controlling both vessels above and below the injury. Repair both vessels as described previously, with the vein first.

Closed arterial injury

- may be due to spasm, thrombus or intimal tear. Make a diagnosis of
- spasm only after exclusion of all other causes of occlusion. The
- spasm usually disappears after reduction of the fracture. If it persists,
  —inject the isolated segment with saline under pressure. If
  —spasm persists, or the artery is thrombosed,
  —remove the thrombus with a Fogarty catheter,
  —resect the damaged segment, and repair it as described previously.
  Do not wait. If the
- artery is blocked but appears normal at surgery, open it longitudinally.
  Rolled-up intima can be resected, and thrombus can be removed
  from the vessel and its branches.

Postoperative care

- no encircling bandage or cast;
- elevate the limb to prevent edema;
- keep the limb warm to prevent reflex vasoconstriction. If the
- crush syndrome is likley to develop, give
  —sodium bicarbonate intravenously (IV) to counter acidosis, and
  —correct hypotension and oliguria to prevent renal failure secondary
  to myohemoglobinemia;
- prophylactic antibiotics;
- failure of arterial repair postoperatively is an indication for
  —immediate reexploration.

Associated skeletal injury

- less than 0.3% of long bone fractures have associated arterial injury but
  up to
- half of all peripheral arterial injuries have an associated fracture, and
  this is
- 5 times more common in the leg than in the arm;
- the following arteries lying close to bone are the most vulnerable:
  —subclavian artery behind the clavicle,
  —brachial artery at the elbow, especially with extension type supracondylar fracture of the humerus,
  —femoral artery with femoral shaft fracture, particularly in the distal third where the artery goes through the adductor opening,
  —popliteal artery with supracondylar fracture of the femur, dislocation or hyperextension injury of the knee,
  —tibial artery with fracture of the proximal tibial metaphysis, grossly displaced
  —fracture or dislocation of the ankle or talus and
  —midtarsal or tarsometatarsal injuries;

- always examine the neurovascular status of a fractured limb;
- a large hematoma or recurrent bleeding may be the sign of a vascular injury;
- internal fixation before or after vascular repair is ideal, but it
  —prolongs wound exposure, may
  —damage collateral circulation, and may
  —increase the risk of infection;
- external stabilization with splints or, better still, external fixation is usually adequate;
- do not use circumferential bandages or casts for a patient with known or suspected vascular injury;
- prognosis for the patient with fracture and associated vascular injury is worsened by
  —venous injury,
  —open fracture,
  —delay in repair, and
  —infection.

Compartmental Syndromes

ANATOMOPATHOLOGY

- anterior and posterior compartments of the forearm and anterior, lateral, superficial and deep posterior compartments of the leg are surrounded by tight, inelastic fascial sleeves;
- when pressure in the compartment surpasses capillary pressure, about 30 mm Hg, the muscular capillaries are compressed and
- muscle bellies become ischemic. Muscle damage is related to duration of ischemia;
- nerves in the compartment may also become ischemic with resultant hypoesthesia or anesthesia of the distal limb. Nerve damage depends on pressure in the compartment;
- major arteries passing through the compartment will still carry blood distally because arterial blood pressure is higher than capillary pressure. Therefore,
- distal pulses will still be present and the hand or foot will not be ischemic unless intracompartmental pressure eventually rises above arterial pressure;
- the skin of the forearm or leg is not affected because it is outside the fascia;
- the end result of compartmental syndrome is
  —muscle death;
  —part may regenerate, but the rest is
  —replaced by fibrous tissue which contracts with resultant classical

- Volkmann's ischemic contracture,
  —wrist flexion,
  —metacarpophalangeal (MP) hyperextension and
  —interphalangeal (IP) flexion in the upper limb, or
- equinocavus deformity and claw toes in the foot.

ETIOLOGY

- fracture of the forearm or leg is the commonest cause;
- a tightly applied bandage or cast on a fractured forearm or leg also causes local skin necrosis. When the bandage is very tight, arterial compression and gangrene may occur;
- arterial repair with revascularization of previously ischemic muscles causes
  —reactive hyperemia and
  —intracellular and extracellular edema with consequent
  —pressure increase within the compartment, hence the rationale for fasciotomy with arterial repair;
- impaired venous return, direct trauma to muscles, and vigorous muscular exercise increase intracompartmental pressure.

CLINICAL FEATURES

- the syndrome may be
- mild and occurs particularly in the anterior tibial compartment with pain on vigorous exercise and relief on resting. Occasionally, fasciotomy is necessary.
- moderate, with some pain and swelling. This is often unrecognized, especially when the limb is in a plaster cast, because clinical features are not classical and may be dismissed as being normal after a fracture;
- severe, caused by trauma, and characterized by the 5 Ps:
- pain
  —key sign;
  —unrelenting pain in muscles in spite of reduction and stabilization of the fracture and powerful analgesics;
  —exacerbated by passive extension of the fingers or toes;
  —muscles in the compartment are firm and tender. If this is
  —untreated, the pain gradually subsides as the
  —nerves die!
- paresthesia or anesthesia;
- paralysis or weakness, a late sign. Whenever you
  —pass a patient with a cast or bandage, ask him to
  —move the fingers or toes.
- pallor with
  —pale, cool skin in the finger pulp, not the nail bed. This sign is
  —unreliable because major and collateral arteries may function normally;

—similarly unreliable are the temperature of the limb and the distal
- pulse.
- Wick catheter measures intracompartmental pressure. Use this and the
- Doppler pulse meter to differentiate compartment syndrome from
  —arterial or nerve injury, a
  —frightened and lonely patient or the
  —Mediterranean syndrome with a heightened response to pain.

PREVENTION
- avoid tight or elastic bandages;
- pad plasters well;
- do not put a circular cast on a fresh or recently manipulated or operated fracture;
- elevate the limb for 48 hours after manipulation or surgery;
- instruct the patient to move the fingers or toes actively every hour, and see that he does it;
- evaluate vascular status regularly.

TREATMENT

Early
- treat the problem before damage is irreversible;
- it is better to perform
  —too many fasciotomies
  —than too few!
- remove dressings,
- split the entire length of a cast to the skin,
- extend the joint if this is flexed and
- elevate the limb to the level of the heart;
- if there is no improvement within 30 minutes or compartment pressure exceeds 30 mm Hg, perform a
  —fasciotomy and leave both
  —skin and fascia open. In the
  —forearm, both compartments can be decompressed through a medial incision, but two incisions are better. Decompress deep as well as superficial fexors and the carpal tunnel for the median nerve. In the
  —leg two, three or all four compartments may be compressed simultaneously. In this instance in an adult
  —resect the fibula shaft and
  —decompress all compartments through the fibular bed or, better still, use
  —medial and lateral incisions;
- fasciotomy is best performed within 6 hours of injury but is still worth

doing even days later to save what viable tissue remains and, in particular, to permit nerve regeneration.
- prevent late fixed deformities by
  —physiotherapy and
  —padded splints.

Late

- treatment after irreversible damage and consequent contractures.

Upper limb

- serial static and dynamic splints may improve mild contractures;
- for successful reconstructive surgery of the upper limb, the severe claw hand must have
  —good sensation in the hand,
  —good passive mobility of the fingers and
  —some remaining muscle power;
- Scaglietti-Page flexor muscle slide gives the best results;
- ischemic nerves will require grafting.

Lower limb

- correction of fixed deformities by soft tissue or bony operation may be combined with
- tendon transfers to provide a
- stable, balanced, plantigrade foot and to
- eliminate abnormal pressure areas.

Venous Injuries

- etiology is similar to that of arterial injuries;
- a vein bleeds longer than an artery,
  —slow hemorrhage, but the patient may lose
  —considerable quantity, so anticipate shock;
- veins do not go into spasm;
- should be repaired surgically but
- venous repair is difficult because the vein wall is thin and friable and
- thrombus often forms at the site of the repair. However, even the
- temporary restoration of venous flow is beneficial;
- veins which should be repaired are
  —femoral and
  —popliteal because collateral flow is inadequate;
- do fasciotomy too and
- elevate the leg postoperatively;
- other veins can be ligated.
- widespread venous damage may later cause
  —edema of the distal limb with
  —hard, pigmented skin and sometimes
  —ulceration, especially in the leg and foot.

Suggested Further Reading

Charnley J: *The Closed Treatment of Common Fractures*, ed 3. Edinburgh, Churchill Livingstone, 1961.

Edmonson AS, Crenshaw AH (eds): *Campbell's Operative Orthopaedics*, ed 6. St Louis, CV Mosby, 1980.

Lewis RC: *Handbook of Traction, Casting and Splinting Techniques.* Philadelphia, JB Lippincott, 1977.

Ogden JA: *Skeletal Injury in the Child.* Philadelphia, Lea & Febiger, 1982.

Rang M: *Children's Fractures*, ed 2. Philadelphia, JB Lippincott, 1983.

Wilson JN (ed): *Watson-Jones Fractures and Joint Injuries*, ed 6. Edinburgh, Churchill Livingstone, 1982.

INDEX